OCULAR DISEASES

Edited by **Adedayo Adio**

Ocular Diseases
http://dx.doi.org/10.5772/1678
Edited by Adedayo Adio

Contributors

A. Triviño, R. de Hoz, B. Rojas, B.I. Gallego, A.I. Ramírez, J.J. Salazar, J.M. Ramírez, Linjing Li, Ozge Yildiz, Manisha Anand, Hemant Khanna, Retno Supriyanti, Hitoshi Habe, Masatsugu Kidode, Emina Alimanović Halilović, Maria Jesus Giraldez, Eva Yebra-Pimentel, Wan Jin Jahng, Covadonga Pañeda, Tamara Martínez, Natalia Wright, Ana Isabel Jimenez

Published by InTech

Janeza Trdine 9, 51000 Rijeka, Croatia

Publishing Process Manager Dragana Manestar
Technical Editor InTech DTP team
Cover InTech Design team

Additional hard copies can be obtained from orders@intechopen.com

Ocular Diseases, Edited by Adedayo Adio
p. cm.
ISBN 978-953-51-0761-3

For EU product safety concerns:
IN TECH d.o.o., Prolaz Marije Krucifikse Kozulić 3, 51000 Rijeka, Croatia,
info@intechopen.com or visit our website at intechopen.com.

Meet the editor

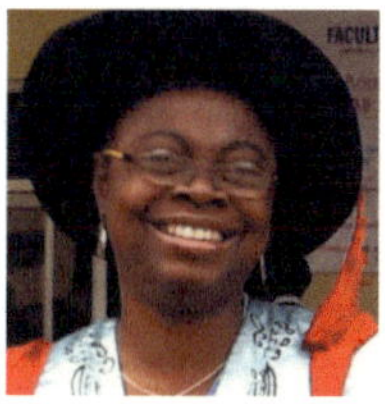

Dr Adedayo Omobolanle Adio (Nee Omoni) FWACS, FMCOPHTH, FCIA is a Senior Lecturer and Consultant Ophthalmologist in the Department of Ophthalmology, University of Port Harcourt with her area of Specialty/ Sub-specialty being Paediatric Ophthalmology, glaucoma and strabismus. She completed Medical school education in 1990 at the University of Ilorin and Kwara state and obtained post graduate fellowships in Ophthalmology in 2000 in both, the West African college and the National Postgraduate Medical Colleges of Nigeria. She is an Examiner for both colleges and a national and international reviewer of Medical Journals. Currently she is in charge of Paediatric Ophthalmology services in the University of Port Harcourt Teaching Hospital. She is also the Coordinator of the Rivers state Prevention of Blindness(PBL) Committee since 2008, the South -South Zonal Facilitator for the Nigerian Prevention of Blindness Committee since 2005 and recently appointed (2012) the South south coordinator for Ophthalmological society of Nigeria OSN. She has given several public lectures and is actively engaged in awareness and public enlightenment programs in the print media and electronic media. She has also been actively engaged in Community volunteer activities, notably in the State PBL committee organized cataract surgical eye camp of 2010. She is actively engaged in research with over 36 publications in local and international journals.

Contents

Preface IX

Chapter 1 **Effects of Hypercholesterolaemia in the Retina 1**
A. Triviño, R. de Hoz, B. Rojas, B.I. Gallego,
A.I. Ramírez, J.J. Salazar and J.M. Ramírez

Chapter 2 **Photoreceptor Sensory Cilium and Associated Disorders 43**
Linjing Li, Ozge Yildiz, Manisha Anand and Hemant Khanna

Chapter 3 **Utilization of Portable Digital Camera for Detecting Cataract 61**
Retno Supriyanti, Hitoshi Habe and Masatsugu Kidode

Chapter 4 **Clinical Application of Photodisruptors in Ophthalmology 79**
Emina Alimanović Halilović

Chapter 5 **Hydrogel Contact Lenses Surface Roughness and Bacterial Adhesion 95**
Maria Jesus Giraldez and Eva Yebra-Pimentel

Chapter 6 **New Biomarkers in the Retina and RPE Under Oxidative Stress 121**
Wan Jin Jahng

Chapter 7 **Recent Advances in Ocular Nucleic Acid-Based Therapies: The Silent Era 157**
Covadonga Pañeda, Tamara Martínez,
Natalia Wright and Ana Isabel Jimenez

Preface

This comprehensive resource on ocular diseases will provide you with a better and more practical understanding of the science behind eye disease and help you to relate it with treatment. Some of the contributors to this book are some of the world's leading and most experienced scientists in this major area of interest and they have provided great insight into this often difficult to understand aspect of ophthalmology. Its unique blend of basic science and clinical applications will serve you as a clinical guide to understanding the cause and management of ocular disease.

Adedayo Adio
University of Port Harcourt teaching Hospital Rivers State,
Nigeria

Chapter 1

Effects of Hypercholesterolaemia in the Retina

A. Triviño, R. de Hoz, B. Rojas, B.I. Gallego,
A.I. Ramírez, J.J. Salazar and J.M. Ramírez

Additional information is available at the end of the chapter

http://dx.doi.org/10.5772/48359

1. Introduction

A cholesterol-rich diet causes postprandial hyperlipaemia with an accumulation of chylomicrons. This accumulation leads to a redistribution of the very-low-density lipoproteins (VLDL), thereby determining the elimination of the coarsest particles, the residual chylomicrons, which promote the onset of atherogenesis [1].

For some years, cholesterol-rich food has been associated with the subsequent development of complications such as the formation of atheromatous plaque and lipid deposits at the ocular level. These findings have been reproduced in an experimental rabbit model [2,3], this animal being particularly sensitive to the induction of atheromatous lesions, which faithfully reproduce those caused in human atherosclerosis [4-6].

One of the main barriers of the eye is Bruch's membrane, which, for its strategic situation between the choroidal vascular membrane and the outer retina, constitutes a semi-permeable filtration zone, through which the nutrients pass from the choriocapillaris towards the photoreceptors, while the cell-degradation products of the retina pass in the opposite direction. The accumulation of these waste products thickens Bruch's membrane and the basal layer of the retinal pigment epithelium (RPE) [7]. These changes in the outer retina may be the consequence of metabolic stress associated with the metabolism of fatty acids or of the changes in choroidal perfusion due to atherosclerosis [8]. In any case, the lipids that accumulate in a structurally altered Bruch's membrane cause a hydrophobic barrier that can hamper the free metabolic exchange between the choriocapillaris and the RPE, on interfering with the passage of nutrients and oxygen to the retina. This situation could contribute to the loss of retinal sensitivity and play a pathogenic role in the development of age-related macular degeneration (AMD) [9], the leading cause of blindness among people over 65 years in developed countries. On the other hand, the deposits that accumulate underneath the RPE, which contains unsaturated fatty acids, are oxidized by the light, strengthening lipid peroxidation [10,11] and negatively influencing retinal function.

The changes in the RPE-Bruch's membrane complex contribute to the death of multiple retinal neurons, this translating as a thinning and disorganization of its layers.

Cholesterol is essential for cell functioning. The main cholesterol source for the photoreceptors and the RPE comes from extracellular lipid metabolism, as has been demonstrated on detecting native low-density lipoprotein (LDL) receptors at the RPE level [12], which could be involved in the local production of apolipoprotein E (apoE). The retina also locally produces lipoprotein particles that contain apoE. These particles are secreted fundamentally by the Müller glia to the extracellular retinal compartment and to the vitreous, from which they are transported to the optic nerve [13]. Also, the retinal astrocytes associated with the axons of the ganglion cells participate in the secretion of apoE. This cholesterol transport is essential to supply the retinal neurons the lipids needed for the maintenance and remodelling of their cell membrane.

Studies in apoE-deficient mice have demonstrated the presence of alterations in Müller glia and in amachrine cells, these generating aberrations in the retinal circuit as a consequence of the local disruption of cholesterol homeostasis [14]. In a hypercholesterolaemic rabbit model, cell loss in the inner nuclear layer and in the ganglion-cell layer of the retina has been demonstrated [15,16]. This cell loss probably results from the deprivation of the neurotrophic support [17] and of the CNTF (ciliary neurotrophic factor) and glial fibrillary acidic protein (GFAP) upregulation secondary to the reactivation of the Müller cells [18,19]. In hypercholesterolaemic rabbits, added to the situation of ischaemia at the level of the outer retina induced by the alterations in Bruch's membrane and in the choriocapillaris, is the thickening of the basal membranes of the retinal vessels, which by hampering the passage of oxygen and nutrients towards the inner retina would generate a prolonged situation of ischaemia [15,20]. This chronic ischaemia could increase the concentration of extracellular glutamate, conditioning oxidative damage by a neuronal cytotoxic mechanism [21,22]. This situation can be counteracted so long as the astrocytes maintain their capacity to eliminate cytotoxic neurotransmitters and to supply growth factors and cytokines [23].

In summary, in the present chapter, the structural and ultrastructural changes in the retina of an experimental model of hypercholesterolaemia are described, specifically changes in Bruch's membrane, RPE, and retinal layers as well as the vascular changes responsible for chronic ischaemia. Further on, the effects of the diet-induced normalization of the plasma-cholesterol levels in the retinal structures are discussed. The comparison between the two scenarios suggests that hypercholesterolaemia is a risk factor for the development of chronic ischaemia in the retina and therefore for neuronal survival.

2. Anatomy and physiology of the Bruch's membrane-retinal complex

Bruch's membrane, the innermost layer of the choroid, fuses with RPE as a 5-layered structure consisting of (from outer to inner): a basement membrane of the choriocapillaris, an outer collagenous layer, an elastic layer, an inner collagenous layer, and a basement membrane of the RPE [7,24] (Figure 1, 3A, 4A). Fine filaments from the basement membrane of the RPE merge with the fibrils of the inner collagenous zone, contributing to the tight adhesion between choroid and the RPE. The basement membrane of the choriocapillaris is discontinuous and is absent in the intercapillary spaces [25]. The collagenous layers surround the elastic layer [7]. Some collagen fibres are arranged parallel to the tissue plane, especially at the inner collagenous zone; others cross from one side of the elastic fibre layer to another, interconnecting the two collagenous layers [7]. Collagen fibres pass through the disruption of the basement membrane to join the collagen fibres of the intercapillary septae. This arrangement may help Bruch's membrane to attach to the choriocapillaris. Vesicles, linear structures, and dense bodies occur in the collagenous and elastic zones but predominantly in the inner collagenous layer [26]. The elastic layer is made up of inter-woven bands of elastic fibres with irregular spaces between them, through which the collagen fibres pass [7,26] (Figure 3A, 4A). The exchange of substances between the choroid and retina (both directions) must traverse Bruch's membrane [7]. The importance of this process is evident in situations in which this membrane is disrupted. During aging, Bruch's membrane gradually thickens [27]. The collagenous layers thicken from the accumulation of membranous lipidic debris [28], abnormal extracellular matrix components (collagen fibres "cross-linking") and the advanced glycation end-product [29]. This decreases the porosity of Bruch's membrane, presumably heightening resistance to the movement of water through it [30]. Also, it has been found that this thickening of Bruch's membrane is accompanied by lower membrane permeability [31]. Although this thickening with aging is relatively minor, greater increases can appear in specific regions. The accumulation of material in the inner collagenous layer bulging toward the retina, is what is known by the term "drusen" [32]. These drusen will deprive the photoreceptors of their nutrition from the choriocapillaris.

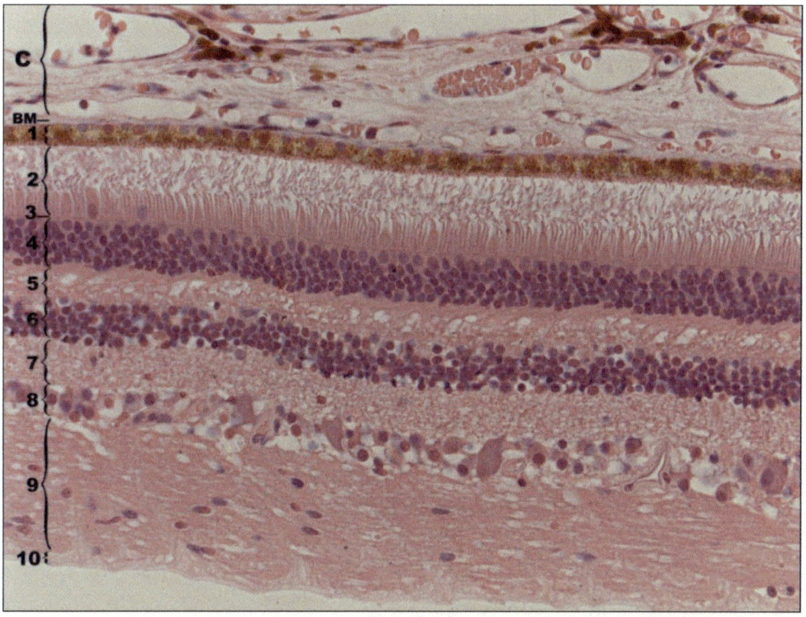

Figure 1. Histological section of the human retina. Retinal layers. Hematoxylin/eosin. 1: retinal pigment epithelium; 2: photoreceptor layer; 3: outer limiting membrane; 4: outer nuclear layer; 5: outer plexiform layer; 6: inner nuclear layer; 7: inner plexiform layer; 8: ganglion-cell layer; 9: nerve-fibre layer; 10: inner limiting membrane. [Bruch's membrane (BM); choroidal vascular layers (C)].

The elastic layer also suffers a disruption with aging, namely, an increase in density and calcification [33]. These aged-related changes could cause cracks and holes in Bruch's membrane. Major breaks in Bruch's membrane are associated with oedema, leading to the accumulation of fluid between the RPE and photoreceptors, and hence to a retinal detachment. This association between the discontinuity of Bruch's membrane and retinal oedema suggests that, under normal conditions, Bruch's membrane could play a role in limiting fluid movement to and from the retina [25].

2.1. Anatomy of the retina

The primary function of the retina is to convert light into nerve impulses which are transferred to the brain via the optic nerve. The retina comprises the retinal pigment epithelium and the neurosensory retina, the latter containing neurons, glial cells and components of the vascular system. Various types of neurons are present, such as: photoreceptors, bipolar cells, ganglion cells, amacrine cells and horizontal cells [34]. The coding function of the retina depends not only on photoreceptors but also on neurons, glial cells and RPE, which amplify the signal [35]. The photoreceptors are the cells that capture light and are situated at the most external side of the neurosensory retina, in the vicinity of the RPE. These cells are of two types: rods (for scotopic vision) and cones (for photopic vision) [34]. The ability of photoreceptors to convert light photons into an electrical signal is due to the presence of a photopigment in their outer segments. These segments consist of a stack of disk membranes that are synthesised in the proximal portion of the outer segment and shed at its apical size [35]. Photoreceptors form contacts with horizontal and bipolar cells in the outer plexiform layer (OPL). Coupling between neighbouring rods and cones in OPL allows the first stage of visual processing. The inner nuclear layer (INL) contains cell bodies of Müller glial, bipolar, amacrine, and horizontal cells. The inner plexiform layer (IPL) consists of a synaptic connection between the axons of bipolar cells and dendrites of ganglion and amacrine cells. The ganglion-cell layer (GCL) contains the cell bodies of retinal ganglion cells, certain displaced amacrine cells, and astrocytes. Inside the eye, ganglion-cell axons run along the retinal surface toward the optic-nerve head forming nerve-fibre layer (NFL) [34,35] (Figure 1).

The neural retina also contains two types of macroglial cells: Müller cells and astrocytes (Figure 2).

Müller cells are long, radially oriented cells which span the width of the neural retina from the outer limiting membrane (OLM), where their apical ends are located, to the inner limiting membrane (INL), where their basal endfeet terminate (Figure 2A). In the nuclear layers, the lamellar processes of the Müller cells can be seen to form basket-like structures which envelope the cell bodies of photoreceptors and neural cells. In plexiform layers, fine processes of these cells are interwoven between the synaptic processes of neural cells. In both the plexiform and nuclear layers, Müller cell processes cover most but not all neural surfaces [36].

Astrocytes are located mainly in the NFL and GCL in most mammals (human, rabbit, rats and mouse, among others) [37-39] (Figure 2B). Astrocyte morphology differs between species. In humans, two types of astrocytes can be distinguished: elongated (located in the NFL) and star-shaped (located in GCL) astrocytes. In mice and rats the astrocytes are stellate (Figure 2B). The greatest variety of retinal astroglial cell morphologies is found in the rabbit, which possesses two large astrocyte groups: astrocytes associated with the nerve-fibre bundles (AANFB) which are aligned parallel to the axonal bundles in the NFL (Figure 10G), and perivascular astrocytes (PVA), associated with the retinal and vitreous blood vessels (Figure 10A,D). PVA can be further subdivided into: i) type I PVA, which have numerous sprouting, hair-like processes, associated with medium-sized epiretinal vessels, and with capillaries located over the inner limiting membrane (ILM) (Figure 10A), and ii) type II star-shaped PVA, which are located on and between larger and medium-sized epiretinal vessels [15,38,40-42] (Figure 10D). The morphology of retinal astrocytes in different animal species is determined by the way their processes adapt to the surrounding structures [43].

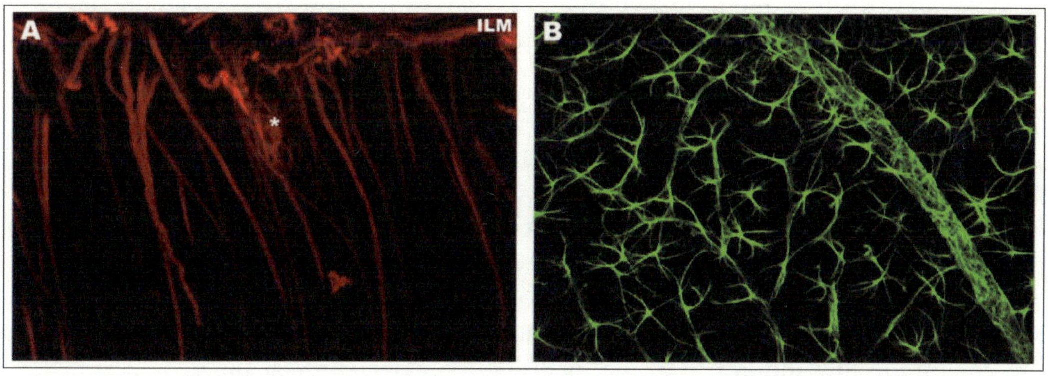

Figure 2. Immunohistochemistry anti-GFAP in mouse retinal whole-mount. A: GFAP+ Müller cells after 15 days of laser-induced ocular hypertension. The pressure exerted by the cover glass on the retinal whole-mount, produced a retinal-like section effect in some retinal borders. Müller cells exhibit a radial morphology that creates a columnar matrix that maintains the laminar structure of the retina [Astrocyte (*); inner limiting membrane (ILM)]. B: Confocal microscopy of normal retinal astrocytes. These cells form a homogeneous plexus on the nerve-fibre-RCG layer constituted by stellate cells. (Modified from Gallego et al [39]).

Macroglial cells perform a variety of essential roles for the normal physiology of the retina, maintaining a close and permanent relationship with the neurons [43]. Thus every aspect of the development, homeostasis, and function of the visual system involves a neuron-glia partnership. Glial cells insulate neurons, provide physical support, and supplement them with several metabolites and growth factors. These cells also play important roles in axon guidance and control of synaptogenesis [44]. Under normal conditions, astrocytes and Müller cells maintain the homeostasis of extracellular ions, glucose, and other metabolites, water, pH and neurotransmitters such as glutamate and GABA [45]. These cells also produce a great quantity of growth factors and cytokines, which may contribute both to neurotoxic as well as neuroprotective effects. It has also been demonstrated that macroglial cells are more resistant to oxidative damage than are the neurons, this trait protecting them against such damage. This potential is due to the fact that these cells contain high concentrations of antioxidants such as reduced glutathione and vitamin C. Consequently, a depression of these cellular activities could lead to neuronal dysfunction [46]. Macroglial cells induce the properties of barrier in the endothelial cells of retinal capillaries (the blood-retinal barrier), securing immune privilege to protect neurons from potentially damaging effects of an inflammatory immune response. Finally, glial cells can play fundamental roles in local immune responses and immunosurveillance [44].

Macroglial cells also play a part in pathological processes in central nervous system (CNS). Glial cells in the CNS have been cited as participants in the pathological course of neuronal damage after mechanical, ischaemic, and various other insults. Glial cell activation is a hallmark of CNS injury, characterized by an increase in size and number of glial cells and upregulation of GFAP, with additional cellular changes that may cause or relieve neuronal impairment. These reactive cells also have higher metabolic activity. After injury, reactive glial cells participate in the formation of a glial scar, in which there is an accumulation of enlarged astrocyte bodies and a thick network of processes with increased expression of GFAP and vimentin. Macroglial cells become reactive in response to a wide variety of stimuli, including inflammation and oxidative and mechanical stress [47].

Other components of the retina are the blood vessels. Photoreceptors receive nutrients via the choriocapillaris. The inner retinal layers have their own blood supply coming from the blood vessels entering the retina at the optic-nerve head. For its protection, the retina is physiologically and immunologically segregated from the rest of the body by tight junctions between vascular endothelial cells (inner blood-retinal barrier) and RPE cells (outer blood-retinal barrier). This fact is responsible for intraocular tissue to be an immune privileged site, thus protecting the eye from the innocent-bystander effect of inflammation [34]. In addition, only small molecules can cross these barriers, making it difficult for many drugs to reach ocular tissue.

The outermost retinal layer is the RPE (Figure 1), which is formed by a single layer of pigmented hexagonal cells. These cells provide the supportive role necessary to sustain the high metabolic demands of photoreceptors. RPE cells supply nutrients and oxygen, regenerate phototransduction products, and digest debris shed by the photoreceptors. The basal aspect of RPE cells contains numerous infoldings and is adjacent to Bruch's membrane. The apical surface is adjacent the neural retina. The RPE cells contain numerous pigment granules (melanosomes), lipofuscin granules, and degradation products of phagocytosis, which grow in number with age (Figure 4A) [7]. The RPE had several intercellular junctions: zonula occludens, zonula adherents, desmosomes, and gap junctions. The latter allow the cell electrical coupling and provide a low-resistance pathway for the passage of ions and metabolites [48]. The RPE fosters the health of the neural retina and choriocapillaris in several ways: the zonula occludens joining the RPE cells are part of the blood-retinal barrier and selectively control movement of nutrients and metabolites from choriocapillaris into the retina and removal of waste products from the retina into the choriocapillaris [49]. RPE cells phagocytose fragments of the photoreceptor outer segment discs, metabolise and store vitamin A, and produce growth factors, helping to maintain choriocapillaris and retinal function. Other, less well-characterized functions of the RPE are the absorption of stray light and the scavenging of free radicals by the melanin pigment in the epithelium and the drug detoxification by the smooth endoplasmic reticulum cytochrome p-450 system [50]. From the several functions displayed by RPE, it can be easily concluded that dysfunction of RPE cells has serious consequences on the health of photoreceptors [34].

2.2. The metabolism of lipids in the retina

Recent studies have demonstrated that fatty acids are fundamental for normal visual function [51]. Humans are unable to synthesise essential fatty acids (EFAs) and must acquire them through the food intake. Dietary EFAs are transformed into the endoplasmic reticulum of hepatic and retinal cells [52] into long-chain polyunsaturated fatty acids (LCPUFAs). LCPUFAs perform various functions, e.g. serving as ligands for gene-transcription factors for cell growth and differentiation, to participate in the metabolism of lipids, carbohydrates, and proteins, and to intervene in the inter- and intracellular signal cascades that influence vascular, neural, and immune functions [51].

In the neural retina, the richest LCPUFA-containing lipids are the phospholipids of the cell membranes [53], and the most abundant LCPUFAs in the retina are docosahexaenoic acid (DHA) and arachidonic acid (AA). DHA is a long-chain polyunsaturated fatty acid from the omega 3 series. It is present at high levels in the neurosensory retina [54]. DHA improves the kinetics of the photocycle by creating specific intermolecular associations with rhodopsin [35]. Brain astrocytes [55] and retinal tissue [34] can produce DHA, but in a limited way [56], given that the synthesis process is slow [57] and restricted to the RPE and the endothelial cells of the retinal vessels [58]. Consequently, retinal requirements of LCPUFAs depend on input from the liver (the main site of LCPUFA biosynthesis) [59] and hence on transportation of LCPUFAs from the choriocapillaris to the outer segments of the RPE-photoreceptor.

Cell-membrane permeability is thought to depend on the balance between LCPUFAs and cholesterol [60,61]. Ocular DHA levels are lower in high-cholesterol diets, a fact that could influence the development of ocular disease [62]. Recently, it has been reported the relationship between lipid intake and AMD in patients with low intake of linoleic acid (a LCPUFA) [63].

Cholesterol is present exclusively as the free form in the neurosensory retina, and distributed in all cell layers [54,64]. Cholesterol in the neuroretina originates from *in situ* synthesis and extra-retinal sources. RPE, Müller cells and rods express 3-hydroxy-3-methyl-glutaryl-CoA reductase, the rate-limiting enzyme in the cholesterol biosynthetic pathway [65]. RPE cells express various lipoprotein and scavenger receptors which can promote the recognition of cholesterol-rich lipoprotein and enhance the entry of cholesterol in the neurosensory retina [65]. Indeed, cholesterol bound to LDL can reach the RPE and enter the neurosensory retina [66]. Neurosensory retina and RPE cells express proteins which participate to cholesterol export in tissues other than the retina, such as ABCA1, apoE, ApoA1 or SR-BI [65]. RPE cells have the capacity to synthesise lipoprotein-like particles which may also play a role in these mechanisms of efflux and influx of cholesterol in the retina [67].

Similar to the brain [68,69], the neurosensory retina expresses cholesterol-24S-hydroxylase (CYP46A1) [70]. CYP46A1 is a microsomal cytochrome P450 enzyme which catalyses the hydroxylation of cholesterol at position C24. It has been suggested that CYP46A1 represents a mechanism of cholesterol removal from neurons [71] and strongly induces oxidative stress as well the inflammatory response in RPE cells. RGC specifically express CYP46A1 [70], a hydroxylase that might promote apoptosis of RGC in glaucoma. Cholesterol-27-hydroxylase (CYP27A1) shows a property the similar to that of CYP46A1, converting cholesterol into a more polar metabolite [72]).

7-ketocholesterol is a non-enzymatic-oxidation product of cholesterol. The formation of 7-ketocholesterol in the retina has been thoroughly studied in the retina, in connection with oxidative stress, aging and AMD [73].

With age, the diffusion characteristics of the choriocapillaris-Bruch's membrane-RPE-photoreceptor complex [74,75] change, RPE density decreases [76], and the cytoarchitecture of RPE cells transforms [77]. Such morphological and functional changes lead to AMD in some patients. Additionally, there may be age-related changes in the specific activities of the lysosomal enzymes of the RPE and it has been reported that animals fed a fish-oil-enriched diet presented higher activity of lysosomal acid lipase [78,79]. This could augment the hydrolysis of the intralysosomal lipids of the RPE, thus reducing lipofuscin deposits and oxidative damage of the RPE, this in turn preventing the development of AMD.

Recent studies have demonstrated the relationships between dietary fat and the promotion of vascular disease [51]. Lipoprotein metabolism has also been associated with neurodegenerative disorders in rats [14] but preliminary results showed no marked changes in apo-E knockout mice [80]. Eukaryotic cells require sterols to achieve normal structure and function of their plasma membranes, and deviations from normal sterol composition can perturb these features and compromise cell and organism viability [81]. Given that cholesterol is required by neurons, an intimate relationship could exist between cholesterol homeostasis and the development, maintenance, and repair of these cells [14].

The particular spatial arrangement of retinal macroglial cells (astrocytes and Müller cells) that are intercalated between vasculature and neurons points to their importance in the uptake of nutrients from the circulation, metabolism, and transfer of energy to neurons [37,40,82]. Moreover, apoE lipoprotein, which plays a central role in serum-cholesterol homeostasis through its ability to bind cholesterol with other lipids and to mediate their transport into cells, is produced by glial cells [83]. Müller cells express HMGcoA reductase. Glia is also known to support neurons in the formation and maintenance of synapses in which cholesterol is crucial [84]. Therefore, all together, these data suggest that glial Müller cells may also help deliver cholesterol to neurons [35].

As mentioned above, associations between 24S-hydroxycholesterol in glaucoma and other neurodegenerative diseases are suspected. Glial expression of CYP46A1 has also been reported in the brain of Alzheimer's patients [85,86]. Glia may compensate for the loss of neurons while expressing CYP46A1. Meanwhile, Müller cells play a key role in the maintenance of RGC bodies in the retina, besides participating in lipid metabolism, including fatty acid oxidation [86].

Reactive gliosis, a general response to injury and inflammation in the adult brain [87,88], is characterized by up-regulation of various kinds of molecules, the best known being GFAP [89]. The *de novo* expression of GFAP by retinal Müller cells is indicative of retinal impairment, whether induced by glaucoma [39,90,91] (Figure 2A), retinal detachment [88,92-94], diabetic retinopathy [88,94], or AMD ([74]. By contrast, retinal astrocytes may not only acquire gliotic features but may also diminish in number when there is either vessel damage with greater permeability of the blood-retinal barrier [95] or a massive loss of neurons [96].

Given the intricate metabolic interdependence between vessels, macroglial cells, and neurons, high cholesterol levels could deregulate a number of cell functions in both macroglial and neuronal cells.

3. Hypercholesterolaemia as a risk factor for retinal ischaemia

Most of the information available on vascular diseases is based mainly on studies of ischaemic heart disease [97] and cerebrovascular diseases [98]. In both, the underlying phenomenon is artherosclerosis, a general term referring to any vascular degeneration causing the thickening and loss of arterial-wall elasticity and that encompasses atherosclerotic and non-atherosclerotic conditions. Atherosclerosis involves a hardening of the arterial intima due to a lipid build-up in artery, a condition that appears in humans at an early age and develops progressively over the aging process [99].

Schematically, we can point to various types of long-recognized vascular risk factors: i) non-reversible factors, such as age, male gender or family history of early atherosclerosis; ii) reversible factors such as smoking, hypertension, obesity or hypercholesterolaemia; iii) partially reversible factors such as hypertriglyceridaemia and other forms of hyperlipidaemia, hyperglycaemia, and diabetes mellitus; and iv) potential risk factors such as physical inactivity or emotional stress. Some new factors can be added to the aforementioned vascular risk factors, including lipoprotein A, homocysteine, coagulation factors and C-reactive protein [99,100].

It bears noting that the importance of hypercholesterolaemia as a cardiovascular risk factor lies not only in its direct effect on the pathogenesis of coronary or cerebrovascular disease, but also in the influence exerted on the course of other pathologies. For ocular diseases, epidemiological studies have demonstrated that hypercholesterolaemia is a risk factor for several pathologies despite not being considered the primary cause of the process.

In the case of retinal lesions, classical risk factors for atherosclerosis seem to lose influence. The Atherosclerosis Risk in Communities Study (ARIC) has suggested that changes in the retinal vessels (arteriolar narrowing, arteriovenous index, and abnormalities where the arterioles cross or arteriovenous nicking) are closely linked to hypertension but not to other factors [101], although the presence of retinal lesions is associated with a higher prevalence of ischaemic heart disease, myocardial infarction, stroke, or carotid plaques in patients over 65 years [102,103]. It has been suggested that the retinal lesions could reflect the persistence of small-vessel damage due to hypertension and possibly inflammation and endothelial dysfunction, although they have little relation to large-vessel damage [103].

Another work of the ARIC study found that retinal arteriolar narrowing intensifies the risk of ischaemic heart disease in women but not men after adjusting the population for other known risk factors such as blood pressure, diabetes, smoking, and lipids. The authors speculated that the difference between sexes may be due to the fact that microvascular lesions may have a greater role in women than in men. Hormones protect women from macrovascular injury but it is not clear whether small vessels receive the same protection [104].

The examination of the retinal vasculature offers a unique opportunity to investigate cerebral microcirculation [105], which can be of outstanding importance to clarify the role of microcirculation in stroke [106]. The presence of retinal microvascular abnormalities is linked to the incidence of any stroke and also to the presence of high blood pressure, not only at the time of diagnosis, but also beforehand. Furthermore, stroke has been associated with markers of inflammation and endothelial dysfunction, suggesting the possibility of a significant microvascular component in stroke that a retinal examination might reveal [107]. Notably, although the importance of the association between brain and retinal microvascular lesions is still unknown, the prediction of a stroke provided by the white-matter lesions multiply in the presence of retinal lesions [108].

In conclusion, epidemiological studies have shown an association between vascular changes in the retina and elsewhere. This association appears to be related to common factors of microvasculature damage, the role of which, both in ischaemic heart disease and stroke, may be greater than suspected.

4. Animal models of hypercholesterolaemia

Animal models provide a controlled environment in which to study disease mechanisms and to devise technologies for diagnosis and therapeutic intervention for human atherosclerosis. Different species have been used for experimental purposes (cat, pig, dog, rabbit, rat, mouse, zebra fish). The larger animal models more closely resemble human situations of atherosclerosis and transplant atherosclerosis and can also be easily used in (molecular) imaging studies of cardiovascular disease, in which disease development and efficacy of (novel) therapies can be monitored objectively and non-invasively. Imaging might also enable early disease diagnosis or prognosis [109]. On the other hand, the benefits of genetically modified inbred mice remain useful, especially in quantitative trait locus (QTL)-analysis studies (a genetic approach to examine correlations between genotypes and phenotypes and to identify (new) genes underlaying polygenic traits [109].

4.1. Mice

Wild-type mice are quite resistant to atherosclerosis as a result of high levels of anti-atherosclerotic HDL and low levels of pro-atherogenic LDL and very-low-density-lipoproteins (VLDL). All of the current mouse models of atherosclerosis are therefore based on perturbations of lipoprotein metabolism through dietary or genetic manipulations [110].

ApoE-knockout mice

In apoliprotein-deficient mice (apoE-/-) the homozygous delection of the apoE gene results in a pronounced rise in the plasma levels of LDL and VLDL attributable to the failure of LDL-receptor (LDLr-) and LDL-related proteins (LRP-) mediated clearance of these lipoproteins. As a consequence, apoE-/- mice develop spontaneous atherosclerosis. Of the genetically engineered models, the apoE-deficient model is the only one that develops extensive atherosclerotic lesions on a low-fat cholesterol-free chow diet (<40g/kg). The development of atherosclerosis lesion can be strongly accelerated by a high-fat, high-cholesterol (HFC) diet [111].

ApoE-knockout mice have played a pivotal role in understanding the inflammatory background of atherosclerosis, a disease previously thought to be mainly degenerative. The apoE-deficient mouse model of atherosclerosis can be used to: i) identify atherosclerosis-susceptibility-modifying genes; ii) define the role of various cell types in atherogenesis; iii) characterize environmental factors affecting atherogenesis; and iv) to assess therapies [112].

Because of the rapid development of atherosclerosis and the resemblance of lesion to human counterparts, the apoE-/- model have been widely used. However, some drawbacks are associated with the complete absence of apoE proteins: i) the model is dominated by high levels of plasma cholesterol; ii) most plasma levels are confined to VLDL and not to LDL particles, as in humans; and iii) apoE protein has additional antiatherogenic properties besides regulating the clearance of lipoproteins such as antioxidant, antiproliferative (smooth-muscle cells, lymphocytes), anti-inflammatory, antiplatelet, and also has NO-generating properties or immunomodulatory effects [113-115]. The study of the above processes and the effects of drugs thereupon is restricted in this model.

LDLreceptor-deficient mice (LDLr-/- mice)

In humans, mutations in the gen for the LDLr cause familial hypercholesterolaemia. Mice lacking the gene for LDL receptor (LDLr-/- mice), develops atherosclerosis, especially when fed a lipid-rich diet [116]. The morphology of the lesions in LDLr-/- mice is comparable to that in apoE-/-, while the main plasma lipoprotein in LDLr-/- mice are LDL and high-density-lipoprotein (HDL) [117].

*ApoE*3Leiden (E3L) transgenic mouse*

ApoE*3Leiden (E3L) transgenic mice are being generated by introducing a human ApoE*3-Leiden construct into C57B1/6 mice. E3L mice develop atherosclerosis on being fed cholesterol. Because they are highly responsive to diets containing fat, sugar, and cholesterol, plasma lipid levels can easily be adjusted to a desired concentration by titrating the amount of cholesterol and sugar in the diet. E3L mice have a hyperlipidaemic phenotype with a prominent increase in VLDL- and LDL-sized lipoproteins fractions [118] and are more sensitive to lipid-lowering drugs than are apoE-/- and LDLr-/- mice [110].

4.2. Minipigs

Because of their well-known physiological and anatomical similarities to humans, swine are considered to be increasingly attractive toxicological and pharmacological models. Pigs develop plasma cholesterol levels and atherosclerotic lesions similar to those of humans, but their maintenance is more difficult and expensive than that of smaller animals [109]. The minipig, smaller than the domestic swine, has served as a model of hypercholesterolaemia for more than two decades now. In 1986, the ref. [119] reported that the Göttingen strain had more susceptibility to alimentary hypercholesterolaemia and experimental atherosclerosis than did domestic swine of the Swedish Landrace. Clawn, Yucatan, Sinclair, and Handford are among other general minipigs used for experimental use [120-122].

Down-sized Rapacz pigs are minipigs with familial hypercholesterolaemia caused by a mutation in the low-density lipoprotein receptor. It is a model of advanced atherosclerosis with human like vulnerable plaque morphology that has been used to test an imaging modality aimed at vulnerable plaque detection [123].

The Microminipig (MMP) is the smallest of the minipigs used for experimental atherosclerosis [124]. One of its advantages is that in 3 months an atherosclerosis very similar in location, pathophysiology and pathology to that in humans can be induced [125]. The easy handling and mild character of the MMP make it possible to draw blood and conduct CT scanning under non-anaesthesized conditions.

4.3. Zebra fish

Cholesterol-fed zebra fish represent a novel animal model in which to study the early events involved in vascular lipid accumulation and lipoprotein oxidation [126,127]. Feeding zebra fish a high-cholesterol diet results in hypercholesterolaemia, vascular lipid accumulation, myeloid cell recruitment, and other pathological processes characteristic of early atherogenesis in mammals [128]. The advantages of the zebra-fish model include the optical transparency of the larvae, which enables imaging studies.

4.4. Rabbits

Investigation has continued on hypercholesterolaemic rabbits since 1913, when Anitschkow demonstrated that, in rabbits fed a hypercholesterolaemic diet underwent atherosclerotic changes at the level of the arterial intima similar to those in atherosclerotic humans. The atheromatose lesions in this animal are similar to those in humans also in sequence, as confirmed in aortic atherosclerosis [3], making this animal a universal model for studying the anti-atherogenic activity of many drugs [129-132].

For the characteristics detailed below, the New Zealand rabbit is an excellent model to reproduce human atheromatosis because: i) it is possible to induce hypercholesterolaemia in a few days after administration of a high-cholesterol diet [2]; ii) it is sensitive to the induction of atheromatose lesions [3]; iii) hypercholesterolaemia results from excess LDL [133]; iv) excess cholesterol is eliminated from the tissues to be incorporated in HDL [134]; vi) it is capable of forming cholesterol-HDL complexes associated with apoE which are transported by the blood to the liver [134]; vii) the lipoprotein profile is similar in size to that of humans in the highest range, with HDL being practically the same [135]; viii) it presents postprandial hyperlipaemia for the existence of chilomicron remnants [136]; ix) the hyperlipaemic diet increases apoE [4]; and x) the sustained alteration of lipids after feeding with a cholesterol-rich diet is reversible when the diet [130] is replaced by a normal one [2].

Studies on hypercholesterolaemic rabbits have improved our knowledge of human atherosclerosis by delving into different aspects of the disease such as lipoproteins, mitogenes, growth factors, adhesion molecules, endothelial function, and different types of receptors. At the vascular level, the importance of endothelial integrity and cell adhesion has been investigated [137]. It has been demonstrated that the high levels of lysosomal iron start the oxidation of the LDL, spurring the formation of lesions [138]. In addition, the expression of VCAM-1 preceding the infiltration of the subendothelial space by macrophages has been studied [139], as have the proteins, including MCP-1. In hypercholesterolaemic rabbits, this protein is over-expressed when the serum-cholesterol levels rise in macrophages and smooth-muscle cells, contributing to the development of fatty streaks [140].

In hypercholesterolaemic rabbits, the expression of Fas-L in cells of the arterial wall help us to understand the progression of the atherosclerotic lesion, as this expression indicates an increase in cell injury, as well as a greater accumulation in the intima of smooth-muscle cells [141]. Also, a hyperlipaemic diet causes a selective alteration of the functioning of certain regulatory proteins that are involved in gene expression, as occurs with the nuclear B factor, which stimulates the proliferation of macrophages and smooth-muscle cells [142].

In this model, a study was also made of the pre-thrombosis state triggered by the platelet aggregation in an altered endothelium and the possibilities of its inhibition [143], as well as the interactions of the LDL with the extracellular matrix to form aggregates that accumulate in the intima of the artery wall [144].

The consequences of hypercholesterolaemia in ischaemic cardiopathy and cerebrovascular pathology are well known. The same does not occur with the functional repercussions of the hypercholesterolaemia at the ocular level, partly because the underlying structural changes are not well known.

The hypercholesterolaemic rabbit constitutes a useful model to explore the repercussions of excess lipids at the ocular level. This is because rabbits are susceptible to both systemic as well as ocular alterations. One of the broadest contributions made to the implications of experimental hypercholesterolaemia at the ocular level was that of ref. [145]. These authors, apart from analysing the changes in the liver, spleen, adrenaline glands, heart, aorta, and supraaortic trunk, described the most significant ocular findings, such as the accumulation of lipids in the choroid, retinal disorganization, and lipid keratopathy. With respect to the retinal macroglia, the synthesis of the apoE by the Müller cells, its subsequent secretion in vitro, and its being taken up by the axons and transported by the optic nerve enabled the detection of apoE in the latter geniculate body and in the superior colliculus [13].

Studies with electron microscopy on hypercholesterolaemic rabbits have revealed hypercellularity and optically empty spaces in the corneal stroma. These optically empty spaces, with an elongated or needle shape, were previously occupied by crystals of cholesterol monohydrate or crystals of cholesterol esters [146]. In other studies, the analysis in the form adopted for the crystallizations of the different types of lipids revealed that the needles corresponded to esterified cholesterol, and the short, thin ones to triglycerides [134]. Both crystallizations appear to be associated with other components such as collagen.

It had been recently reported that hypercholesterolaemic rabbis had a build-up of lipids (foam cells and cholesterol clefts) mainly at the suprachoroidea and to a lesser extent at the choroidal vascular layers. This lipids compressed the choroidal vessels and causes hypertrophy of the vascular endothelial- and vascular smooth-muscle cells. The ultrastructural analysis of these vascular structures demonstrated numerous sings of necrosis and a severe damage of the cytoplasmic organelles and caveolar system [16,147].

Recently, it has been reported that in comparison with normal control animals, hypercholesterolaemic rabbits had a reduction of the amplitudes of the first negative peak of the visually evoked potentials, the density of the RGCs, and the thickness of the INL and photoreceptor-cell layer. Additionally, the immunoreactivity to eNOS was reduced and increased to iNOSs. Enhanced activity of iNOS in hypercholesterolaemic rabbits might be involved in impaired visual function and retinal histology. Downregulation of eNOS activity might be one of the causes for impairment of the autoregulation [148].

The formation of foam cells is a consequence of phagocytes from the macrophage-oxidized LDL [16], with the retention of cholesterol in the vascular wall and the activation of ACAT (acetyl-cholesterol-acyl-transferase) [149], this point being key to the role of macrophages in the progression or regression of the lesions [134].

Watanabe

The Watanabe heritable hyperlipidaemic (WHHL) rabbit is an animal model for hypercholesterolaemia due to genetic defects in LDL receptors [150] and a lipoprotein metabolism very similar to that of humans [150,151]. These features make WHHL rabbits a true model of human familial hypercholesterolaemia. The first paper on the WHHL rabbit was published in 1980 [152]. The original WHHL rabbits had a very low incidence of coronary atherosclerosis and did not develop myocardial infarction. Several years of selective breeding led to the development of coronary atherosclerosis-prone WHHL rabbits, which showed metabolic syndrome-like features, and myocardial infarction-prone WHHLMI rabbits. WHHL rabbits have been used in studies of several compounds with hypocholesterolaemic and/or anti-atherosclerotic effects with special relevance for statins [151]. Recently, WHHLMI rabbits have been used in studies of the imaging of atherosclerotic lesions by MRI [153], PET [154] and intravascular ultrasound [155].

5. Hypercholesterolemia induced ultrastructural changes in the Bruch's membrane-retinal complex

Few experimental studies examine the effects of hypercholesterolaemia on the posterior segment of the eye [14,15,145,156-158]. Hypercholesterolaemic rabbits constitute a useful model to delve into the repercussions of excess lipids at the ocular level. Rabbits fed a 0.5% cholesterol-enriched diet for 8 months showed a statistical increase in total serum cholesterol [15,16,147,158,159]. In these animals, the hypercholesterolaemia caused numerous changes in the Bruch's membrane-retinal complex. Bruch's membrane was thicker than in normal animals (Figure 3A,B) due to the build-up of electrodense and electrolucent particles (Figure 3B) in the inner and outer collagenous layers [15]. As in hypercholesterolaemic animals, thickening and lipid accumulation in Bruch's membrane has been described in human AMD [160,161]. These deposits of lipids or lipid-rich material could add resistance to the flow of solutes and water through the Bruch's membrane-RPE complex, as demonstrated by the studies that have measured the hydraulic conductivity of isolated Bruch's membranes [162,163]. The local metabolism and transport of cholesterol, impaired in hypercholesterolaemic rabbits as a result of a thickened Bruch's membrane with changes in its collagenous layers, could play an important role in the contribution of lipids required for retinal neurons to maintain and remodel their membranes.

The cholesterol source for RPE and photoreceptors are the plasma lipids. Given that there is no direct contact between the photoreceptors and the choroidal circulation, adjacent cell types (RPE cells and Müller cells) must facilitate the transfer of lipids to the photoreceptors. In fact, the expression of native receptors for LDL on RPE cells has been reported [12,164]; this could be related to local production of apoE by RPE cells. An abnormal metabolism of lipids secondary to a cholesterol-enriched diet and/or apoE deficiencies could upset the cholesterol balance in RPE and photoreceptors. This could be the situation in hypercholesterolaemic rabbits in which ERP changes have been reported [15]. In this experimental model, RPE showed numerous hypertrophic cells and some nuclei were absent. The cytoplasm of these cells showed numerous dense bodies, debris from cell membranes, and numerous clumps of lipids (Figure 4B) filling the cytoplasm and replacing the nucleus and organelles that could be contributing to the hypertrophy and degeneration of the RPE [15]. Additionally, the basal zone of some RPE cells revealed autophagic vesicles, vacuoles, electrodense deposits, and debris from cell membranes [15] that could correspond to the laminar deposits described by [165] (Figure 4B). As in human AMD, changes of RPE could contribute to the degeneration of the photoreceptors [164] whose metabolism depends on normal RPE function and integrity [15,166].

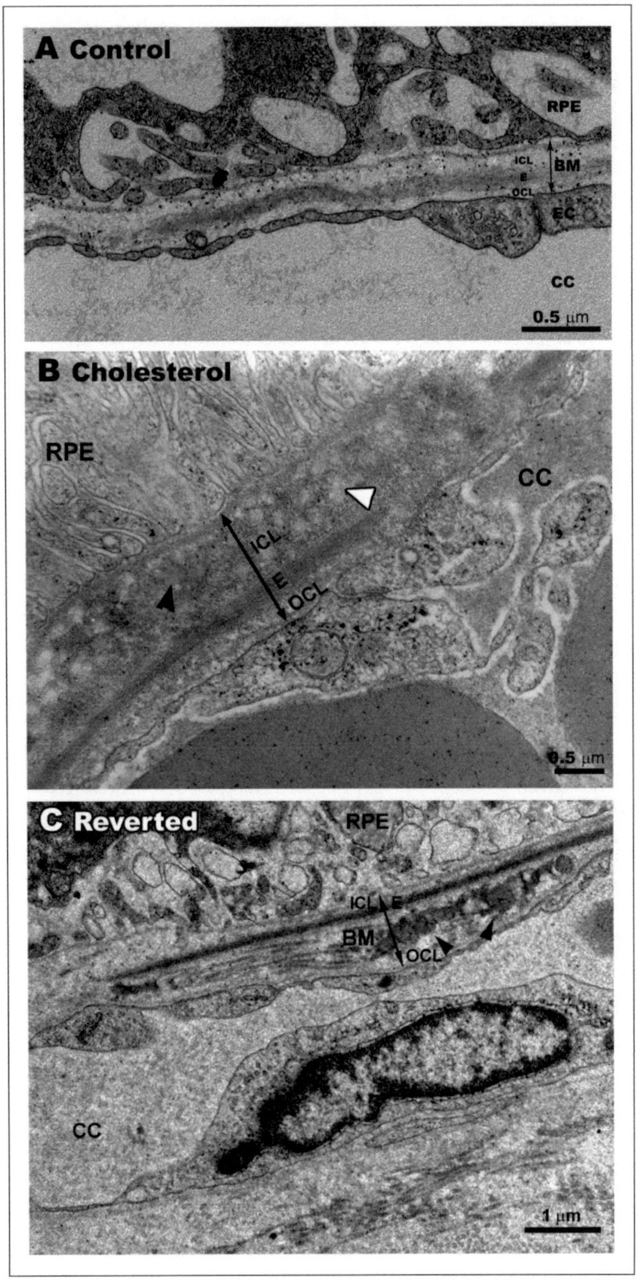

Figure 3. Transmission electron microscopy of Bruch's membrane and choriocapillaris. A: Control rabbit. B: Hypercholesterolaemic rabbit. Electrodense (black arrowhead) and electroluminescent (white arrowhead) particles at the inner collagenous layer Modified from Triviño et al. [15]). C: Reverted rabbit. Bruch's membrane with electrodense particles (black arrowheads) at the outer collagenous layer. [Bruch's membrane (BM); choriocapillaris (CC); retinal pigment epithelium (RPE); inner collagenous layer (ICL); elastic layer (E); outer collagenous layer (OCL); endothelial cell (EC)]. (Modified from Ramírez et al. [158])

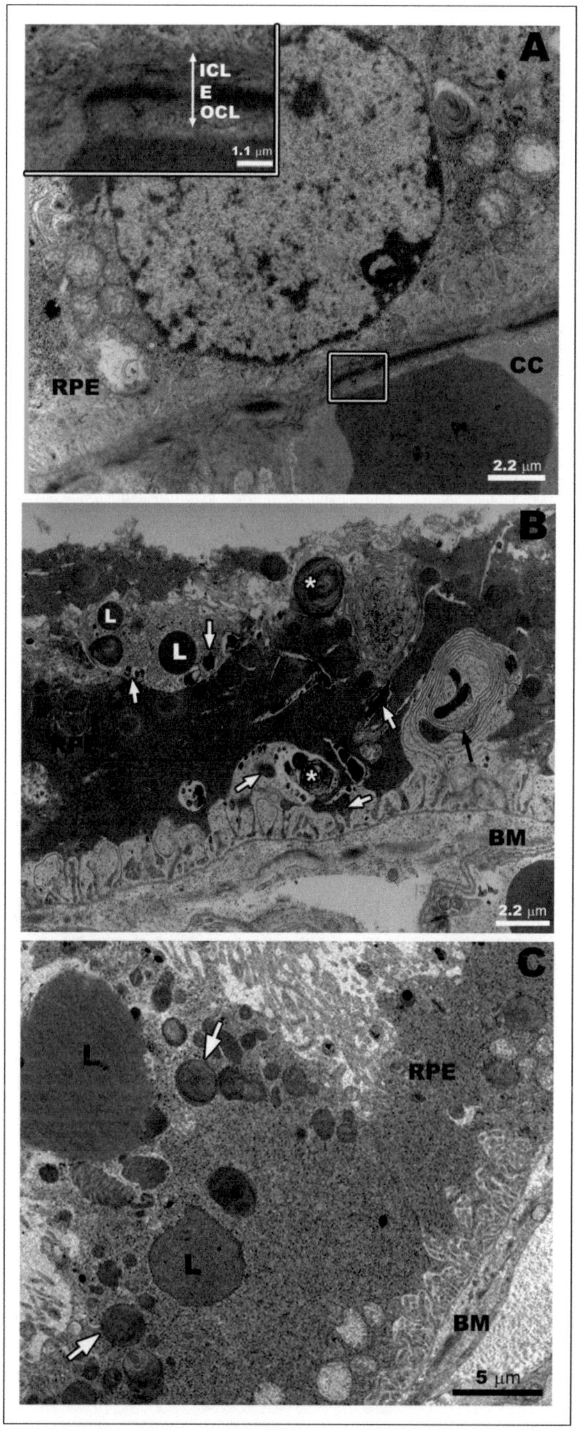

Figure 4. Transmission electron microscopy of Bruch's membrane and retinal pigment epithelium cells (RPE). A: Choriocapillaris - Bruch's membrane - RPE complex from control rabbit. Detail of Bruch's

membrane (insert) showing the outer collagenous layer, elastic layer and inner collagenous layer. B: The cytoplasm of RPE cell in hypercholesterolaemic rabbit shows dense bodies (white arrows), debris from cell membranes (*) and droplets of lipids. The apical microvilli have disappeared and the basal infolding forms lamellar structures (black arrow). C: RPE cells in reverted rabbit. Few lipids, dense bodies (white arrows) and some lamellar structures are visible in the cytoplasm. [Choriocapillaris (CC); retinal pigment epithelium (RPE); Bruch's membrane (BM); inner collagenous layer (ICL); elastic layer (E); outer collagenous layer (OCL); lipids (L)]. (Modified from Ramírez et al. [158] and Triviño et al. [15]).

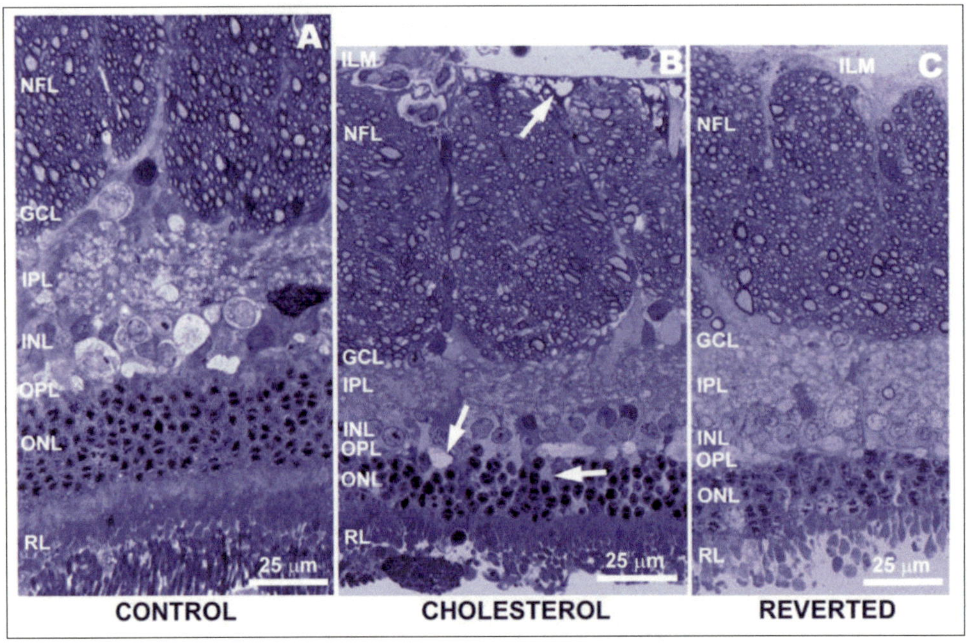

Figure 5. Retinal semi-thin sections (light microscopy). Retinal-layer changes. A: Control rabbit. B: Hypercholesterolaemic rabbit. C: Reverted rabbit. The figure illustrates the overall thinning of the retinal layers in hypercholesterolaemic and reverted animals with respect to control. The empty spaces (arrows) secondary to cell loss and degeneration observed in hypercholesterolaemic (B) are less evident in reverted rabbit (C). [Ganglion-cell layer (GCL); inner nuclear layer (INL); inner plexiform layer (IPL); inner limiting membrane (ILM); nerve-fibre layer (NFL); outer nuclear layer (ONL); outer plexiform layer (OPL); photoreceptor layer (RL)]. (Modified from Ramírez et al. [158]).

The nutrition of the outer retina depends on the integrity of the choriocapillaris vessels and on the diffusion of plasma through the Bruch's membrane-RPE complex. The alterations in the endothelium of the choriocapillaris and the build-up of lipids (hydrophobic barrier) detected in the Bruch's membrane-RPE complex of hypercholesterolaemic rabbits [15] could interfere with oxygen and nutrient transportation, leading to an ischaemic state [30].

The conditions of hypoxia-ischaemia lead to higher glutamate levels in the extracellular fluid, and thereby could cause oxidative damage by excitotoxic mechanisms in the neurons [21,22]. In hypercholesterolaemic rabbits, neurosensory retinal changes were detected (Figure 5A,B) [15].

These changes were not uniformly distributed throughout the retina, being more intense in the retinal areas overlying the most altered RPE cells. In these areas, the photoreceptor discs were mostly absent. The thickness of the retinal layers (ONL, OPL, INL, IPL, GCL and NFL) were reduced (Figure 5B) and empty spaces were visible at different retinal levels that consisted of different stages of cell degeneration due to necrosis and apoptosis (Figure 6A,7A,B). In necrotic cells, the nucleoplasm, cytoplasm, and cytoplasmic organelles underwent progressive hydropic degeneration (swelling, vacuolization, and disappearance of specific ultrastructural features) (Figure 6A). The nuclear and cytoplasm membranes ruptured and released their contents into the intercellular space (Figure 6A). The remains were taken up and absorbed by neighbouring cells –essentially Müller cells (Figure 6A,7A) and astrocytes -, the latter only in the NFL. The apoptotic cells showed progressive condensation and shrinkage of the nucleoplasm and cytoplasm (Figure 7A,B). Cells in more advanced stages of apoptosis shed part of their substance, which was observed as dense inclusion bodies in neighbouring cells (Figure 6A,7A). The compact bodies appeared surrounded by or engulfed in Müller cells and astrocytes [15,158].

Changes found in the nuclear layers of the retina of hypercholesterolaemic rabbits resemble those described in human AMD [74]. As in human AMD, hypercholesterolaemic rabbits exhibited a loss of ganglion cells and had cell features of apoptosis and necrosis as well as electrodense inclusions (probably lipofuscin) in the cytoplasm of this cell type (Figure 7B). This ganglion-cell loss could be caused, at least partly, by a local disruption of cholesterol homeostasis [14]. A reduced population of ganglion cells could secondarily impair the neurotrophic support of the retinal neurons as a consequence of reduced secretion of brain-derived neurotrophic factor (BDNF) by ganglion cells. This scenario is feasible, given that amacrine cells express the TrkB receptor for BDNF [17] and that BDNF improves the survival of bipolar cells upon activation of the p75 receptor, which then induces the secretion of fibroblast growth factor b (bFGF) [167]. The situations described could contribute to the axon loss observed in hypercholesterolaemic rabbits [158]; this loss parallels human AMD, in which a considerable axonal degeneration has been reported [74].

In hypercholesterolaemic rabbits, the capillaries in the NFL and in the vitreous humour had a thickening of the basal membrane, dense bodies, and cytoplasm vacuoles (Figure 8A,B). These alterations have also been reported in hypercholesterolaemic rats [156].

In summary, the thickening of the basal membrane together with the alterations of the endothelial cells of the intraretinal and epiretinal capillaries, combined with the changes in Bruch's membrane and the build-up of lipids in the outer retina, could contribute to a situation of chronic ischaemia observed in the retina of hypercholesterolaemic rabbits.

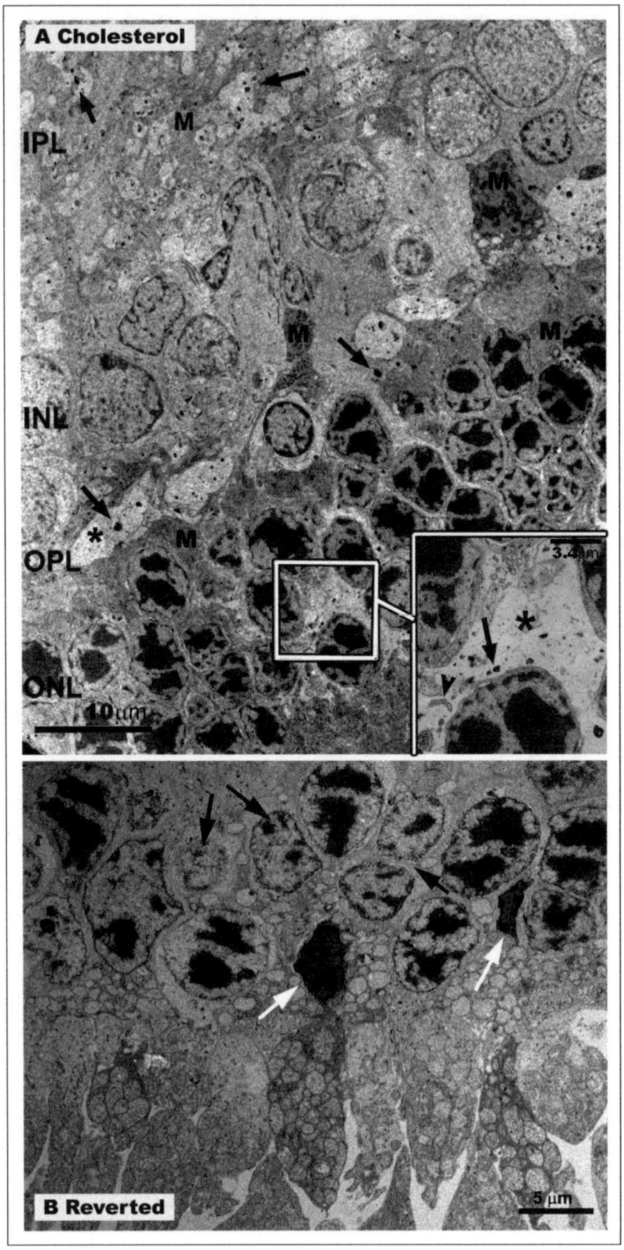

Figure 6. Ultrastructural retinal changes in outer nuclear layer and outer plexiform layer. A: Hypercholesterolaemic rabbit. Numerous dense bodies (black arrows) and empty spaces (*) are visible in these layers. The processes of Müller cells fill the empty spaces left by degenerated cells. Insert: at greater magnification the empty spaces consist of degenerated cytoplasm with numerous dense bodies (black arrow) and cell debris (black arrowhead). B: Reverted rabbit. Apoptosis (white arrows) and necrosis (black arrows) of photoreceptors are visible in the ONL. [Müller cells (M); inner nuclear layer (INL); inner plexiform layer (IPL); outer nuclear layer (ONL); outer plexiform layer (OPL)]. (Modified from Ramírez et al. [158] and Triviño et al. [15]).

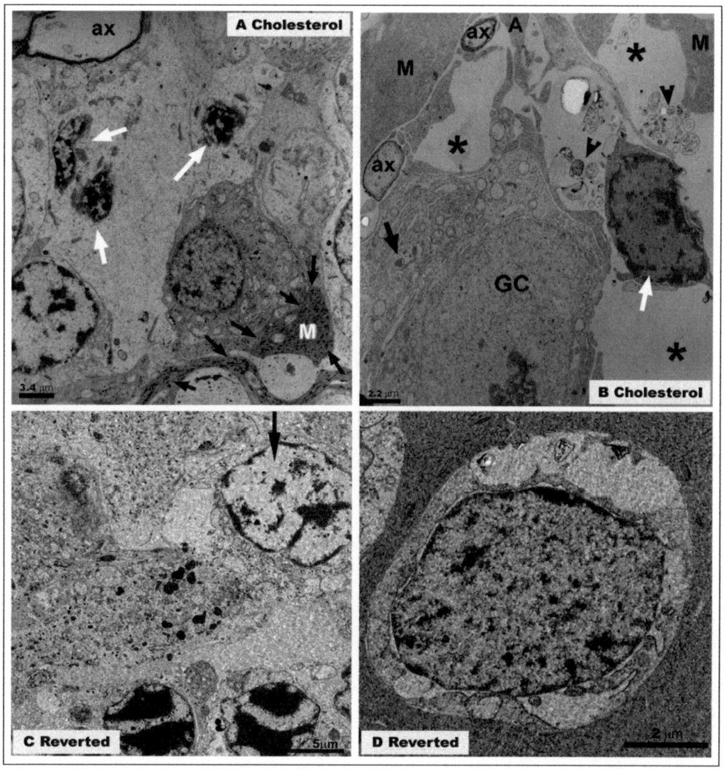

Figure 7. Ultrastructural retinal changes in inner nuclear layer and ganglion-cell layer.
A-B: Hypercholesterolaemic rabbit. A: Cells in apoptosis (white arrows) in the inner nuclear layer. Dense bodies (black arrows) inside the Müller cell processes. B: Apoptosis (white arrow) in the ganglion-cell layer. Cell debris (black arrowheads) and dense bodies (black arrow). [Müller cell (M); axon (ax); ganglion cell (GC)]. C-D: Reverted rabbit. C: Cell necrosis (black arrow) in the inner nuclear layer.
D: Ganglion cell in advanced stage of necrosis. (Modified from Ramírez et al. [158] and Triviño et al. [15])

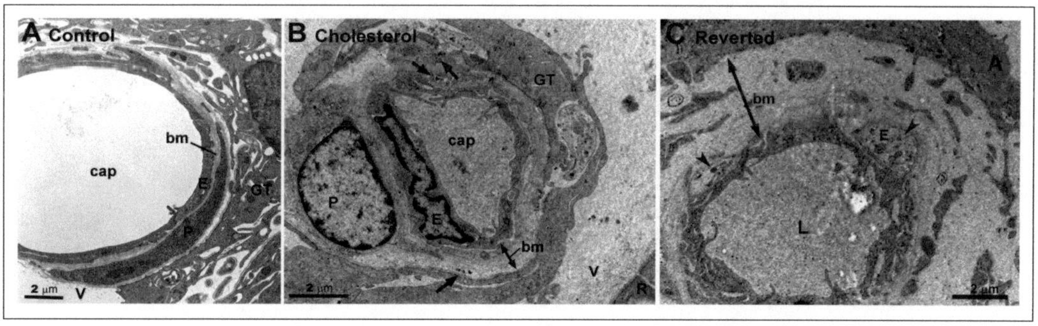

Figure 8. Transmission electron microscopy of capillaries in the vitreous humour. A: Control rabbit.
B: Hypercholesterolaemic rabbit. The basal membrane is thickened with respect the control. C: Reverted rabbit. The basal membrane is thicker than control and cholesterol animals. Necrotic features (arrowhead) are visible in some endothelial cells. [Basal membrane (bm); capillary (cap); endothelial cell (E); glial tuft (GT); pericyte (P); vitreous humour (V); dense bodies (black arrows); retina (R); vascular lumen (L); astrocyte (A)]. (Modified from Ramírez et al. [158] and Triviño et al. [15])

6. Hypercholesterolaemia-induced changes in the retinal macroglia

An abnormal metabolism of lipids secondary to a cholesterol-enriched diet and/or apoE deficiencies could upset the cholesterol balance in the retinal layers, as mentioned above. However, it appears that other retinal components can produce heterogeneous particles locally containing apoE [13]. These particles are synthesised mainly by Müller cells, although astrocytes associated with ganglion cells axons could be involved in their production [13]. Müller cells are radially oriented cells that along their course, extend branches that interdigitate with every type of retinal neuron, with other types of glia (Figure 2A), and with the blood vessels of vascularized retinas [168]. Its participation in the cholesterol metabolism (supplying heterogeneous lipoprotein particles and apoE) and transport (due to its anatomical position in the retina) determines its importance as a source of the lipids needed by neurons for maintaining and restructuring their cell membranes [13,168].

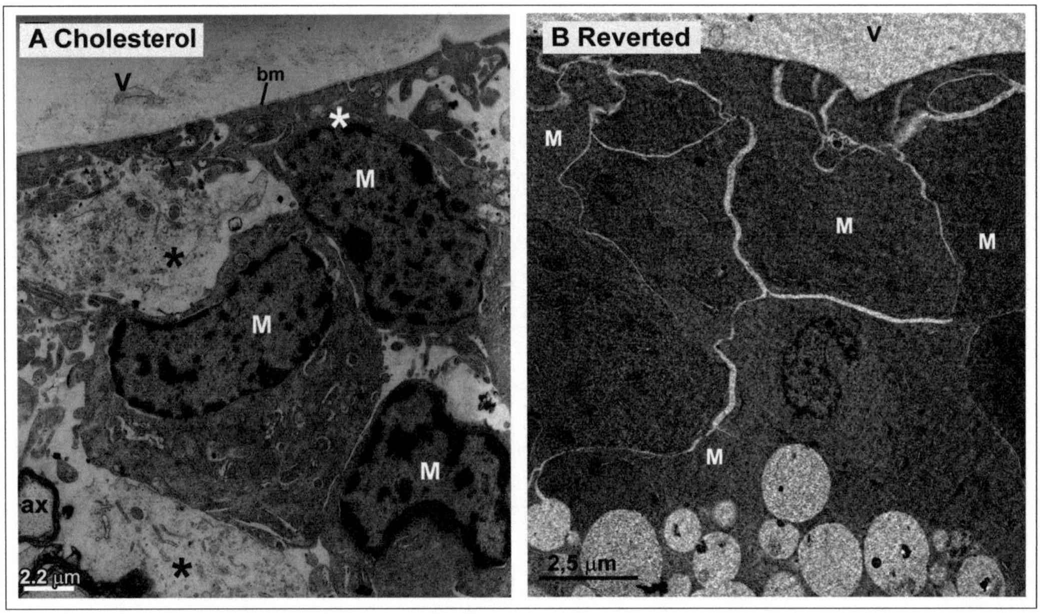

Figure 9. Transmission electron microscopy of retinal astrocytes and Müller cells.
A: Hypercholesterolaemic rabbit. Three nuclei of Müller cells displaced to the nerve-fibre layer. One of the Müller cells participates in the formation of the inner limiting membrane (white asterisk). Astrocytes in advanced stage of necrosis (black asterisk). B: Reverted rabbit. The empty spaces left by degenerated axons in the medullated nerve-fibre region are occupied only by the Müller cells in the retinal periphery. [Axon (ax); basal membrane of the ILM (bm); Müller cell (M); vitreous humour (V)]. (Modified from Ramírez et al. [158] and Triviño et al. [15]).

In situations of sustained hypercholesterolaemia, alterations of lipid metabolism could take place, potentially influencing the glial response. In fact, in hypercholesterolaemic rabbits Müller cells were reactive, exhibiting large amounts of rough endoplasmic reticulum and abundant glial filaments in their cytoplasm (Figure 9A), manifested by a more intense immunoreaction to GFAP (Figure 10H) [158]. Normally, GFAP is expressed at a low level or is not detectable in mammalian Müller cells (Figure 10G). In pathological situations, the major intermediate filament expressed by reactive Müller cells appears to be GFAP. The loss of retinal integrity as a result of mechanical injury, detachment, photoreceptor degeneration or glaucoma (Figure 2A) provokes intense GFAP immunoreactivity in Müller cells and increases the GFAP content of the retina [39,91,169-171]. This over-expression of GFAP is due to the activation of the transcriptional gene for GFAP in Müller cells [168]. Additionally, Müller cell reactivity transduces an increase in cell metabolism [168].

Another consequence of the reactivity of Müller cells is their capacity to form glial scars, most probably in an attempt to restore the blood-retinal barrier [172]. These scars, formed by hypertrophic cells in which the nuclei were displaced to the NFL, were detected in hypercholesterolaemic rabbits (Figure 9A). In addition, hypertrophic Müller cells occupied some of the empty spaces left by degenerated neurons in the INL, ONL, IPL, and NFL (Figure 6A) [15,158,173]. This type of cell response, which has also been described in human AMD [74] resembles that following photoceptor degeneration, which induces the processes of Müller cells to extend into and fill the empty spaces [168]. Another similarity between human AMD and experimental hypercholesterolaemia are the ultrastructural changes affecting the outer and inner retina. In both instances, the bodies of Müller cells are displaced from the INL to the vitreous in the case of human AMD [74] and to the NFL and ILM in hypercholesterolaemic rabbits [15,158]. It is possible that in both situations Müller cells migrate in an attempt to reach the metabolic reserve in the vitreous. This could be an adaptive system for transporting nutrients and energy substrates to those areas of the retina exposed to the chronic ischaemic insult.

Like Müller cells, astrocytes are related to apoE secretion [174,175], making these cells susceptible to alteration in long-term hypercholesterolaemia. Müller cells and astrocytes are intermediate between neurons and vessels; they are located on the basal membrane of capillaries separating them from neurons [37,82,95,168]. The thickening of the basal membrane and the presence of dense bodies and vacuoles in the endothelial cytoplasm of the retinal blood vessel in hypercholesterolaemic rabbits (Figure 8A) [15] could indicate impaired transport of oxygen and nutrients to the retinal tissue as well as the removal of cellular debris, thus contributing to a situation of chronic ischaemia [20] in the inner retina. It is known that astrocytes protect neurons from ischaemia by different mechanisms: they remove excitotoxic neurotransmitters and ions from the perineural space, doing so partly by glutamine synthetase, which also provides glutamine to neurons ([176,177]. In addition, astrocytes store glycogen, have the potential to provide lactate, and produce growth factors as well as cytokines [23]. Moreover, it has been shown that astrocytes are more resistant to oxidative damage because they possess antioxidant mechanisms such as high concentrations of reduced glutathione and vitamin C [21]. Therefore, a reduction in the protective function of astrocytes could contribute to neural dysfunction.

Differences between rabbit and human retinas and astrocytes must be taken into account when comparing the two species [38,41,42,82]. The rabbit retina has epiretinal vascularization and possesses perivascular astrocytes which are absent in humans. However, in both species, astrocytes are located at the NFL and GCL. The rabbit retina had two main groups of astrocytes: astrocytes associated with the nerve-fibre bundles (Figure 10A) and perivascular astrocytes (type I and type II) (Figure 10A,D), associated with the vitreous blood vessels [40].

As mentioned above, astrocytes are essential for the maintenance of neural homeostasis, and their susceptibility to alteration in long-term hypercholesterolaemia has been reported [15]. Thus, in hypercholesterolaemic rabbits, all retinal types of astrocytes were reactive, having large amounts of rough endoplasmic reticulum and upregulation of GFAP immunoreactivity (Figure 10B,E,H). The altered lipid homeostasis, in conjunction with increased astrocyte activity, could explain the build-up of electrodense particles, probably lipofuscin and lipids, found in their cytoplasm. The exposure of these electrodense particles to light and high oxygen concentrations provide ideal conditions for the formation of reactive oxygen species that damage cellular proteins and lipid membranes [178], a situation that could impair the mechanism of protection from ischaemia. If we add to this the higher concentrations of extracellular toxic substances (e.g. glutamate) which could damage the neurons by cytotoxic mechanisms [21,22], the possibilities of keeping the cellular machinery intact against ischaemia diminish in favour of neuronal death. All the above-mentioned conditions could contribute to macroglial swelling and subsequent breakdown of intermediate filaments (loss of GFAP staining) and ultimately macroglial death [23]. In fact, hypercholesterolaemic rabbits showed apoptosis and necrosis affecting Müller cells and astrocytes (Figure 7B,9A), resulting in a statistically significant loss of all types of astrocytes in comparison with control animals (Figure 10A,B, 11) [15].

In summary, long-term hypercholesterolaemia lowers the astrocyte number and their antioxidant activity as well as the capability to remove glutamate from the extracellular space; it may also contribute to neuronal dysfunction [15,158]. The reactivation and migration of retinal Müller cells may be reflecting an adaptive system to supply nutrients to those areas of the retina exposed to the chronic ischaemia generated by the hyperlipidaemia.

7. Changes in Bruch's membrane retinal complex after the normalization of hypercholesterol levels

It has been established that the atherosclerotic lesions can undergo regression in experimental animals such as rabbits, dogs, and non-human primates [179]; and the lack of progression or even regression can occur in humans, especially with the introduction of new therapeutic options [180].

Animal models are useful for studying lesion regression after the normalization of cholesterol serum values. When high levels of cholesterol are withdrawn from the diet, rabbits recover some of the biochemical and histological parameters altered in cholesterol-fed animals [16,181]. Serum concentration of total cholesterol, triglycerides, phospholipids, VLDL, HDL, LDL, and intermediate-density lipoprotein (IDL) have reported to increase in rabbits fed with a 0.5% cholesterol-enriched diet for eight months. When the same animals are then fed a standard diet for another 6 months, (reverted rabbits), lipid values returned to normal [158]. Notably, the normalization of serum values was not followed by a complete recovery of the thoracic aorta, choroid [16], or histology of the retina (Figure 5C) [158]. Specifically, in reverted rabbits, Bruch's membrane (Figure 3C) and RPE alterations (Figure 4C) were still present although to a lesser extent than in hypercholesterolaemic animals (Figure 3B, 4B). Bruch's membrane was thicker in some areas due to collagenous and electrodense material in the outer collagenous layer (Figure 3C). This contrasted with the observations in hypercholesterolaemic rabbits in which the thicker Bruch's membrane resulted from the build-up of electrodense and electrolucent particles, mainly at the inner collagenous layer (Figure 3B) [15]. The cytoplasm of RPE cells contained a considerably lower quantity of lipids in reverted animals (Figure 4C), although in some instances the lamellar structures (the plasma membrane of basal infolding back on itself) described in hypercholesterolaemic rabbits were also seen. This partial structural recovery could improve the diffusion of nutrients from the choriocapillaris and removal of cell debris from RPE, thus exerting a possible effect on the retina. However, reverted rabbits retained features observed in hypercholesterolaemic animals, such as an apparent decrease in retinal thickening (Figure 5C), intense cell degeneration due to necrosis and apoptosis in the ONL, INL, and GCL and axonal degeneration at the NFL (Figure 6B, 7CD). The empty spaces following neuronal death observed in hypercholesterolaemic animals were occupied by Müller cells (in OPL, IPL, NFL) and by astrocytes (in NFL) in reverted rabbits (Figure 6A) [158].

It bears mentioning that the retinal vessel in reverted rabbits showed greater damage than in hypercholesterolaemic animals such as: thickening of the basal membrane with numerous dense bodies, necrosis of endothelial cells, hypertrophy of the muscle layer, and increase in the collagen tissue of the adventitia (Figure 8C) [158]. The maintenance of retinal damage observed in reverted animals could be at least partly due to the greater alterations of retinal vessels and the persistence of the choriocapillaris alterations [16]. The vascular retinal alterations, which extended from the endothelium to the adventitia, could contribute to sustain an ischaemic situation despite the diet-induced normalization of lipid levels. Another factor that could contribute to the maintenance of retinal damage would be the role of Müller cells in neuronal swelling and apoptosis. During ischaemia, over-excitation of ionotropic glutamate receptors not only leads to neuron depolarization, which causes excess Ca^{2+} influx into the cells, but also activates the apoptosis machinery. The ion fluxes in the retinal neurons, associated with water movements that are mediated by aquaporin-4 water channels expressed by Müller cells, can result in neuronal swelling [182]. Thus, during ischaemic episodes in the rabbit retina, the plexiform layers and the cytoplasm of neurons become oedematous.

In summary, normalization of the lipid level is not followed by a complete normalization of the retinal histology. The remaining changes in the retina are due mainly to the sustained chronic ischaemia caused by the alterations in the retinal vessel, Bruch's membrane, and RPE. Such ischaemic situations exert a detrimental impact on the neurons of the different layers of the retina.

8. Changes in the retinal macroglia after normalization of hypercholesterol levels

As described for the Bruch's membrane-retinal complex, the normalization of the blood-lipid levels by the substitution of 8 months of a hypercholesterolaemic diet by 6 months of a standard one, do not reverse the changes in the retinal macroglial population of hypercholesterolaemic rabbits [158].

In reverted animals, Müller cells were hypertrophic and filled up the empty spaces left by degenerated neurons and axons (Figure 9B). This hypertrophy could be due to the osmotic swelling of Müller cells. A significant correlation between Müller cell hypertrophy and the extent of osmotic Müller cell swelling has been reported in rat retina during retinal inflammation, suggesting that the alterations of swelling properties is characteristic of Müller cell gliosis [183]. It has also been proposed that Müller cell swelling in the post-ischaemic retina is caused by inflammatory mediators, due to the activation of phospholipase A2 by osmotic stress [182]. In both hypercholesterolaemic and reverted rabbits, the hyperlipaemic diet could have caused an imbalance in long-chain polyunsaturated fatty acids (in the neural retina, these are present mainly in the phospholipids of the cell membranes [53]) which could prompt an increase in inflammatory elements such as reactive oxygen species from macrophages, TNF-α, IL-1β, IL-6, Natural Killer, cytotoxic T lymphocyte activation, and lymphocyte proliferation [51]. Therefore, ischaemic and inflammatory processes could trigger Müller cell hypereactivity in hypercholesterolaemic animals and reverted rabbits and provoke the hypertrophy and swelling of this cell type.

The astrocytes of reverted rabbits displayed changes with respect to hypercholesterolaemic animals. The area occupied by the astrocytes associated with the nerve-fibre bundles was significantly lower than in the hypercholesterolaemic group (Figure 10H,I,11). With respect PVA (perivascular astrocytes), a striking feature was the absence of type I PVA, thus the intense GFAP immunoreactivity found in the retinal blood vessels was due mainly to type II PVA (Figure 10C,F). The processes of these cells formed a network similar to that exhibited by the type I PVA of the normal rabbits [158]. The maintenance of the area occupied by the PVA in reverted animals (Figure 11) could be due to the hyperplasia of type II PVA as an attempt to compensate for the loss of type I PVA (Figure 10C,F). This cell proliferation is presumably a response to the sustained retinal ischaemia undergone by reverted rabbits despite of normalization of cholesterol levels. Type II PVA of reverted animals were reactive, hypertrophic, and had an enlargement of their cell bodies and processes (Figure 10F) [158]. These features plus the above-mentioned hyperplasia are typical changes of glial cells in response to nerve damage [184].

The specific function of reactive gliosis is unknown. It has been reported that glial cells undergoing reactive gliosis up-regulate the production of cytokines and neurotrophic factors which may be crucial for the viability of injured neurons [168]. Additionally, it is presumed that reactive gliosis is involved in phagocytosis of debris and in restoring breaches in the blood-brain barrier by scar formation [185]. Müller cells and astrocytes from hypercholesterolaemic and reverted rabbits had cell debris in their cytoplasm [158]. It has been reported that astrocytes [186] as well as Müller cells [187] can exert phagocytic functions and that the microglia (the main phagocytic cell of the nervous system) intervene only when the build-up of debris in the nervous tissue is abundant [188]. Phagocytosis of exogenous particles, cell debris, and hemorrhagic products may be an important scavenging function of Müller cells [168]. It has been suggested that the phagocytic process of these cells is similar to that associated with macrophages and that in addition they can function as antigen-presenting cells [39,168].

From the above, it can be concluded that the substitution of a hyperlipaemic diet by a standard one in an experimental rabbit model normalizes the blood-lipid levels. However, the progressive and irreversible chronic retinal ischaemia secondary to cholesterol-induced changes in the choroid [16,147] as well as the retinal blood vessels trigger a sustained reactive gliosis that could be exerting neurotrophic, phagocytic or immune-related functions among others.

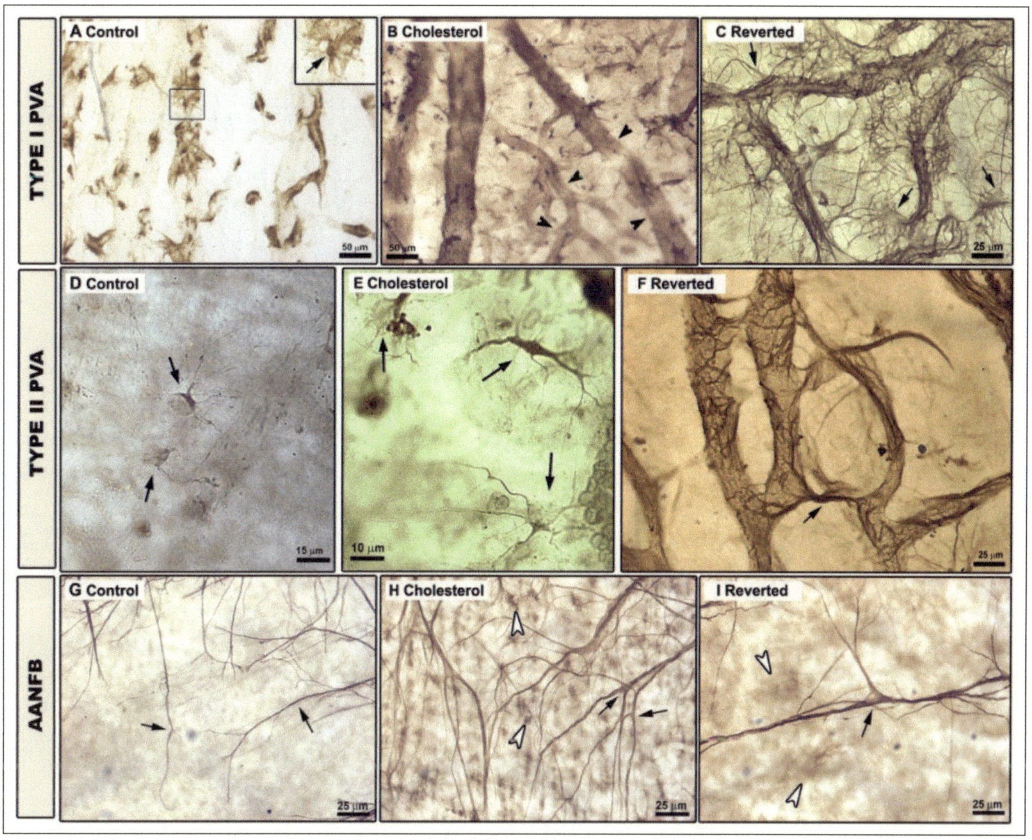

Figure 10. Immunohistochemistry anti-GFAP in rabbit retinal whole-mount. A-C: Type I perivascular astrocytes (PVA). D-F: Type II PVA. G-I: Astrocytes associated with the nerve-fibre bundles (AANFB). A, D, G: Control rabbits. B, E, H: Hypercholesterolaemic rabbits. C, F, I: Reverted rabbits. A-C: In hypercholesterolaemic animals Type I PVA have a higher GFAP+ immunoreactivity than in control animals; these cells are absent from many retinal vessels. In reverted animals a striking feature is the absence of type I PVA. D-F: In hypercholesterolaemic animals Type II PVA have higher GFAP immunoreactivity, robust cell bodies and thicker processes than in control. In reverted animals the intense GFAP+ cells are morphologically similar to the reactive type II PVA of hypercholesterolaemic animals. G-I: In hypercholesterolaemic and reverted animals the AANFB show high GFAP+ immunoreactivity, robust cell bodies, and thick processes. [Astrocytes cell bodies (arrow); vessel free of type I PVA (arrowhead); GFAP immunorectivity of Müller cells (empty arrow)]. (Modified from Ramírez et al. [158]).

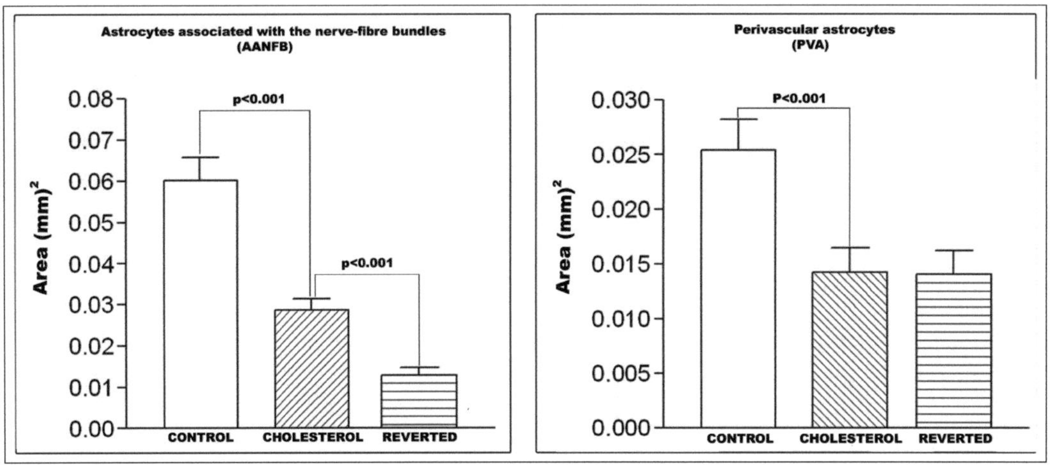

Figure 11. Area occupied by astrocytes per zone measured (0.1899mm2) in Control, hypercholesterolaemic, and reverted animals. (Modified from Ramírez et al. [158]).

9. Conclusions and perspectives

Hypercholesterolaemia is a risk factor for the development of chronic ischaemia in the retina and therefore for neuronal survival [15,158]. It is now recognized that lipids play a key role as structural and signalling molecules. Given that lipid intake is most dependent on food composition, the dietary regimen could contribute to induction or prevention of retinal diseases. In relation to this, a pertinent question would be whether or not the normalization of the plasma-cholesterol levels could restore the retinal changes that take place during hypercholesterolaemia and reverse the chronic ischaemia process generated by this situation. The answer to this question seems to be no, since, although it is true that the lipid accumulations in the choroid and Bruchs' membrane are reduced with the normalization of the blood-lipid level, some structural changes do not reverse [16,158], implying an irreversibly chronic situation and very probably progressive ischaemia in retina.

Author details

A. Triviño, B. Rojas and J.M. Ramírez
Instituto de Investigaciones Oftalmológicas Ramón Castroviejo,
Universidad Complutense de Madrid, Madrid, Spain
Departamento de Oftalmología, Facultad de Medicina,
Universidad Complutense de Madrid, Madrid, Spain

R. de Hoz, B.I. Gallego, A.I. Ramírez and J.J. Salazar
Instituto de Investigaciones Oftalmológicas Ramón Castroviejo,
Universidad Complutense de Madrid, Madrid, Spain
Escuela Universitaria de Óptica,
Universidad Complutense de Madrid, Madrid, Spain

Acknowledgement

The authors would like to thank David Nesbitt for correcting the English version of this work. This work was supported by RETICs Patología Ocular del Envejecimiento, Calidad Visual y Calidad de Vida (Grant ISCIII RD07/0062/0000, Spanish Ministry of Science and Innovation); Fundación Mutua Madrileña (Grant 4131173); BSCH-UCM GR35/10-A Programa de Grupos de Investigación Santander-UCM. Beatriz Gallego is currently supported by a predoctoral fellowship from the Universidad Complutense de Madrid.

10. References

[1] Zilversmit DB. Atherogenesis: a postprandial phenomenon. Circulation 1979;60(3) 473-485.

[2] Finking G, Hanke H. Nikolaj Nikolajewitsch Anitschkow (1885-1964) established the cholesterol-fed rabbit as a model for atherosclerosis research. Atherosclerosis 1997;135(1) 1-7.

[3] Yanni AE. The laboratory rabbit: an animal model of atherosclerosis research. Laboratory Animals 2004;38(3) 246-256.

[4] Reddy C, Stock EL, Mendelsohn AD, Nguyen HS, Roth SI, Ghosh S. Pathogenesis of experimental lipid keratopathy: corneal and plasma lipids. Investigative Ophthalmology & Visual Science 1987;28(9) 1492-1496.

[5] Roth SI, Stock EL, Siel JM, Mendelsohn A, Reddy C, Preskill DG, Ghosh S. Pathogenesis of experimental lipid keratopathy. An ultrastructural study of an animal model system. Investigative Ophthalmology & Visual Science 1988;29(10) 1544-1551.

[6] Garibaldi BA, Goad ME. Lipid keratopathy in the Watanabe (WHHL) rabbit. Veterinary Pathology 1988;25(2) 173-174.

[7] Hogan MJ, Alvarado JA, Weddell JE. Histology of the human eye: an atlas and textbook.. Toronto: W.B. Saunders Company Ed; 1971.

[8] Miceli MV, Newsome DA, Tate DJ,Jr, Sarphie TG. Pathologic changes in the retinal pigment epithelium and Bruch's membrane of fat-fed atherogenic mice. Current Eye Research 2000;20(1) 8-16.

[9] Mullins RF, Russell SR, Anderson DH, Hageman GS. Drusen associated with aging and age-related macular degeneration contain proteins common to extracellular deposits associated with atherosclerosis, elastosis, amyloidosis, and dense deposit disease. FASEB Journal 2000;14(7) 835-846.

[10] Connor WE, Neuringer M, Reisbick S. Essential fatty acids: the importance of n-3 fatty acids in the retina and brain. Nutrition Reviews 1992;50(4) 21-29.

[11] Cousins SW, Espinosa-Heidmann DG, Alexandridou A, Sall J, Dubovy S, Csaky K. The role of aging, high fat diet and blue light exposure in an experimental mouse model for basal laminar deposit formation. Experimental Eye Research 2002;75(5) 543-553.

[12] Hayes KC, Lindsey S, Stephan ZF, Brecker D. Retinal pigment epithelium possesses both LDL and scavenger receptor activity. Investigative Ophthalmology & Visual Science 1989;30(2) 225-232.

[13] Amaratunga A, Abraham CR, Edwards RB, Sandell JH, Schreiber BM, Fine RE. Apolipoprotein E is synthesized in the retina by Muller glial cells, secreted into the vitreous, and rapidly transported into the optic nerve by retinal ganglion cells. Journal of Biological Chemistry 1996;271(10) 5628-5632.

[14] Ong JM, Zorapapel NC, Rich KA, Wagstaff RE, Lambert RW, Rosenberg SE, Moghaddas F, Pirouzmanesh A, Aoki AM, Kenney MC. Effects of cholesterol and apolipoprotein E on retinal abnormalities in ApoE-deficient mice. Investigative Ophthalmology & Visual Science 2001;42(8) 1891-1900.

[15] Triviño A, Ramírez AI, Salazar JJ, de Hoz R, Rojas B, Padilla E, Tejerina T, Ramírez JM. A cholesterol-enriched diet induces ultrastructural changes in retinal and macroglial rabbit cells. Experimental Eye Research 2006;83(2) 357-366.

[16] Salazar JJ, Ramírez AI, de Hoz R, Rojas B, Ruiz E, Tejerina T, Triviño A, Ramírez JM. Alterations in the choroid in hypercholesterolemic rabbits: reversibility after normalization of cholesterol levels. Experimental Eye Research 2007;84(3) 412-422.

[17] Cusato K, Bosco A, Linden R, Reese BE. Cell death in the inner nuclear layer of the retina is modulated by BDNF. Brain research.Developmental Brain Research 2002;139(2) 325-330.

[18] Ju WK, Lee MY, Hofmann HD, Kirsch M, Chun MH. Expression of CNTF in Muller cells of the rat retina after pressure-induced ischemia. Neuroreport 1999;10(2) 419-422.

[19] Honjo M, Tanihara H, Kido N, Inatani M, Okazaki K, Honda Y. Expression of ciliary neurotrophic factor activated by retinal Muller cells in eyes with NMDA- and kainic acid-induced neuronal death. Investigative Ophthalmology & Visual Science 2000;41(2) 552-560.

[20] Rivard A, Fabre JE, Silver M, Chen D, Murohara T, Kearney M, Magner M, Asahara T, Isner JM. Age-dependent impairment of angiogenesis. Circulation 1999;99(1) 111-120.

[21] Wilson JX. Antioxidant defense of the brain: a role for astrocytes. Canadian Journal of Physiology and Pharmacology 1997;75(10-11) 1149-1163.

[22] Iadecola C. Mechanisms of cerebral ischemic damage In: Walz W. (ed.) Cerebral Ischemia. Molecular and Cellular Pathophysiology. Totowa: Humana Press Inc.; 1999. p3-32.

[23] Liu D, Smith CL, Barone FC, Ellison JA, Lysko PG, Li K, Simpson IA. Astrocytic demise precedes delayed neuronal death in focal ischemic rat brain. Brain Research.Molecular Brain Research 1999;68(1-2) 29-41.

[24] Alexander RA, Garner A. Elastic and precursor fibres in the normal human eye. Experimental Eye Research 1983;36(2) 305-315.

[25] Oyster CW. The human eye. Structure and function. Sunderland (Massachusetts): Sinauer Associates; 1999.

[26] Bron AJ, Tripathi RC, Tripathi BJ. The choroid and uveal vessels. In: Bron AJ, Tripathi RC, Tripathi BJ. (ed.) Wolff's Anatomy of the Eye and Orbit (Eighth edition). London: Chapman & Hall Medical; 1997. p371-410.

[27] Ramrattan RS, van der Schaft TL, Mooy CM, de Bruijn WC, Mulder PG, de Jong PT. Morphometric analysis of Bruch's membrane, the choriocapillaris, and the choroid in aging. Investigative Ophthalmology & Visual Science 1994;35(6) 2857-2864.

[28] Bird AC. Bruch's membrane change with age. British Journal of Ophthalmology 1992;76(3) 166-168.

[29] Handa JT, Verzijl N, Matsunaga H, Aotaki-Keen A, Lutty GA, te Koppele JM, Miyata T, Hjelmeland LM. Increase in the advanced glycation end product pentosidine in Bruch's membrane with age. Investigative Ophthalmology & Visual Science 1999;40(3) 775-779.

[30] Marshall J, Hussain AA, Starita C, Moore DJ, Patmore AL. Ageing and Bruch's membrane In: Marmor MF, Wolfensberger TJ. (ed.) Retinal pigment epithelium: function and disease. New York: Oxford University Press; 1998. p669-692.

[31] Hillenkamp J, Hussain AA, Jackson TL, Cunningham JR, Marshall J. The influence of path length and matrix components on ageing characteristics of transport between the choroid and the outer retina. Investigative ophthalmology & visual science 2004 May;45(5)1493-1498.

[32] Green WR, Key SN,3rd. Senile macular degeneration: a histopathologic study. Transactions of The American Ophthalmological Society 1977;75 180-254.

[33] Sarks SH. Ageing and degeneration in the macular region: a clinico-pathological study. British Journal of Ophthalmology 1976;60(5) 324-341.

[34] Sharma RK. Molecular Neurobiology of Retinal Degeneration. In: Lajtha A, Johnson D. (ed.) Handbook of Neurochemistry and Molecular Neurobiology: Sensory Neurochemistry (3rd ed). New York: Springer US; 2007. p47-92.

[35] Fourgeux C, Bron A, Acar N, Creuzot-Garcher C, Bretillon L. 24S-hydroxycholesterol and cholesterol-24S-hydroxylase (CYP46A1) in the retina: from cholesterol homeostasis to pathophysiology of glaucoma. Chemistry and Physics of Lipids 2011;164(6) 496-499.

[36] Newman EA. The Müller cell. In: Federoff S, Vernadakis A. (ed.) Development, morphology and regional specialization of astrocytes. London: Academic Press; 1986. p. 149-171.

[37] Ramírez JM, Triviño A, Ramírez AI, Salazar JJ, García-Sánchez J. Immunohistochemical study of human retinal astroglia. Vision Research 1994;34(15) 1935-1946.

[38] Triviño A, Ramírez JM, Ramírez AI, Salazar JJ, García-Sánchez J. Comparative study of astrocytes in human and rabbit retinae. Vision Research 1997;37(13) 1707-1711.

[39] Gallego B, Salazar JJ, De Hoz R, Rojas B, Ramírez AI, Salinas-Navarro M, Ortín-Martínez A, Valiente-Soriano FJ, AvilésTrigueros M, Villegas-Perez MP, Vidal-Sanz,M.,Triviño,A., Ramírez JM. IOP induces upregulation of GFAP and MHC-ii and microglia reactivity in mice retina contralateral to experimental glaucoma.Journal of Neuroinflammation 2012 in press.

[40] Triviño A, Ramírez JM, Ramírez AI, Salazar JJ, García-Sánchez J. Retinal perivascular astroglia: an immunoperoxidase study. Vision research 1992;32(9) 1601-1607.

[41] Haddad A, Ramírez AI, Laicine EM, Salazar JJ, Triviño A, Ramírez JM. Immunohistochemistry in association with scanning electron microscopy for the morphological characterization and location of astrocytes of the rabbit retina. Journal of Neuroscience Methods 2001;30;106(2) 131-137.

[42] Haddad A, Salazar JJ, Laicine EM, Ramírez AI, Ramírez JM, Triviño A. A direct contact between astrocyte and vitreous body is possible in the rabbit eye due to discontinuities in the basement membrane of the retinal inner limiting membrane. Brazilian Journal of Medical and Biological Research 2003;36(2) 207-211.
[43] Ramírez JM, Triviño A, Ramírez AI, Salazar JJ. Organization and function of astrocytes in human retina. In: Castellano B, Gonzalez B, Nieto-Sampedro M. (ed.) Understanding glial cells. Boston: Kluwer Academic Publishers; 1998. p47-62.
[44] Tezel G, the Fourth ARVO/Pfizer Ophthalmics Research Institute Conference,Working Group. The role of glia, mitochondria, and the immune system in glaucoma. Investigative Ophthalmology Visual Science 2009;50(3) 1001-1012.
[45] Johnson EC, Morrison JC. Friend or foe? Resolving the impact of glial responses in glaucoma. Journal of Glaucoma 2009;18(5) 341-353.
[46] Triviño A, Ramírez AI, Salazar JJ, Rojas B, De Hoz R, Ramírez JM. Retinal changes in age-related macular degeneration. In: Ioseliane OR. (ed.) Focus on Eye Research. New York: Nova science publishers; 2005. p1-37.
[47] Zhong YS, Leung CK, Pang CP. Glial cells and glaucomatous neuropathy. Chinese Medical Journal 2007;120(4) 326-335.
[48] Hudspeth AJ, Yee AG. The intercellular junctional complexes of retinal pigment epithelia. Investigative Ophthalmology 1973;12(5) 354-365.
[49] Cunha-Vaz JG. The blood-ocular barriers: past, present, and future. Documenta ophthalmologica. Advances in Ophthalmology 1997;93(1-2) 149-157.
[50] La Cour M, Tezel T. The retinal pigment epithelium. In: Fischbarg J. (ed.) The biology of the eye. Amsterdam: Elsevier; 2006. p253-272.
[51] SanGiovanni JP, Chew EY. The role of omega-3 long-chain polyunsaturated fatty acids in health and disease of the retina. Progress in Retinal and Eye Research 2005;24(1) 87-138.
[52] Su HM, Bernardo L, Mirmiran M, Ma XH, Corso TN, Nathanielsz PW, Brenna JT. Bioequivalence of dietary alpha-linolenic and docosahexaenoic acids as sources of docosahexaenoate accretion in brain and associated organs of neonatal baboons. Pediatric Research 1999;45(1) 87-93.
[53] Gordon WC, Bazan NG. Retina In: Harding JJ. (ed.) Biochemistry of the Eye. London: Chapman and Hall; 1997. p144-275.
[54] Bretillon L, Thuret G, Grégoire S, Acar N, Joffre C, Bron AM, Gain P, Creuzot-Garcher CP. Lipid and fatty acid profile of the retina, retinal pigment epithelium/choroid, and the lacrimal gland, and associations with adipose tissue fatty acids in human subjects. Experimental Eye Research 2008;87(6) 521-528.
[55] Moore SA. Polyunsaturated fatty acid synthesis and release by brain-derived cells in vitro. Journal of Molecular Neuroscience 2001;16(2-3) 195-200.
[56] Wang N, Anderson RE. Synthesis of docosahexaenoic acid by retina and retinal pigment epithelium. Biochemistry 1993;32(49) 13703-13709.
[57] Wetzel MG, Li J, Alvarez RA, Anderson RE, O'Brien PJ. Metabolism of linolenic acid and docosahexaenoic acid in rat retinas and rod outer segments. Experimental Eye Research 1991;53(4) 437-446.

[58] Delton-Vandenbroucke I, Grammas P, Anderson RE. Polyunsaturated fatty acid metabolism in retinal and cerebral microvascular endothelial cells. Journal of Lipid Research 1997;38(1) 147-159.

[59] Li F, Chen H, Anderson RE. Biosynthesis of docosahexaenoate-containing glycerolipid molecular species in the retina. Journal of Molecular Neuroscience 2001;16(2-3) 205-214.

[60] Serougne C, Lefevre C, Chevallier F. Cholesterol transfer between brain and plasma in the rat: a model for the turnover of cerebral cholesterol. Experimental Neurology 1976;51(1) 229-240.

[61] Hussain ST, Roots BI. Effect of essential fatty acid deficiency & immunopathological stresses on blood brain barrier (B-BB) in Lewis rats: a biochemical study. Biochemical Society Transactions 1994;22(3) 338S.

[62] Puskas LG, Bereczki E, Santha M, Vigh L, Csanadi G, Spener F, Ferdinandy P, Onochy A, Kitajka K. Cholesterol and cholesterol plus DHA diet-induced gene expression and fatty acid changes in mouse eye and brain. Biochimie 2004;86(11) 817-824.

[63] Seddon JM, Rosner B, Sperduto RD, Yannuzzi L, Haller JA, Blair NP, Willett W. Dietary fat and risk for advanced age-related macular degeneration. Archives of Ophthalmology 2001;119(8) 1191-1199.

[64] Bretillon L, Acar N, Seeliger MW, Santos M, Maire MA, Juaneda P, Martine L, Gregoire S, Joffre C, Bron AM, Creuzot-Garcher C. ApoB100,LDLR-/- mice exhibit reduced electroretinographic response and cholesteryl esters deposits in the retina. Investigative Ophthalmology & Visual Science 2008;49(4) 1307-1314.

[65] Fliesler SJ, Bretillon L. The ins and outs of cholesterol in the vertebrate retina. Journal of Lipid Research 2010;51(12) 3399-3413.

[66] Tserentsoodol N, Sztein J, Campos M, Gordiyenko NV, Fariss RN, Lee JW, Fliesler SJ, Rodriguez IR. Uptake of cholesterol by the retina occurs primarily via a low density lipoprotein receptor-mediated process. Molecular Vision 2006;12 1306-1318.

[67] Curcio CA, Johnson M, Huang J, Rudolf M. Aging, age-related macular degeneration, and the response-to-retention of apolipoprotein B-containing lipoproteins. Progress in Retinal and Eye Research 2009;28(6) 393-422.

[68] Bjorkhem I, Lutjohann D, Diczfalusy U, Stahle L, Ahlborg G, Wahren J. Cholesterol homeostasis in human brain: turnover of 24S-hydroxycholesterol and evidence for a cerebral origin of most of this oxysterol in the circulation. Journal of Lipid Research 1998;39(8) 1594-1600.

[69] Lund EG, Guileyardo JM, Russell DW. cDNA cloning of cholesterol 24-hydroxylase, a mediator of cholesterol homeostasis in the brain. Proceedings of the National Academy of Sciences of the United States of America 1999;96(13) 7238-7243.

[70] Bretillon L, Diczfalusy U, Bjorkhem I, Maire MA, Martine L, Joffre C, Acar N, Bron A, Creuzot-Garcher C. Cholesterol-24S-hydroxylase (CYP46A1) is specifically expressed in neurons of the neural retina. Current Eye Research 2007;32(4) 361-366.

[71] Bjorkhem I, Lutjohann D, Breuer O, Sakinis A, Wennmalm A. Importance of a novel oxidative mechanism for elimination of brain cholesterol. Turnover of cholesterol and

24(S)-hydroxycholesterol in rat brain as measured with 18O2 techniques in vivo and in vitro. Journal of Biological Chemistry 1997;272(48) 30178-30184.

[72] Pikuleva IA, Babiker A, Waterman MR, Bjorkhem I. Activities of recombinant human cytochrome P450c27 (CYP27) which produce intermediates of alternative bile acid biosynthetic pathways. Journal of Biological Chemistry 1998;273(29) 18153-18160.

[73] Rodriguez IR, Larrayoz IM. Cholesterol oxidation in the retina: implications of 7KCh formation in chronic inflammation and age-related macular degeneration. Journal of Lipid Research 2010;51(10) 2847-2862.

[74] Ramírez JM, Ramírez AI, Salazar JJ, de Hoz R, Triviño A. Changes of astrocytes in retinal ageing and age-related macular degeneration. Experimental Eye Research 2001;73(5) 601-615.

[75] Ambati J, Ambati BK, Yoo SH, Ianchulev S, Adamis AP. Age-Related Macular Degeneration: Etiology, Pathogenesis, and Therapeutic Strategies. Survey of Ophthalmology 2003;48(3) 257-293.

[76] Panda-Jonas S, Jonas JB, Jakobczyk-Zmija M. Retinal pigment epithelial cell count, distribution, and correlations in normal human eyes. American Journal of Ophthalmology 1996;121(2) 181-189.

[77] Watzke RC, Soldevilla JD, Trune DR. Morphometric analysis of human retinal pigment epithelium: correlation with age and location. Current Eye Research 1993;12(2) 133-142.

[78] Boulton M, Moriarty P, Jarvis-Evans J, Marcyniuk B. Regional variation and age-related changes of lysosomal enzymes in the human retinal pigment epithelium. British Journal of Ophthalmology 1994;78(2) 125-129.

[79] Elner VM. Retinal pigment epithelial acid lipase activity and lipoprotein receptors: effects of dietary omega-3 fatty acids. Transactions of the American Ophthalmological Society 2002;100 301-338.

[80] Fliesler SJ, Richards MJ, Miller CY, Cenedella RJ. Cholesterol synthesis in the vertebrate retina: effects of U18666A on rat retinal structure, photoreceptor membrane assembly, and sterol metabolism and composition. Lipids 2000;35(3) 289-296.

[81] Berring EE, Borrenpohl K, Fliesler SJ, Serfis AB. A comparison of the behavior of cholesterol and selected derivatives in mixed sterol-phospholipid Langmuir monolayers: a fluorescence microscopy study. Chemistry and Physics of Lipids 2005;136(1) 1-12.

[82] Ramírez JM, Triviño A, Ramírez AI, Salazar JJ, García-Sánchez J. Structural specializations of human retinal glial cells. Vision Research 1996;36(14) 2029-2036.

[83] Mahley RW. Apolipoprotein E: cholesterol transport protein with expanding role in cell biology. Science 1988;240(4852) 622-630.

[84] Pfrieger FW. Role of glial cells in the formation and maintenance of synapses. Brain Research Reviews 2010;63(1-2) 39-46.

[85] Brown J,3rd, Theisler C, Silberman S, Magnuson D, Gottardi-Littell N, Lee JM, Yager D, Crowley J, Sambamurti K, Rahman MM, Reiss AB, Eckman CB, Wolozin B. Differential

expression of cholesterol hydroxylases in Alzheimer's disease. Journal of Biological Chemistry 2004;279(33) 34674-34681.

[86] Atsuzawa K, Nakazawa A, Mizutani K, Fukasawa M, Yamamoto N, Hashimoto T, Usuda N. Immunohistochemical localization of mitochondrial fatty acid beta-oxidation enzymes in Muller cells of the retina. Histochemistry and Cell Biology 2010;134(6) 565-579.

[87] Norton WT, Aquino DA, Hozumi I, Chiu FC, Brosnan CF. Quantitative aspects of reactive gliosis: a review. Neurochemical Research 1992;17(9) 877-885.

[88] Rungger-Brandle E, Dosso AA, Leuenberger PM. Glial reactivity, an early feature of diabetic retinopathy. Investigative Ophthalmology & Visual Science 2000;41(7) 1971-1980.

[89] Laping NJ, Teter B, Nichols NR, Rozovsky I, Finch CE. Glial fibrillary acidic protein: regulation by hormones, cytokines, and growth factors. Brain Pathology 1994;4(3) 259-275.

[90] Tanihara H, Hangai M, Sawaguchi S, Abe H, Kageyama M, Nakazawa F, Shirasawa E, Honda Y. Up-regulation of glial fibrillary acidic protein in the retina of primate eyes with experimental glaucoma. Archives of Ophthalmology 1997;115(6) 752-756.

[91] Ramírez AI, Salazar JJ, de Hoz R, Rojas B, Gallego BI, Salinas-Navarro M, Alarcón-Martínez L, Ortín-Martínez A, Avilés-Trigueros M, Vidal-Sanz M, Trivino A, Ramírez JM. Quantification of the effect of different levels of IOP in the astroglia of the rat retina ipsilateral and contralateral to experimental glaucoma. Investigative Ophthalmology & Visual Science 2010;51(11) 5690-5696.

[92] Okada M, Matsumura M, Ogino N, Honda Y. Muller cells in detached human retina express glial fibrillary acidic protein and vimentin. Graefe's Archive for Clinical and Experimental Ophthalmology 1990;228(5)467-474.

[93] Lewis GP, Chapin EA, Luna G, Linberg KA, Fisher SK. The fate of Muller's glia following experimental retinal detachment: nuclear migration, cell division, and subretinal glial scar formation. Molecular Vision 2010;16 1361-1372.

[94] Agardh E, Bruun A, Agardh CD. Retinal glial cell immunoreactivity and neuronal cell changes in rats with STZ-induced diabetes. Current Eye Research 2001;23(4) 276-284.

[95] Chan-Ling T, Stone J. Degeneration of astrocytes in feline retinopathy of prematurity causes failure of the blood-retinal barrier. Investigative Ophthalmology & Visual Science 1992;33(7) 2148-2159.

[96] Pournaras CJ, Rungger-Brändle E, Riva CE, Hardarson SH, Stefansson E. Regulation of retinal blood flow in health and disease. Progress in Retinal and Eye Research 2008;27(3) 284-330.

[97] Sierra A, García R. Epidemiología y prevención de la cardiopatía isquémica. In: Piedrola G. (ed.) Medicina preventiva y salud pública. Barcelona: Masson; 2001. p663-678.

[98] Rodríguez F, Banegas JR, Guallar P, Gutiérrez JL. Enfermedad cerebrovascular e hipertensión arterial. In: Piédrola G (ed.) Medicina preventiva y salud pública. Barcelona: Masson; 2001. p679-688.

[99] Peterson ED, Gaziano JM. Cardiology in 2011--amazing opportunities, huge challenges. JAMA 2011;306(19) 2158-2159.

[100] Selvarajah S, Haniff J, Kaur G, Guat Hiong T, Chee Cheong K, Lim CM, Bots ML. Clustering of cardiovascular risk factors in a middle-income country: a call for urgency. European Journal of Preventive Cardiology in press, first published on January 24, 2012 doi:10.1177/2047487312437327

[101] Klein R, Klein BEK, Tomany SC, Wong TY. The relation of retinal microvascular characteristics to age-related eye disease: the Beaver Dam eye study. American Journal of Ophthalmology 2004;137(3) 435-444.

[102] Edwards MS, Wilson DB, Craven TE, Stafford J, Fried LF, Wong TY, Klein R, Burke GL, Hansen KJ. Associations between retinal microvascular abnormalities and declining renal function in the elderly population: the Cardiovascular Health Study. American Journal of Kidney Diseases 2005;46(2) 214-224.

[103] Wong TY, McIntosh R. Systemic associations of retinal microvascular signs: a review of recent population-based studies. Ophthalmic and Physiological Optics 2005;25(3) 195-204.

[104] Wong TY, Klein R, Sharrett AR, Duncan BB, Couper DJ, Tielsch JM, Klein BEK, Hubbard LD. Retinal Arteriolar Narrowing and Risk of Coronary Heart Disease in Men and Women. JAMA 2002;287(9) 1153-1159.

[105] Wong TY, Klein R, Nieto FJ, Klein BE, Sharrett AR, Meuer SM, Hubbard LD, Tielsch JM. Retinal microvascular abnormalities and 10-year cardiovascular mortality: a population-based case-control study. Ophthalmology 2003;110(5) 933-940.

[106] Wong TY, Duncan BB, Golden SH, Klein R, Couper DJ, Klein BE, Hubbard LD, Sharrett AR, Schmidt MI. Associations between the metabolic syndrome and retinal microvascular signs: the Atherosclerosis Risk In Communities study. Investigative Ophthalmology & Visual Science 2004;45(9) 2949-2954.

[107] Wong TY, Klein R, Couper DJ, Cooper LS, Shahar E, Hubbard LD, Wofford MR, Sharrett AR. Retinal microvascular abnormalities and incident stroke: the Atherosclerosis Risk in Communities Study. Lancet 2001;358(9288) 1134-1140.

[108] Wong TY, Klein R, Sharrett AR, Couper DJ, Klein BEK, Liao D, Hubbard LD, Mosley TH, for the ARIC Investigators. Cerebral White Matter Lesions, Retinopathy, and Incident Clinical Stroke. JAMA 2002;288(1) 67-74.

[109] Donners MMPC, Heeneman S, Daemen MJAP. Models of atherosclerosis and transplant arteriosclerosis: the quest for the best. Drug Discovery Today: Disease Models 2004;1(3) 257-263.

[110] Zadelaar S, Kleemann R, Verschuren L, de Vries-Van der Weij J, van der Hoorn J, Princen HM, Kooistra T. Mouse Models for Atherosclerosis and Pharmaceutical Modifiers. Arteriosclerosis, Thrombosis, and Vascular Biology 2007;27(8) 1706-1721.

[111] Nakashima Y, Plump AS, Raines EW, Breslow JL, Ross R. ApoE-deficient mice develop lesions of all phases of atherosclerosis throughout the arterial tree. Arteriosclerosis and Thrombosis 1994;14(1) 133-140.

[112] Jawien J. The role of an experimental model of atherosclerosis: apoE-knockout mice in developing new drugs against atherogenesis. Current Pharmaceutical Biotechnology 2012 Jan 20 [Epub ahead of print]. PMID:22280417

[113] Davignon J. Apolipoprotein E and atherosclerosis: beyond lipid effect. Arteriosclerosis, Thrombosis, and Vascular Biology 2005;25(2) 267-269.

[114] Ali K, Middleton M, Pure E, Rader DJ. Apolipoprotein E suppresses the type I inflammatory response in vivo. Circulation Research 2005;97(9) 922-927.

[115] Grainger DJ, Reckless J, McKilligin E. Apolipoprotein E modulates clearance of apoptotic bodies in vitro and in vivo, resulting in a systemic proinflammatory state in apolipoprotein E-deficient mice. Journal of Immunology 2004;173(10) 6366-6375.

[116] Knowles JW, Maeda N. Genetic modifiers of atherosclerosis in mice. Arteriosclerosis, Thrombosis, and Vascular Biology 2000;20(11) 2336-2345.

[117] Ishibashi S, Goldstein JL, Brown MS, Herz J, Burns DK. Massive xanthomatosis and atherosclerosis in cholesterol-fed low density lipoprotein receptor-negative mice. Journal of Clinical Investigation 1994;93(5) 1885-1893.

[118] van Vlijmen BJ, van den Maagdenberg AM, Gijbels MJ, van der Boom H, HogenEsch H, Frants RR, Hofker MH, Havekes LM. Diet-induced hyperlipoproteinemia and atherosclerosis in apolipoprotein E3-Leiden transgenic mice. Journal of Clinical Investigation 1994;93(4) 1403-1410.

[119] Jacobsson L. Comparison of experimental hypercholesterolemia and atherosclerosis in Gottingen mini-pigs and Swedish domestic swine. Atherosclerosis 1986;59(2) 205-213.

[120] Kamimura R, Miura N, Suzuki S. The hemodynamic effects of acute myocardial ischemia and reperfusion in Clawn miniature pigs. Experimental Animal 2003;52(4) 335-338.

[121] Turk JR, Henderson KK, Vanvickle GD, Watkins J, Laughlin MH. Arterial endothelial function in a porcine model of early stage atherosclerotic vascular disease. International Journal of Experimental Pathology 2005;86(5) 335-345.

[122] Liang Y, Zhu H, Friedman MH. The correspondence between coronary arterial wall strain and histology in a porcine model of atherosclerosis. Physics in Medicine and Biology 2009;54(18) 5625-5641.

[123] Thim T. Human-like atherosclerosis in minipigs: a new model for detection and treatment of vulnerable plaques. Danish Medical Bulletin 2010;57(7) B4161.

[124] Miyoshi N, Horiuchi M, Inokuchi Y, Miyamoto Y, Miura N, Tokunaga S, Fujiki M, Izumi Y, Miyajima H, Nagata R, Misumi K, Takeuchi T, Tanimoto A, et al. Novel microminipig model of atherosclerosis by high fat and high cholesterol diet, established in Japan. In Vivo 2010;24(5) 671-680.

[125] Kawaguchi H, Miyoshi N, Miura N, Fujiki M, Horiuchi M, Izumi Y, Miyajima H, Nagata R, Misumi K, Takeuchi T, Tanimoto A, Yoshida H. Microminipig, a non-rodent experimental animal optimized for life science research:novel atherosclerosis model

induced by high fat and cholesterol diet. Journal of Pharmacological Sciences 2011;115(2) 115-121.

[126] Fang L, Harkewicz R, Hartvigsen K, Wiesner P, Choi SH, Almazan F, Pattison J, Deer E, Sayaphupha T, Dennis EA, Witztum JL, Tsimikas S, Miller YI. Oxidized cholesteryl esters and phospholipids in zebrafish larvae fed a high cholesterol diet: macrophage binding and activation. Journal of Biological Chemistry 2010;285(42) 32343-32351.

[127] Fang L, Green SR, Baek JS, Lee SH, Ellett F, Deer E, Lieschke GJ, Witztum JL, Tsimikas S, Miller YI. In vivo visualization and attenuation of oxidized lipid accumulation in hypercholesterolemic zebrafish. Journal of Clinical Investigation 2011;121(12) 4861-4869.

[128] Stoletov K, Fang L, Choi SH, Hartvigsen K, Hansen LF, Hall C, Pattison J, Juliano J, Miller ER, Almazan F, Crosier P, Witztum JL, Klemke RL, et al. Vascular lipid accumulation, lipoprotein oxidation, and macrophage lipid uptake in hypercholesterolemic zebrafish. Circulation Research 2009;104(8) 952-960.

[129] Daugherty A, Zweifel BS, Schonfeld G. Probucol attenuates the development of aortic atherosclerosis in cholesterol-fed rabbits. British Journal of Pharmacology 1989;98(2) 612-618.

[130] Del Rio M, Chulia T, Merchan-Perez A, Remezal M, Valor S, Gonzalez J, Gutierrez JA, Contreras JA, Lasuncion MA, Tejerina T. Effects of indapamide on atherosclerosis development in cholesterol-fed rabbits. Journal of Cardiovascular Pharmacology 1995;25(6) 973-978.

[131] Huff MW, Carroll KK. Effects of dietary protein on turnover, oxidation, and absorption of cholesterol, and on steroid excretion in rabbits. Journal of Llipid Research 1980;21(5) 546-548.

[132] Zauberman H, Livni N. Experimental vascular occlusion in hypercholesterolemic rabbits. Investigative Ophthalmology & Visual Science 1981;21(2) 248-255.

[133] Redgrave TG, Dunne KB, Roberts DCK, West CE. Chylomicron metabolism in rabbits fed diets with or without added cholesterol. Atherosclerosis 1976;24(3) 501-508.

[134] Crispin S. Ocular lipid deposition and hyperlipoproteinaemia. Progress in Retinal and Eye Research 2002;21(2) 169-224.

[135] Chapman MJ. Animal lipoproteins: chemistry, structure, and comparative aspects. Journal of Lipid Research 1980;21(7) 789-853.

[136] Roth RI, Gaubatz JW, Gotto AM,Jr, Patsch JR. Effect of cholesterol feeding on the distribution of plasma lipoproteins and on the metabolism of apolipoprotein E in the rabbit. Journal of Lipid Research 1983;24(1) 1-11.

[137] Holm P, Andersen HL, Arroe G, Stender S. Gender gap in aortic cholesterol accumulation in cholesterol-clamped rabbits: role of the endothelium and mononuclear-endothelial cell interaction. Circulation 1998;98(24) 2731-2737.

[138] Ponraj D, Makjanic J, Thong PS, Tan BK, Watt F. The onset of atherosclerotic lesion formation in hypercholesterolemic rabbits is delayed by iron depletion. FEBS letters 1999;459(2) 218-222.

[139] Hanyu M, Kume N, Ikeda T, Minami M, Kita T, Komeda M. VCAM-1 expression precedes macrophage infiltration into subendothelium of vein grafts interposed into

carotid arteries in hypercholesterolemic rabbits--a potential role in vein graft atherosclerosis. Atherosclerosis 2001;158(2) 313-319.

[140] Chen Y, Chang Y, Jyh Jiang M. Monocyte chemotactic protein-1 gene and protein expression in atherogenesis of hypercholesterolemic rabbits. Atherosclerosis 1999;143(1) 115-123.

[141] Schneider DB, Vassalli G, Wen S, Driscoll RM, Sassani AB, DeYoung MB, Linnemann R, Virmani R, Dichek DA. Expression of Fas Ligand in Arteries of Hypercholesterolemic Rabbits Accelerates Atherosclerotic Lesion Formation. Arteriosclerosis, Thrombosis, and Vascular Biology 2000;20(2) 298-308.

[142] Kálmán J, Kudchodkar BJ, Krishnamoorthy R, Dory L, Lacko AG, Agarwal N. High cholesterol diet down regulates the activity of activator protein-1 but not nuclear factor-kappa B in rabbit brain. Life Sciences 2001;68(13) 1495-1503.

[143] de la Peña NC, Sosa-Melgarejo JA, Ramos RR, Méndez JD. Inhibition of platelet aggregation by putrescine, spermidine, and spermine in hypercholesterolemic rabbits. Archives of Medical Research 2000;31(6) 546-550.

[144] Öörni K, Pentikäinen MO, Ala-Korpela M, Kovanen PT. Aggregation, fusion, and vesicle formation of modified low density lipoprotein particles: molecular mechanisms and effects on matrix interactions. Journal of Lipid Research 2000;41(11) 1703-1714.

[145] Francois J, Neetens A. Vascular manifestations of experimental hypercholesteraemia in rabbits. Angiologica 1966;3(1) 1-20.

[146] Sebesteny A, Sheraidah GA, Trevan DJ, Alexander RA, Ahmed AI. Lipid keratopathy and atheromatosis in an SPF laboratory rabbit colony attributable to diet. Laboratory Animals 1985;19(3) 180-188.

[147] Rojas B, Ramírez AI, Salazar JJ, de Hoz R, Redondo A, Raposo R, Mendez T, Tejerina T, Trivino A, Ramírez JM. Low-dosage statins reduce choroidal damage in hypercholesterolemic rabbits. Acta Ophthalmologica 2011;89(7) 660-669.

[148] Shibata M, Sugiyama T, Hoshiga M, Hotchi J, Okuno T, Oku H, Hanafusa T, Ikeda T. Changes in optic nerve head blood flow, visual function, and retinal histology in hypercholesterolemic rabbits. Experimental Eye Research 2011;93(6) 818-824.

[149] Rong JX, Shen L, Chang YH, Richters A, Hodis HN, Sevanian A. Cholesterol Oxidation Products Induce Vascular Foam Cell Lesion Formation in Hypercholesterolemic New Zealand White Rabbits. Arteriosclerosis, Thrombosis, and Vascular Biology 1999;19(9) 2179-2188.

[150] Yamamoto T, Bishop RW, Brown MS, Goldstein JL, Russell DW. Deletion in cysteine-rich region of LDL receptor impedes transport to cell surface in WHHL rabbit. Science 1986;232(4755) 1230-1237.

[151] Shiomi M, Ito T. The Watanabe heritable hyperlipidemic (WHHL) rabbit, its characteristics and history of development: A tribute to the late Dr. Yoshio Watanabe. Atherosclerosis 2009;207(1) 1-7.

[152] Watanabe Y. Serial inbreeding of rabbits with hereditary hyperlipidemia (WHHL-rabbit). Atherosclerosis 1980;36(2) 261-268.

[153] Steen H, Lima JA, Chatterjee S, Kolmakova A, Gao F, Rodriguez ER, Stuber M. High-resolution three-dimensional aortic magnetic resonance angiography and quantitative

vessel wall characterization of different atherosclerotic stages in a rabbit model. Investigative Radiology 2007;42(9) 614-621.

[154] Ogawa M, Ishino S, Mukai T, Asano D, Teramoto N, Watabe H, Kudomi N, Shiomi M, Magata Y, Iida H, Saji H. (18)F-FDG accumulation in atherosclerotic plaques: immunohistochemical and PET imaging study. Journal of Nuclear Medicine 2004;45(7) 1245-1250.

[155] Iwata A, Miura S, Imaizumi S, Zhang B, Saku K. Measurement of atherosclerotic plaque volume in hyperlipidemic rabbit aorta by intravascular ultrasound. Journal of Cardiology 2007;50(4) 229-234.

[156] Yamakawa K, Bhutto IA, Lu Z, Watanabe Y, Amemiya T. Retinal vascular changes in rats with inherited hypercholesterolemia--corrosion cast demonstration. Current Eye Research 2001;22(4) 258-265.

[157] Kouchi M, Ueda Y, Horie H, Tanaka K. Ocular lesions in Watanabe heritable hyperlipidemic rabbits. Veterinary Ophthalmology 2006;9(3) 145-148.

[158] Ramírez AI, Salazar JJ, de Hoz R, Rojas B, Ruiz E, Tejerina T, Ramírez JM, Triviño A. Macroglial and retinal changes in hypercholesterolemic rabbits after normalization of cholesterol levels. Experimental Eye Research 2006;83(6) 1423-1438.

[159] Torres RJ, Maia M, Precoma DB, Noronha L, Luchini A, Precoma LB, Souza GK, Muccioli C. Evaluation of early abnormalities of the sensory retina in a hypercholesterolemia experimental model: an immunohistochemical study. Arquivos Brasileiros de Oftalmologia 2009;72(6) 793-798.

[160] Curcio CA, Millican CL, Bailey T, Kruth HS. Accumulation of cholesterol with age in human Bruch's membrane. Investigative Ophthalmology & Visual Science 2001;42(1) 265-274.

[161] Curcio CA, Presley JB, Malek G, Medeiros NE, Avery DV, Kruth HS. Esterified and unesterified cholesterol in drusen and basal deposits of eyes with age-related maculopathy. Experimental Eye Research 2005;81(6) 731-741.

[162] Moore DJ, Hussain AA, Marshall J. Age-related variation in the hydraulic conductivity of Bruch's membrane. Investigative ophthalmology & Visual Science 1995;36(7) 1290-1297.

[163] Starita C, Hussain AA, Pagliarini S, Marshall J. Hydrodynamics of ageing Bruch's membrane: implications for macular disease. Experimental Eye Research 1996;62(5) 565-572.

[164] Gordiyenko N, Campos M, Lee JW, Fariss RN, Sztein J, Rodriguez IR. RPE cells internalize low-density lipoprotein (LDL) and oxidized LDL (oxLDL) in large quantities in vitro and in vivo. Investigative Ophthalmology & Visual Science 2004;45(8) 2822-2829.

[165] Curcio CA, Millican CL. Basal linear deposit and large drusen are specific for early age-related maculopathy. Archives of Ophthalmology 1999;117(3) 329-339.

[166] Green WR. Histopathology of age-related macular degeneration. Molecular Vision 1999;5 27.

[167] Wexler EM, Berkovich O, Nawy S. Role of the low-affinity NGF receptor (p75) in survival of retinal bipolar cells. Visual Neuroscience 1998;15(2) 211-218.

[168] Sarthy V, Ripps H. The Retinal Müller Cell: Structure and Function. New York: Kluwer Academic Publishers NY; 2001.
[169] Erickson PA, Fisher SK, Anderson DH, Stern WH, Borgula GA. Retinal detachment in the cat: the outer nuclear and outer plexiform layers. Investigative Ophthalmology & Visual Science 1983;24(7) 927-942.
[170] Guerin MB, Donovan M, McKernan DP, O'Brien CJ, Cotter TG. Age-dependent rat retinal ganglion cell susceptibility to apoptotic stimuli: implications for glaucoma. Clinical & Experimental Ophthalmology 2011;39(3) 243-251.
[171] Tyler NK, Burns MS. Alterations in glial cell morphology and glial fibrillary acidic protein expression in urethane-induced retinopathy. Investigative Ophthalmology & Visual Science 1991;32(2) 246-256.
[172] Murabe Y, Ibata Y, Sano Y. Morphological studies on neuroglia. IV. Proliferative response of non-neuronal elements in the hippocampus of the rat to kainic acid-induced lesions. Cell and Tissue Research 1982;222(1) 223-226.
[173] Lindsey RM. Reactive gliosis In: Fedoroff S, Vernadakis A. (ed.) Astrocytes, Orlando: Academic Press; 1986. p231-262.
[174] Baskin F, Smith GM, Fosmire JA, Rosenberg RN. Altered apolipoprotein E secretion in cytokine treated human astrocyte cultures. Journal of the Neurological Sciences 1997;148(1) 15-18.
[175] Goritz C, Mauch DH, Pfrieger FW. Multiple mechanisms mediate cholesterol-induced synaptogenesis in a CNS neuron. Molecular and Cellular Neurosciences 2005;29(2) 190-201.
[176] Kettenmann H, Faissener A, Trotter J. Neuron-glia interactions in homeostasis and degeneration. In: Greger R and Windhorst U. (ed.) Comprehensive Human Physiology. From cellular mechanisms to integration. Berlin: Springer-Verl; 1996. p533-543.
[177] Nieto-Sampedro M, Verdú E. Lesiones del sistema nervioso: respuesta neuronal y reparación. In: Delgado JM, Ferrús A, Mora F, Rubia FJ. (ed.) Manual de neurociencia. Madrid: Síntesis S.A.; 1998. p929-969.
[178] Winkler BS, Boulton ME, Gottsch JD, Sternberg P. Oxidative damage and age-related macular degeneration. Molecular Vision 1999;5 32.
[179] Malinow MR. Experimental models of atherosclerosis regression. Atherosclerosis 1983;48(2) 105-118.
[180] Lusis AJ. Atherosclerosis. Nature 2000;407(6801) 233-241.
[181] Saso Y, Kitamura K, Yasoshima A, Iwasaki HO, Takashima K, Doi K, Morita T. Rapid induction of atherosclerosis in rabbits. Histology and Histopathology 1992;7(3) 315-320.
[182] Bringmann A, Pannicke T, Grosche J, Francke M, Wiedemann P, Skatchkov SN, Osborne NN, Reichenbach A. Muller cells in the healthy and diseased retina. Progress in Retinal and Eye Research 2006;25(4) 397-424.
[183] Pannicke T, Uckermann O, Iandiev I, Wiedemann P, Reichenbach A, Bringmann A. Ocular inflammation alters swelling and membrane characteristics of rat Muller glial cells. Journal of Neuroimmunology 2005;161(1-2) 145-154.
[184] Ridet J, Privat A. Reactive astrocytes, their roles in CNS injury, and repair mechanisms. Advances in Structural Biology: JAI. p147-185.

[185] Reier PJ. Gliosis following CNS injury: The anatomy of astrocytic scars and their influences on axonal elongation. In: Fedoroff S, Vernadakis A, editors. Astrocytes Orlando: Academic. Press; 1996. p. 263-324.

[186] Penfold PL, Provis JM. Cell death in the development of the human retina: phagocytosis of pyknotic and apoptotic bodies by retinal cells. Graefe's archive for clinical and experimental ophthalmology 1986;224(6) 549-553.

[187] Mano T, Puro DG. Phagocytosis by human retinal glial cells in culture. Investigative Ophthalmology & Visual Science 1990;31(6) 1047-1055.

[188] Cook RD, Wisniewski HM. The role of oligodendroglia and astroglia in Wallerian degeneration of the optic nerve. Brain Research 1973;61 191-206.

Chapter 2

Photoreceptor Sensory Cilium and Associated Disorders

Linjing Li, Ozge Yildiz, Manisha Anand and Hemant Khanna

Additional information is available at the end of the chapter

http://dx.doi.org/10.5772/48387

1. Introduction

The primary cilium is a microtubule-based extension of the plasma membrane, which is present in almost all cell types. Ciliary microtubules extend from a basal body (or mother centriole), which docks at the apical membrane. Elegant studies have been carried out to determine the mechanism that regulates the docking of the mother centriole at the membrane for cilia formation. Cilia function as antennae of the cell to detect chemical and physical changes of the microenvironment [1-5]. Owing to their near-ubiquitous nature, cilia are involved in diverse cellular functions, such as patterning of left-right asymmetry (nodal cilia), limb development, bone morphogenesis, and neurosensory functions (mechanosensation, olfaction, and photoreception). Cilia are also implicated in several developmental cascades, such as Wnt signaling, sonic hedgehog signaling, and platelet derived growth factor receptor signaling pathways. Such functions of cilia are brought about by the ability of the ciliary membrane to concentrate a specific subset of membrane proteins in the ciliary compartment as compared to the rest of the cell membrane [6-8].

Cilia are generated by an elaborate process of formation of multiple protein complexes and molecular motor dependent transport of membrane cargo from the proximal to the distal tip, thereby extending the microtubule-based axoneme and the ciliary membrane. Such transport, called Intraflagellar Transport, was initially identified in green alga *Chlamydomonas reinhardtii* and is composed of more than 20 IFT subunits arranged in two distinct complexes, IFT-A and IFT-B [9-10]. They interact with motors and transport cargo along axoneme [11]. Microtubules are polarized with a plus end (growing tip), and a minus end (at the proximal end of cilia). The anterograde motor Kinesin (heterotrimeric Kinesin-2 or homodimeric Kif17) mobilizes proteins to the distal (plus) end while cytoplasmic dynein 2 carries cargos to the proximal end of cilia [12-15]. Similarly, IFT-A and IFT-B play complementary roles in ciliary transport. The complex B, contributing to anterograde transport, is indispensable for the ciliogenesis and maintenance. In contrast, complex A, involved in the retrograde transport, does not play essential role in ciliary assembly [11]. Defects in IFT disturb the ciliogenesis or ciliary maintenance. Even slight defects in the composition of the ciliary membrane or in the generation and/or maturation of cilia result in developmental and degenerative disorders in humans, such as Bardet-Biedl Syndrome (BBS), Joubert Syndrome (JBTS), Meckel-Gruber Syndrome (MKS), Senior-Løken Syndrome (SLSN), Usher Syndrome (USH), renal cystic diseases, and photoreceptor degeneration and blindness [6-7, 16-18].

2. Photoreceptor sensory cilium and its components

In photoreceptors (rods and cones), cilia are highly specialized and modified into a very distinct part of the cell, which consists multiple membranous discs and initiates phototransduction cascade in response to light. The details of the phototransduction cascade in photoreceptors have been elegantly described elsewhere and will not be covered in this chapter.

There are three major compartments that compose the sensory cilia of photoreceptor: the outer segment (OS), transition zone (TZ) and basal body (Figure 1). Like other primary cilia, photoreceptor cilia are 9+0 microtubule-based structures that are nucleated from the basal body. The mother centriole consists of triplet microtubules and recruits proteins and initiates axoneme assembly. The region adjacent to the basal body is TZ (also called connecting cilium; CC), and consists of doublet microtubules [19-20]. These microtubules are linked to the plasma membrane via transition fibers and Y-linkers, the two distinct structures of TZ [21]. TZ, is a narrow conduit between OS and IS [22]. It is estimated to be 200~500 nm long and 170 nm in diameter. TZ carries out critical transport function by acting as a gate between the IS and the OS. The sensory OS of photoreceptors is enriched in membrane proteins, such as rhodopsin, the cyclic nucleotide gated (CNG) channel, membrane guanylyl cyclases, and peripherin-2 [22-25]. Moreover, the TZ is the only link between the two segments and all proteins need to be transported via this narrow bridge-like structure to the OS. Hence, the TZ serves as a bottleneck as well as a track to generate and maintain the sensory cilium. Several proteins, most of which are associated with human retinal degenerative diseases, are enriched at the TZ of photoreceptors. These include RPGR (retinitis pigmentosa GTPase regulator), CEP290, and Nephrocystin-1 (NPHP1). The microtubules then extend in the form of axoneme. Depending upon the species and cell-type examined, the axoneme can extend to half or full length of the OS. The axoneme is recognized by the fact that it consists of singlet microtubules. Not much is known about the specific function of the axoneme. However, functional analysis of RP1 (retinitis pigmentosa 1) protein that localizes specifically to the axoneme of photoreceptors indicated that it might be involved in stabilizing the OS discs. The membranous discs arranged in a perpendicular orientation to the axoneme and axoneme is believed to prove a structural support to the OS discs.

In addition to maintaining a specific composition of the OS, the photoreceptors also undergo massive protein trafficking. In fact, photoreceptors are most active neurons in the human body and have high-energy demands. This is due to the fact that photoreceptors shed their distal discs at a high rate. It is estimated that 10% of the distal tips of the OS is shed every day by undergoing phagocytosis by the overlying retinal pigmented epithelium (RPE) cells [26]. As no protein synthesis occurs in the OS, all components necessary for the renewal of OS discs are synthesized in the IS and transported to the OS at a very high rate. Approximately 2000 opsins transported to the OS per second in a normal human photoreceptor. Even slight disturbances in the synthesis and transport of proteins to the OS results in photoreceptor degeneration and blindness.

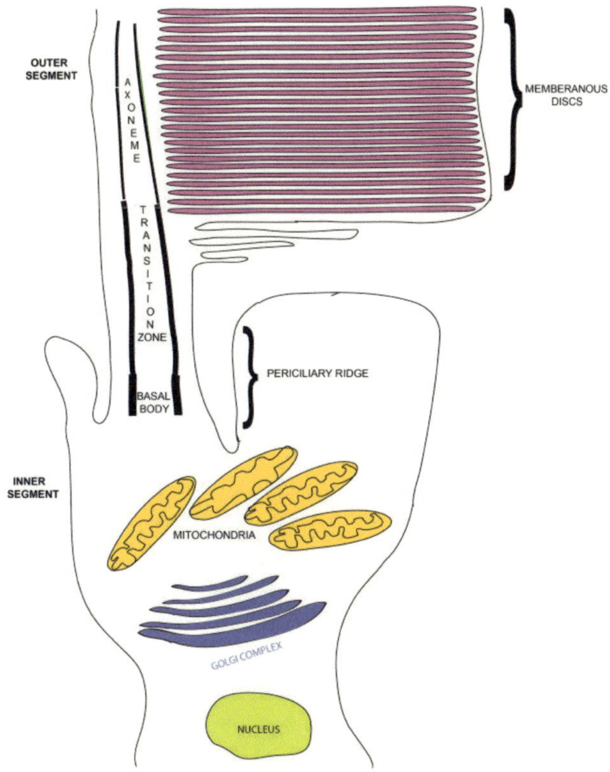

Figure 1. Schematic representation of a rod photoreceptor cell. The membranous discs in the outer segment are enclosed in the plasma membrane. The photoreceptors are rich in mitochondria, which are concentrated around the apical inner segment

3. Docking of cargo and selection at the TZ of photoreceptors

Even though the OS proteins can be targeted to the cilia, they are first docked at the basal body or adjacent membrane. Multiple models have been proposed for the site of docking of the cargo vesicles [27]. These propose docking directly at the basal body, docking at the lateral plasma membrane and then movement of vesicles in the plasma membrane towards to the ciliary compartment, or docking at a privileged domain of the apical plasma membrane. In vertebrate photoreceptors, such a privileged domain was identified as periciliary ridge. Opsin-laden vesicles were identified at this privileged region as well as transiently in the TZ or CC of photoreceptors [25]. More recently, several ciliary disease proteins mutated in Usher Syndrome, were identified at the periciliary ridge and are thought to make a connecting link between the apical plasma membrane and the ciliary membrane [28-29]. If such a domain plays a direct role in cargo docking awaits further investigations, specifically geared towards ascertaining the composition of this microdomain.

After gaining access to the periciliary ridge, the cargo is transported into the TZ, which acts as a 'check post'. Due to its elegant meshwork-like structure with Y-shaped linkers that connect the axonemal microtubules to the plasma membrane, its composition of this structure has been the subject of many recent studies. Remarkable studies identified a network of multiprotein complexes of ciliary disease proteins that are found at the TZ and act as diffusion barrier to limit the trafficking of membrane cargo into the ciliary compartment [22, 30-33]. These proteins include RPGR, RPGR-interacting protein 1 (RPGRIP1) [34-35], CEP290/NPHP6 [36-37], MKS-associated proteins and other JBTS and NPHP-associated proteins [6, 38]. Interestingly, these proteins exist in discrete multiprotein complexes at the TZ. A direct role of TZ proteins in acting as a barrier was established when Witman and colleagues showed that mutation in *Chlamydomonas* CEP290 causes accumulation of non-ciliary membrane proteins to enter cilia and vice versa [39]. However, such a function of CEP290 in photoreceptors still needs to be investigated.

4. Ciliary disorders of retina (retinal ciliopathies)

As the OS of photoreceptors is a sensory cilium, the degenerative diseases that affect the formation or function of the OS can be categorized as a ciliary disorder. However, for simplicity, we will discuss only those cilia-dependent retinopathies that occur due to defects in ciliary TZ proteins and result in defective trafficking of proteins to the OS. Inactivation of the IFT in conditional $Kif3a^{-/-}$ mice and $Tg737^{orpk}$, a hypomorphic allele of IFT88, results in opsin accumulation in the IS [40-41]. Mutations in rhodopsin that affect its trafficking to OS are associated with degenerative blindness disorders of the retina [42-47]. Moreover, ablation of IFT subunit IFT20, which localizes to Golgi and cilia, also results in entrapment of opsins in the IS [48]. Ciliary proteins RP1 and RPGRIP1, mutations in which result in RP/LCA are required for cilia-dependent OS generation [35, 49-50]. Pleiotropic disorders, such as Senior-Loken Syndrome, Joubert Syndrome, and Bardet-Biedl Syndrome, are also caused by mutations in ciliary proteins and share retinal degeneration as a common phenotype [51-53] (Table 1). In this chapter, we will specifically discuss RPGR and RP2, which are mutated in X-linked forms of retinopathies and CEP290, which is a frequent cause of Leber congenital amaurosis (LCA), a childhood blindness disorder (Figure 2).

4.1. Non-syndromic retinal ciliopathies

Retinitis Pigmentosa (RP). RP, detected in 1:3000 people worldwide, is a group of severe blindness disorders that is caused by progressive loss of rod and cone photoreceptors. It is inherited in autosomal recessive, autosomal dominant as well as X-linked manner. Patients exhibit symptoms of night blindness and loss of peripheral vision (due to rod death) in the first two decades of life, which is followed by complete blindness due to loss of cone photoreceptors [54-55]. Loss of cones can either be due to the fact that the causative gene is also expressed in cone photoreceptors or due to starvation or loss of availability of trophic factors secreted from the rods (majority cell type in photoreceptor layer; 95-97%) if the mutation is in a rod-specific gene [56-57].

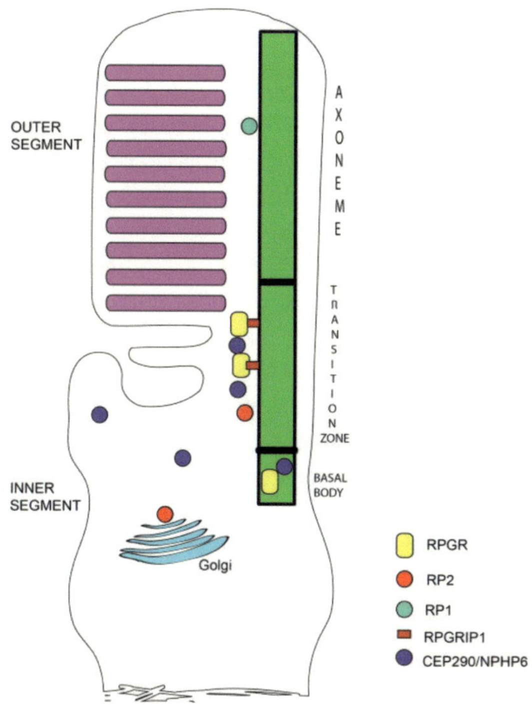

Figure 2. Schematic representation of the localization of the ciliary proteins being discussed in this chapter. As shown, RPGR localizes to the transition zone and basal body and RP1 is concentrated at the distal axoneme, which extends into the outer segment. RPGRIP1 tethers RPGR at the transition zone. RP2 is detected at the Golgi as well as transition zone in photoreceptors. CEP290/NPHP6 is detected at the transition zone, basal body, as well as in the cytosol.

Some forms of RP are caused by defects in genes that encode for ciliary proteins. These include RPGR, RP1, RP2, and TOPORS [50, 56-60]. RP1 and TOPORS are two ciliary proteins mutated in adRP. However, they localize to distinct ciliary compartments: RP1 localizes to the axoneme whereas TOPORS is concentrated in the basal body and transition zone of photoreceptors (Figure 2). The RPGR and RP2 genes are mutated in X-linked forms of RP and together account for more than 90% of XLRP cases [61-64]. Among these, RPGR mutations are found in 70-80% of XLRP and more than 25% of simplex RP males with no family history. On the other hand, RP2 mutations account for 6-10% of XLRP cases. There is considerable clinical heterogeneity among cases of XLRP, which has affected the ability to differentiate between RPGR and RP2 patients in the clinic. This has prompted investigations into genotype-phenotype correlation studies. Such studies are relatively well documented for RPGR patients owing to their majority occurrence as compared to RP2 mutations [65-67].

Nonetheless, recently, a comprehensive analysis of a large group of RP2 patients revealed interesting observations: a majority of RP2 patients seem to exhibit an early involvement of the macula (the central region of the retina) [68].

RPGR: The *RPGR* gene consists of 19 exons and encodes for multiple alternatively spliced transcripts. There are two major transcripts: RPGR$^{1\text{-}19}$ and RPGR^{ORF15}. As the name suggests, the RPGR$^{1\text{-}19}$ isoform consists of exons 1-19 whereas RPGR^{ORF15} isoform consists of exons 1-15 and terminates in intron 15. Both these isoforms therefore, contain a common amino-terminal part comprising of exons 1-15. A part of this region, encoded by exons 2-11 contains a domain of the protein that is homologous to RCC1 (regulator of chromosome condensation 1), a guanine nucleotide exchange factor (GEF) for small GTPases involved in nucleocytoplasmic trafficking of proteins. This domain of RPGR is termed RCC1-like domain (RLD). The carboxyl-terminal region is distinct between these two isoforms. While the RPGR$^{1\text{-}19}$ isoform possesses an isoprenylation motif at the extreme carboxyl-terminus, the RPGR^{ORF15} isoform encodes for an unusual stretch of Glutamic acid and Glycine rich (Glu/Gly rich) domain (Figure 3). At DNA level, the terminal exon of this isoform contains purine-rich repeats [60, 62, 64, 69]. Ablation of the *Rpgr* gene in mice affects opsin trafficking and results in photoreceptor degeneration, starting at around 6 months of age [70]. Similar phenotype was detected in two naturally occurring canine models of RPGR mutation, although the severity of disease was different in the two mutants [71]. First direct correlation of a function of RPGR in cilia was obtained when it was shown that RPGR localizes predominantly to the TZ of photoreceptors and interacts with other ciliary and transport proteins [72-73]. More recently, it was found that silencing of *rpgr* in zebrafish embryos results in shorter cilia and developmental anomalies, reminiscent of ciliary dysfunction [74-75]. These findings indicate that RPGR is involved in regulating the trafficking of proteins at the TZ. Mechanistic insights into RPGR function were obtained when it was shown that RPGR possesses enzymatic activity. RPGR acts as a GEF for the small GTPase RAB8A, which is involved in cilia formation and maturation. As a GEF, RPGR catalyzes the conversion of the inactive, GDP-bound RAB8A to active GTP-RAB8A to facilitate the trafficking of cargo vesicles [76]. The precise function of RPGR as a GEF in photoreceptors still needs to be delineated.

RP2: The RP2 gene is composed of 5 exons and encodes a protein of 350 amino acids. The structure of RP2 reveals two major domains: an amino-terminal domain homologous to tubulin binding cofactor C (TBCC) homology domain and a carboxyl-terminal nucleoside diphosphate kinase domain [77-79] (Figure 3). The purified RP2 protein possesses GTPase activating protein (GAP) activity towards the small GTPase ARL3 (ADP Ribosylation Factor-Like protein 3). As a GAP, RP2 assists in the conversion of GTP-bound ARL3 to ARL3-GDP [80]. Although some human mutations affect this association or activity, the precise role of RP2 as a GAP in photoreceptors is still not clear. The amino terminus of RP2 is palmitoylated and myristoylated and hence, may associate with cell membrane. In fact, RP2 has been found to associate with the plasma membrane of cells and of photoreceptors [81]. In addition, RP2 is also present at the basal body of primary cilia and undergoes trafficking into the cilia like IFT [59]. RP2 interacts with ciliary protein polycystin-2 and assists in the trafficking of polycystin-2 to the cilia. Recent studies have shown that ciliary localization of RP2 is regulated by importins, proteins involved in nucleocytoplasmic trafficking [82]. These data suggest a potential role of such machinery in regulating protein import into the cilia. Silencing of RP2 in cells results in the swelling of the distal tip of the cilium but spares the rate of trafficking of the IFT machinery. Further investigation revealed that RP2 is involved in the secretion of polycystin-2 from ciliary tip to the external microenvironment. One possible scenario is that RP2 may not be directly involved in the secretion rather assists in the trafficking and delivery of an accessory cargo that is required for the secretion of polysystin-2 and other such proteins from the ciliary tip. In photoreceptors, RP2 also localizes to the basal body, TZ as well as Golgi. Silencing of RP2 was also shown to fragment Golgi and may affect Golgi to cilia trafficking in cells [89]. The in vivo effect of ablation of RP2 in photoreceptors will provide critical clues to its involvement in cilia formation, function and protein trafficking.

Leber congenital amaurosis (LCA). LCA is considered the most severe form of retinal degenerative disease that occurs in the childhood or early adulthood, with an incidence of 1 in 30,000 births worldwide. Defective retina exhibits perturbations in the initial development of photoreceptors [83]. Like RP, LCA also exhibits considerable genetic and clinical heterogeneity. To date, mutations in 18 genes have been identified to cause LCA (RetNet, http://www.sph.uth.tmc.edu/Retnet). Of these, four genes, CEP290, RPGR-interacting protein 1 (RPGRIP1), LCA5 or lebercilin and Tubby-like protein 1, encode for ciliary proteins. We will discuss CEP290 and RPGRIP1 below.

CEP290. Mutations in the cilia-centrosomal protein CEP290 are frequently observed in LCA, with an incidence of 22-25% cases [37]. The CEP290 gene consists of 55 exons and encodes a protein of 2,479 amino acids (Figure 3). The CEP290 is a multidomain protein and consists of several coiled-coil domains. Involvement of CEP290 in early onset retinal degeneration was determined when a naturally occurring mouse model called *rd16* (retinal degeneration 16) was identified to carry an in frame deletion in the *Cep290* gene. The *rd16* mouse exhibits early onset severe retinal degeneration, characteristic of LCA in humans, and is accompanied by partial mislocalization of RPGR to the IS. The domain of CEP290 that is deleted in the *rd16* mouse is termed DRD (deleted in rd16 domain) [84]. The deletion renders the CEP290 protein prone to degradation; however, expression of truncated CEP290 protein can be detected in the retina and other tissues in the *rd16* mouse [36]. CEP290 localizes predominantly to the CC/TZ of photoreceptors and interacts with selected ciliary and transport assemblies, including retinal disease proteins Retinitis Pigmentosa GTPase Regulator (RPGR) and RPGR-interacting protein (RPGRIP1), which are mutated in RP and LCA, respectively [36].

In cell culture studies, CEP290 has been shown to regulate cilia assembly program by modulating the localization of RAB8A and Pericentriolar Material 1 (PCM1) [85-86]. Additionally, studies using *Chlamydomonas* CEP290 indicated that it is involved in the stabilization of the diffusion barrier formed by the Y-linkers [39]. It was recently demonstrated that CEP290 interacts with a novel ciliary protein RKIP (Raf-1 Kinase Inhibitory Protein) and modulates its intracellular protein levels. Silencing of *cep290* in zebrafish or mutation in the *rd16* retina results in aberrant accumulation of RKIP; high levels of RKIP subsequently result in mislocalization of RAB8A [84]. Moreover, CEP290 interacts with BBS6; relative dosage of the two proteins seems to be critical in modulating the formation of OS, cochlear cilia, and olfactory cilia [87]. These studies further demonstrated the diverse roles of CEP290 in modulating the formation, maturation, and function of cilia.

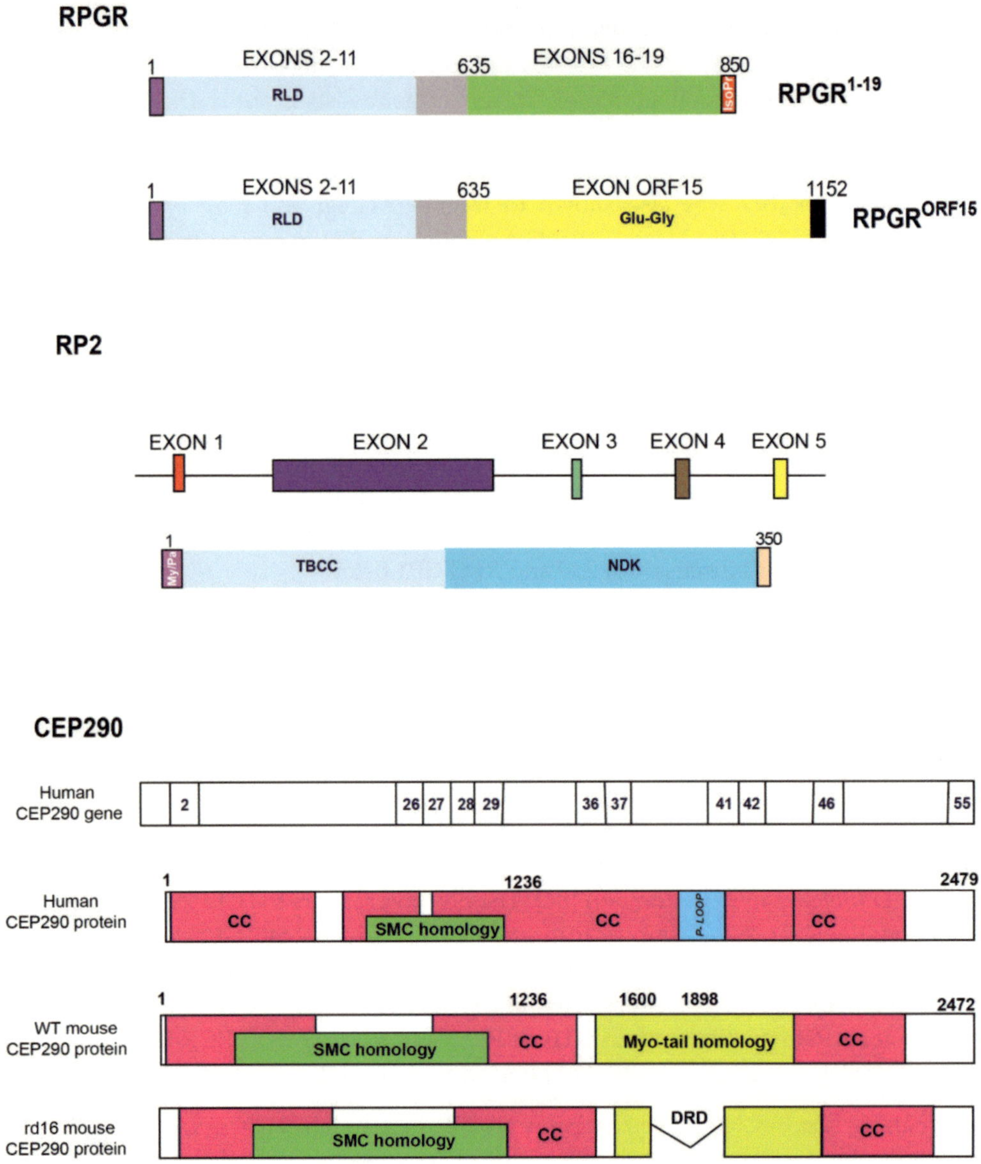

Figure 3. Schematic representation of the primary structure of RPGR, RP2, and CEP290. The two major isoforms of RPGR: $RPGR^{1-19}$ and $RPGR^{ORF15}$ are depicted. The RCC1-like Domain (RLD) is encoded by exons 2-11 of RPGR. The $RPGR^{1-19}$ isoform possesses a carboxyl terminal isoprenylation (IsoPr) site. The RP2 protein consists of amino terminal myristoylation /palmitoylation (My/Pa) site, tubulin binding cofactor C (TBCC) domain and a nucleoside diphosphate kinase (NDK) domain. The CEP290 protein is a multidomain molecule. Both human and mouse CEP290 protein are shown. In rd16 mouse, there is a deletion in the myosin-tail homology domain of the CEP290 protein. SMC: Structural Maintenance of Chromosomes; CC: coiled coil.

RPGRIP1. RPGRIP1 is a ciliary protein that associates directly with the TZ microtubules. Mutations in RPGRIP1 have been identified in a small percentage of LCA cases. In mice, ablation of the *Rpgrip1* gene results in defective OS development and early onset retinal degeneration. RPGRIP1 was identified as an interacting partner of RPGR in photoreceptors. Like *rd16* retina, the *Rpgrip1*$^{-/-}$ mouse retina exhibits mislocalization of RPGR to the IS of photoreceptors and its absence from the TZ. These studies indicate that RPGRIP1 tethers RPGR to the TZ. In addition to RPGR, RPGRIP1 also directly interacts with NPHP4; disease-causing mutations in both these proteins perturb this interaction [35, 88].

Syndromic Ciliopathies. In addition to non-syndromic retinal cilipathies described above, photoreceptor degeneration is a common feature in multiple syndromic ciliopathies, such as Senior-Løken Syndrome (cystic kidneys and retinopathy), Joubert Syndrome (cerebellar vermis hypoplasia, cystic kidneys, and retinal coloboma) and Bardet-Biedl Syndrome (BBS; obesity, mental retardation, polydactyly and retinal degeneration) [6]. Interestingly, some of the proteins described above are also mutated in syndromic ciliopathies and/or associate with other ciliopathy proteins in the cilia. For example, some RPGR patients exhibit extra-retinal phenotypes, such as hearing defects, respiratory infections, sperm dysfunction, and primary cilia dyskinesia. CEP290, on the other hand, is also mutated in syndromic ciliopathies JBTS, MKS, and BBS.

Joubert Syndrome (JBTS). JBTS is an autosomal recessive disorder characterized by cerebellar vermis hypoplasia and retinal coloboma. A characteristic clinical feature of JBTS is the appearance of 'molar tooth sign', which represents a malformation of midbrain-hindbrain junction. Mutations in several ciliary proteins, such as CEP290/NPHP6, NPHP3, RPGRIP1L/NPHP8, AHI1, MKS3, and NPHP1 are associated with JBTS.

Meckel-Gruber Syndrome (MKS). MKS is characterized by embryonic lethality as a result of malformation or malfunction of multiple organs during development. Some characteristic clinical features include microphthalmia (small eye), renal dysplasia, polydactyly, and situs inversus. Interestingly, some of the genes that are mutated in JBTS are also associated with MKS. These include CEP290/NPHP6, RPGRIP1L/NPHP8, MKS1, MKS3, CC2D2A, and TMEM216. It has now been demonstrated that the type of mutation, location of the mutation and the relative combination of the different alleles can determine the outcome of the disorder.

Senior-Løken and Bardet-Biedl Syndromes. Senior-Løken Syndrome (SLSN) is characterized by renal cystic disease Nephronophthisis (NPHP) and retinal degeneration. Mutations in NPHP5 (or nephroretinin) are associated with SLSN; 100% of NPHP5 patients exhibit retinal degeneration. It was demonstrated that NPHP5 localizes to the cilia and interacts with RPGR in the retina. The retinal phenotype is partly attributed to the perturbed interaction of NPHP5 with RPGR in photoreceptors. Bardet-Biedl Syndrome (BBS), on the other hand, involves retinal degeneration, cystic renal disease, cognitive impairment, obesity, infertility and polydactyly as some of the main features. To date, mutations in 16 genes, all of which encode for ciliary proteins have been identified in BBS. These include BBS1-BBS12, MKS1, CEP290, SDCCAG8, and SEPT7.

In addition to the above-mentioned syndromic ciliopathies, there are several other disorders that have been elegantly described elsewhere and are not discussed in this chapter. All these disorders result from defective ciliary development or function. As cilia are involved in regulating numerous signaling cascades, including Wnt signaling, planar cell polarity, hedgehog signaling and cell cycle control, defects in these pathways have also been implicated as a cause of associated disorders. The involvement of signaling cascades in photoreceptor ciliary development and function is not completely understood.

CILIA DEPENDENT RETNOPATHIES

SYNDROMIC FORMS

DISEASE NAME	GENE INVOLVED	PHENOTYPE
USHER SYNDROME	USH1, USH1B, USH1C,USH1D, Pcdh15, PDZ	**Retinal Degeneration** And Hearing disability
SENIOR LOKEN SYNDROME	NPHP1-5, RPGR	**Retinal Degeneration** and Nephronophthisis (NPHP)
JOUBERT SYNDROME	NPHP1, NPHP3, NPHP8/RPGRIP1L, NPHP6/CEP290, RPGRIP1L, AHI1, MKS3	**Retinal degeneration**, Mental Retardation, Renal disease, Liver disease
BARDET BIEDL SYNDROME	BBS1-12, MKS1, NPHP6/CEP290, SDCCAG8, SEPT7	**Retinal Degeneration,** Obesity, Polydactyly, Hypogenitalism, Mental retardation and Renal Abnormalities
MECKEL GRUBER SYNDROME	MKS1, MKS3, NPHP3, NPHP6/CEP290, NPHP8/RPGRIP1L, CC2D2A, TMEM216	**Retinal Degeneration**, Kidney disease, Physical Deformities, Respiratory, infections

NON-SYNDROMIC FORMS

DISEASE NAME	GENE INVOLVED	PHENOTYPE
RETINITIS PIGMENTOSA (RP)	RPGR, RP1, RP2, TOPORS	RETINAL DEGENERATION
LEBER CONGENITAL AMAUROSIS (LCA	RPGRIP1, CEP290	RETINAL DEGENERATION

Table 1. This table depicts selected diseases classified as cilia dependent retinopathies, including non-syndromic as well as syndromic forms. Notably, retinal degeneration is a commonly occurring phenotype in all these disorders.

5. Conclusion

As a number of retinal ciliopathy proteins have now been identified the TZ of photoreceptors, the next step is now to delineate the mechanism by which these proteins modulate the function of the TZ and regulate photoreceptor OS development and function. The existence of discrete multiprotein complexes at the TZ indicates that these complexes are involved in the selection and trafficking of specific cargo moieties to the OS. Mutations in the constituent proteins may impair the function of some of the complexes and trafficking of cognate cargo while other complexes may function normally to extend the life of the photoreceptor. However, if the ciliary protein mutated in disease were involved in the trafficking of proteins regulating the development of OS discs, such as rhodopsin, one would expect a severe and early onset retinal degeneration. It has been shown that RPGR, NPHP proteins and BBS proteins (BBSome) exist in multiprotein complexes and regulate ciliary trafficking.

Some of the TZ proteins possess enzymatic activity. As discussed above, RPGR is a GEF for RAB8A while RP2 is a GAP for ARL3. Such activity of these proteins may impart specificity to the cargo vesicle docking and fusion to the ciliary membrane for crossing the TZ barrier. Moreover, modulating the activity of these proteins may provide insights into developing therapeutic paradigms for associated disorders. It should however, be noted that some TZ proteins are also present in other subcellular compartments of the cell. For example, some RPGR isoforms are detected in the basal body and Golgi; RP2 localizes to Golgi and CEP290 localizes to the cytosol and basal body, in addition to the TZ. These observations beg the question: Are these proteins also involved in extraciliary functions or are these proteins participate in alternative pathways to ultimately regulate cilia dependent cascades. It was recently shown that CEP290 interacts with RKIP, which is involved in modulating MAP Kinase signaling cascades. In addition, CEP290 modulates intracellular levels of RKIP and likely controls its degradation. Hence, CEP290's involvement in intracellular signaling and in protein degradation pathways may be linked to cilia formation or function. However, further investigations are necessary to establish such links and to further delineate the roles of TZ proteins in regulating protein trafficking and photoreceptor OS development and function.

Author details

Linjing Li, Ozge Yildiz, Manisha Anand and Hemant Khanna*
Department of Ophthalmology, University of Massachusetts Medical School, Worcester, MA, USA

Acknowledgement

This work is supported by grants from the National Institutes of Health, Foundation Fighting Blindness, and Worcester foundation (to HK).

6. References

[1] Pazour, G. J. and Bloodgood, R. A. Targeting proteins to the ciliary membrane Curr Top Dev Biol 2008; 85 115-149
[2] Gherman, A., Davis, E. E. and Katsanis, N. The ciliary proteome database: an integrated community resource for the genetic and functional dissection of cilia Nat Genet 2006; 38(9) 961-962

* Corresponding author

[3] Li, J. B., Gerdes, J. M., Haycraft, C. J., Fan, Y., Teslovich, T. M., May-Simera, H., Li, H., Blacque, O. E., Li, L., Leitch, C. C., Lewis, R. A., Green, J. S., Parfrey, P. S., Leroux, M. R., Davidson, W. S., Beales, P. L., Guay-Woodford, L. M., Yoder, B. K., Stormo, G. D., Katsanis, N. and Dutcher, S. K. Comparative genomics identifies a flagellar and basal body proteome that includes the BBS5 human disease gene Cell 2004; 117(4) 541-552

[4] Pazour, G. J. Comparative genomics: prediction of the ciliary and basal body proteome Curr Biol 2004; 14(14) R575-577

[5] Sorokin, S. Centrioles and the formation of rudimentary cilia by fibroblasts and smooth muscle cells J Cell Biol 1962; 15(363-377

[6] Hildebrandt, F., Benzing, T. and Katsanis, N. Ciliopathies N Engl J Med 2011; 364(16) 1533-1543

[7] Singla, V. and Reiter, J. F. The primary cilium as the cell's antenna: signaling at a sensory organelle Science 2006; 313(5787) 629-633

[8] Yoder, B. K. More than just the postal service: novel roles for IFT proteins in signal transduction Dev Cell 2006; 10(5) 541-542

[9] Kozminski, K. G., Johnson, K. A., Forscher, P. and Rosenbaum, J. L. A motility in the eukaryotic flagellum unrelated to flagellar beating Proc Natl Acad Sci U S A 1993; 90(12) 5519-5523

[10] Rosenbaum, J. Intraflagellar transport Curr Biol 2002; 12(4) R125

[11] Ishikawa, H. and Marshall, W. F. Ciliogenesis: building the cell's antenna Nat Rev Mol Cell Biol 2011; 12(4) 222-234

[12] Blacque, O. E., Cevik, S. and Kaplan, O. I. Intraflagellar transport: from molecular characterisation to mechanism Front Biosci 2008; 13(2633-2652

[13] Scholey, J. M. Intraflagellar transport motors in cilia: moving along the cell's antenna J Cell Biol 2008; 180(1) 23-29

[14] Cole, D. G. Intraflagellar transport in the unicellular green alga, Chlamydomonas reinhardtii Protist 2003; 154(2) 181-191

[15] Pedersen, L. B. and Rosenbaum, J. L. Intraflagellar transport (IFT) role in ciliary assembly, resorption and signalling Curr Top Dev Biol 2008; 85(23-61

[16] Badano, J. L., Mitsuma, N., Beales, P. L. and Katsanis, N. The ciliopathies: an emerging class of human genetic disorders Annu Rev Genomics Hum Genet 2006; 7(125-148

[17] Sloboda, R. D. A healthy understanding of intraflagellar transport Cell Motil Cytoskeleton 2002; 52(1) 1-8

[18] Murga-Zamalloa, C. A., Swaroop, A. and Khanna, H. RPGR-containing protein complexes in syndromic and non-syndromic retinal degeneration due to ciliary dysfunction J Genet 2009; 88(4) 399-407

[19] Besharse, J. C., Hollyfield, J. G. and Rayborn, M. E. Photoreceptor outer segments: accelerated membrane renewal in rods after exposure to light Science 1977; 196(4289) 536-538

[20] De Robertis, E. Electron microscope observations on the submicroscopic organization of the retinal rods J Biophys Biochem Cytol 1956; 2(3) 319-330

[21] Silverman, M. A. and Leroux, M. R. Intraflagellar transport and the generation of dynamic, structurally and functionally diverse cilia Trends Cell Biol 2009; 19(7) 306-316

[22] Insinna, C. and Besharse, J. C. Intraflagellar transport and the sensory outer segment of vertebrate photoreceptors Dev Dyn 2008; 237(8) 1982-1992

[23] Huttl, S., Michalakis, S., Seeliger, M., Luo, D. G., Acar, N., Geiger, H., Hudl, K., Mader, R., Haverkamp, S., Moser, M., Pfeifer, A., Gerstner, A., Yau, K. W. and Biel, M. Impaired channel targeting and retinal degeneration in mice lacking the cyclic nucleotide-gated channel subunit CNGB1 J Neurosci 2005; 25(1) 130-138

[24] Baehr, W., Karan, S., Maeda, T., Luo, D. G., Li, S., Bronson, J. D., Watt, C. B., Yau, K. W., Frederick, J. M. and Palczewski, K. The function of guanylate cyclase 1 and guanylate cyclase 2 in rod and cone photoreceptors J Biol Chem 2007; 282(12) 8837-8847

[25] Papermaster, D. S., Schneider, B. G. and Besharse, J. C. Vesicular transport of newly synthesized opsin from the Golgi apparatus toward the rod outer segment. Ultrastructural immunocytochemical and autoradiographic evidence in Xenopus retinas Invest Ophthalmol Vis Sci 1985; 26(10) 1386-1404

[26] Young, R. W. The renewal of photoreceptor cell outer segments J Cell Biol 1967; 33(1) 61-72

[27] Nachury, M. V., Seeley, E. S. and Jin, H. Trafficking to the ciliary membrane: how to get across the periciliary diffusion barrier? Annu Rev Cell Dev Biol 2010; 26 59-87

[28] Maerker, T., van Wijk, E., Overlack, N., Kersten, F. F., McGee, J., Goldmann, T., Sehn, E., Roepman, R., Walsh, E. J., Kremer, H. and Wolfrum, U. A novel Usher protein network at the periciliary reloading point between molecular transport machineries in vertebrate photoreceptor cells Hum Mol Genet 2008; 17(1) 71-86

[29] Yang, J., Liu, X., Zhao, Y., Adamian, M., Pawlyk, B., Sun, X., McMillan, D. R., Liberman, M. C. and Li, T. Ablation of whirlin long isoform disrupts the USH2 protein complex and causes vision and hearing loss PLoS Genet 2010; 6(5) e1000955

[30] Besharse, J. C., Forestner, D. M. and Defoe, D. M. Membrane assembly in retinal photoreceptors. III. Distinct membrane domains of the connecting cilium of developing rods J Neurosci 1985; 5(4) 1035-1048

[31] Horst, C. J., Forestner, D. M. and Besharse, J. C. Cytoskeletal-membrane interactions: a stable interaction between cell surface glycoconjugates and doublet microtubules of the photoreceptor connecting cilium J Cell Biol 1987; 105(6 Pt 2) 2973-2987

[32] Rohlich, P. The sensory cilium of retinal rods is analogous to the transitional zone of motile cilia Cell Tissue Res 1975; 161(3) 421-430

[33] Horst, C. J., Johnson, L. V. and Besharse, J. C. Transmembrane assemblage of the photoreceptor connecting cilium and motile cilium transition zone contain a common immunologic epitope Cell Motil Cytoskeleton 1990; 17(4) 329-344

[34] Dryja, T. P., Adams, S. M., Grimsby, J. L., McGee, T. L., Hong, D. H., Li, T., Andreasson, S. and Berson, E. L. Null RPGRIP1 alleles in patients with Leber congenital amaurosis Am J Hum Genet 2001; 68(5) 1295-1298

[35] Zhao, Y., Hong, D. H., Pawlyk, B., Yue, G., Adamian, M., Grynberg, M., Godzik, A. and Li, T. The retinitis pigmentosa GTPase regulator (RPGR)- interacting protein: subserving RPGR function and participating in disk morphogenesis Proc Natl Acad Sci U S A 2003; 100(7) 3965-3970

[36] Chang, B., Khanna, H., Hawes, N., Jimeno, D., He, S., Lillo, C., Parapuram, S. K., Cheng, H., Scott, A., Hurd, R. E., Sayer, J. A., Otto, E. A., Attanasio, M., O'Toole, J. F., Jin, G., Shou, C., Hildebrandt, F., Williams, D. S., Heckenlively, J. R. and Swaroop, A. In-frame deletion in a novel centrosomal/ciliary protein CEP290/NPHP6 perturbs its interaction with RPGR and results in early-onset retinal degeneration in the rd16 mouse Hum Mol Genet 2006; 15(11) 1847-1857

[37] den Hollander, A. I., Koenekoop, R. K., Yzer, S., Lopez, I., Arends, M. L., Voesenek, K. E., Zonneveld, M. N., Strom, T. M., Meitinger, T., Brunner, H. G., Hoyng, C. B., van den Born, L. I., Rohrschneider, K. and Cremers, F. P. Mutations in the CEP290 (NPHP6) gene are a frequent cause of Leber congenital amaurosis Am J Hum Genet 2006; 79(3) 556-561

[38] Sang, L., Miller, J. J., Corbit, K. C., Giles, R. H., Brauer, M. J., Otto, E. A., Baye, L. M., Wen, X., Scales, S. J., Kwong, M., Huntzicker, E. G., Sfakianos, M. K., Sandoval, W., Bazan, J. F., Kulkarni, P., Garcia-Gonzalo, F. R., Seol, A. D., O'Toole, J. F., Held, S., Reutter, H. M., Lane, W. S., Rafiq, M. A., Noor, A., Ansar, M., Devi, A. R., Sheffield, V. C., Slusarski, D. C., Vincent, J. B., Doherty, D. A., Hildebrandt, F., Reiter, J. F. and Jackson, P. K. Mapping the NPHP-JBTS-MKS Protein Network Reveals Ciliopathy Disease Genes and Pathways Cell 2011; 145(4) 513-528

[39] Craige, B., Tsao, C. C., Diener, D. R., Hou, Y., Lechtreck, K. F., Rosenbaum, J. L. and Witman, G. B. CEP290 tethers flagellar transition zone microtubules to the membrane and regulates flagellar protein content J Cell Biol 2010; 190(5) 927-940

[40] Marszalek, J. R., Liu, X., Roberts, E. A., Chui, D., Marth, J. D., Williams, D. S. and Goldstein, L. S. Genetic evidence for selective transport of opsin and arrestin by kinesin-II in mammalian photoreceptors Cell 2000; 102(2) 175-187

[41] Pazour, G. J., Baker, S. A., Deane, J. A., Cole, D. G., Dickert, B. L., Rosenbaum, J. L., Witman, G. B. and Besharse, J. C. The intraflagellar transport protein, IFT88, is essential for vertebrate photoreceptor assembly and maintenance J Cell Biol 2002; 157(1) 103-113

[42] Deretic, D., Schmerl, S., Hargrave, P. A., Arendt, A. and McDowell, J. H. Regulation of sorting and post-Golgi trafficking of rhodopsin by its C-terminal sequence QVS(A)PA Proc Natl Acad Sci U S A 1998; 95(18) 10620-10625

[43] Deretic, D., Williams, A. H., Ransom, N., Morel, V., Hargrave, P. A. and Arendt, A. Rhodopsin C terminus, the site of mutations causing retinal disease, regulates trafficking by binding to ADP-ribosylation factor 4 (ARF4) Proc Natl Acad Sci U S A 2005; 102(9) 3301-3306

[44] Mazelova, J., Astuto-Gribble, L., Inoue, H., Tam, B. M., Schonteich, E., Prekeris, R., Moritz, O. L., Randazzo, P. A. and Deretic, D. Ciliary targeting motif VxPx directs assembly of a trafficking module through Arf4 EMBO J 2009; 28(3) 183-192

[45] Sung, C. H., Makino, C., Baylor, D. and Nathans, J. A rhodopsin gene mutation responsible for autosomal dominant retinitis pigmentosa results in a protein that is defective in localization to the photoreceptor outer segment J Neurosci 1994; 14(10) 5818-5833

[46] Tai, A. W., Chuang, J. Z., Bode, C., Wolfrum, U. and Sung, C. H. Rhodopsin's carboxy-terminal cytoplasmic tail acts as a membrane receptor for cytoplasmic dynein by binding to the dynein light chain Tctex-1 Cell 1999; 97(7) 877-887

[47] Colley, N. J., Cassill, J. A., Baker, E. K. and Zuker, C. S. Defective intracellular transport is the molecular basis of rhodopsin-dependent dominant retinal degeneration Proc Natl Acad Sci U S A 1995; 92(7) 3070-3074

[48] Keady, B. T., Le, Y. Z. and Pazour, G. J. IFT20 is required for opsin trafficking and photoreceptor outer segment development Mol Biol Cell 2011; 22(7) 921-930

[49] Liu, Q., Lyubarsky, A., Skalet, J. H., Pugh, E. N., Jr. and Pierce, E. A. RP1 is required for the correct stacking of outer segment discs Invest Ophthalmol Vis Sci 2003; 44(10) 4171-4183

[50] Liu, Q., Zuo, J. and Pierce, E. A. The retinitis pigmentosa 1 protein is a photoreceptor microtubule-associated protein J Neurosci 2004; 24(29) 6427-6436

[51] Badano, J. L., Mitsuma, N., Beales, P. L. and Katsanis, N. The Ciliopathies: An Emerging Class of Human Genetic Disorders Annu Rev Genomics Hum Genet 2006;

[52] Badano, J. L., Teslovich, T. M. and Katsanis, N. The centrosome in human genetic disease Nat Rev Genet 2005; 6(3) 194-205

[53] Sayer, J. A., Otto, E. A., O'Toole, J. F., Nurnberg, G., Kennedy, M. A., Becker, C., Hennies, H. C., Helou, J., Attanasio, M., Fausett, B. V., Utsch, B., Khanna, H., Liu, Y., Drummond, I., Kawakami, I., Kusakabe, T., Tsuda, M., Ma, L., Lee, H., Larson, R. G., Allen, S. J., Wilkinson, C. J., Nigg, E. A., Shou, C., Lillo, C., Williams, D. S., Hoppe, B., Kemper, M. J., Neuhaus, T., Parisi, M. A., Glass, I. A., Petry, M., Kispert, A., Gloy, J., Ganner, A., Walz, G., Zhu, X., Goldman, D., Nurnberg, P., Swaroop, A., Leroux, M. R. and Hildebrandt, F. The centrosomal protein nephrocystin-6 is mutated in Joubert syndrome and activates transcription factor ATF4 Nat Genet 2006; 38(6) 674-681

[54] Fishman, G. A., Farber, M. D. and Derlacki, D. J. X-linked retinitis pigmentosa. Profile of clinical findings Arch Ophthalmol 1988; 106(3) 369-375

[55] Heckenlively, J. R., Yoser, S. L., Friedman, L. H. and Oversier, J. J. Clinical findings and common symptoms in retinitis pigmentosa Am J Ophthalmol 1988; 105(5) 504-511

[56] Punzo, C., Kornacker, K. and Cepko, C. L. Stimulation of the insulin/mTOR pathway delays cone death in a mouse model of retinitis pigmentosa Nat Neurosci 2009; 12(1) 44-52

[57] Leveillard, T., Mohand-Said, S., Lorentz, O., Hicks, D., Fintz, A. C., Clerin, E., Simonutti, M., Forster, V., Cavusoglu, N., Chalmel, F., Dolle, P., Poch, O., Lambrou, G. and Sahel, J. A. Identification and characterization of rod-derived cone viability factor Nat Genet 2004; 36(7) 755-759

[58] Chakarova, C. F., Khanna, H., Shah, A. Z., Patil, S. B., Sedmak, T., Murga-Zamalloa, C. A., Papaioannou, M. G., Nagel-Wolfrum, K., Lopez, I., Munro, P., Cheetham, M., Koenekoop, R. K., Rios, R. M., Matter, K., Wolfrum, U., Swaroop, A. and Bhattacharya, S. S. TOPORS, implicated in retinal degeneration, is a cilia-centrosomal protein Hum Mol Genet 2011; 20(5) 975-987

[59] Hurd, T., Zhou, W., Jenkins, P., Liu, C. J., Swaroop, A., Khanna, H., Martens, J., Hildebrandt, F. and Margolis, B. The retinitis pigmentosa protein RP2 interacts with

polycystin 2 and regulates cilia-mediated vertebrate development Hum Mol Genet 2010; 19(22) 4330-4344

[60] Murga-Zamalloa, C., Swaroop, A. and Khanna, H. Multiprotein Complexes of Retinitis Pigmentosa GTPase Regulator (RPGR), a Ciliary Protein Mutated in X-Linked Retinitis Pigmentosa (XLRP) Adv Exp Med Biol 2010; 664(105-114

[61] Meindl, A., Dry, K., Herrmann, K., Manson, F., Ciccodicola, A., Edgar, A., Carvalho, M. R., Achatz, H., Hellebrand, H., Lennon, A., Migliaccio, C., Porter, K., Zrenner, E., Bird, A., Jay, M., Lorenz, B., Wittwer, B., D'Urso, M., Meitinger, T. and Wright, A. A gene (RPGR) with homology to the RCC1 guanine nucleotide exchange factor is mutated in X-linked retinitis pigmentosa (RP3) Nat Genet 1996; 13(1) 35-42

[62] Roepman, R., van Duijnhoven, G., Rosenberg, T., Pinckers, A. J., Bleeker-Wagemakers, L. M., Bergen, A. A., Post, J., Beck, A., Reinhardt, R., Ropers, H. H., Cremers, F. P. and Berger, W. Positional cloning of the gene for X-linked retinitis pigmentosa 3: homology with the guanine-nucleotide-exchange factor RCC1 Hum Mol Genet 1996; 5(7) 1035-1041

[63] Schwahn, U., Lenzner, S., Dong, J., Feil, S., Hinzmann, B., van Duijnhoven, G., Kirschner, R., Hemberger, M., Bergen, A. A., Rosenberg, T., Pinckers, A. J., Fundele, R., Rosenthal, A., Cremers, F. P., Ropers, H. H. and Berger, W. Positional cloning of the gene for X-linked retinitis pigmentosa 2 Nat Genet 1998; 19(4) 327-332

[64] Vervoort, R., Lennon, A., Bird, A. C., Tulloch, B., Axton, R., Miano, M. G., Meindl, A., Meitinger, T., Ciccodicola, A. and Wright, A. F. Mutational hot spot within a new RPGR exon in X-linked retinitis pigmentosa Nat Genet 2000; 25(4) 462-466

[65] Breuer, D. K., Yashar, B. M., Filippova, E., Hiriyanna, S., Lyons, R. H., Mears, A. J., Asaye, B., Acar, C., Vervoort, R., Wright, A. F., Musarella, M. A., Wheeler, P., MacDonald, I., Iannaccone, A., Birch, D., Hoffman, D. R., Fishman, G. A., Heckenlively, J. R., Jacobson, S. G., Sieving, P. A. and Swaroop, A. A comprehensive mutation analysis of RP2 and RPGR in a North American cohort of families with X-linked retinitis pigmentosa Am J Hum Genet 2002; 70(6) 1545-1554

[66] Sharon, D., Bruns, G. A., McGee, T. L., Sandberg, M. A., Berson, E. L. and Dryja, T. P. X-linked retinitis pigmentosa: mutation spectrum of the RPGR and RP2 genes and correlation with visual function Invest Ophthalmol Vis Sci 2000; 41(9) 2712-2721

[67] Sharon, D., Sandberg, M. A., Rabe, V. W., Stillberger, M., Dryja, T. P. and Berson, E. L. RP2 and RPGR mutations and clinical correlations in patients with X-linked retinitis pigmentosa Am J Hum Genet 2003; 73(5) 1131-1146

[68] Jayasundera, T., Branham, K. E., Othman, M., Rhoades, W. R., Karoukis, A. J., Khanna, H., Swaroop, A. and Heckenlively, J. R. RP2 phenotype and pathogenetic correlations in X-linked retinitis pigmentosa Arch Ophthalmol 2010; 128(7) 915-923

[69] Renault, L., Kuhlmann, J., Henkel, A. and Wittinghofer, A. Structural basis for guanine nucleotide exchange on Ran by the regulator of chromosome condensation (RCC1) Cell 2001; 105(2) 245-255

[70] Hong, D. H., Pawlyk, B. S., Shang, J., Sandberg, M. A., Berson, E. L. and Li, T. A retinitis pigmentosa GTPase regulator (RPGR)-deficient mouse model for X-linked retinitis pigmentosa (RP3) Proc Natl Acad Sci U S A 2000; 97(7) 3649-3654

[71] Zhang, Q., Acland, G. M., Wu, W. X., Johnson, J. L., Pearce-Kelling, S., Tulloch, B., Vervoort, R., Wright, A. F. and Aguirre, G. D. Different RPGR exon ORF15 mutations in Canids provide insights into photoreceptor cell degeneration Hum Mol Genet 2002; 11(9) 993-1003

[72] Hong, D. H., Pawlyk, B., Sokolov, M., Strissel, K. J., Yang, J., Tulloch, B., Wright, A. F., Arshavsky, V. Y. and Li, T. RPGR isoforms in photoreceptor connecting cilia and the transitional zone of motile cilia Invest Ophthalmol Vis Sci 2003; 44(6) 2413-2421

[73] Khanna, H., Hurd, T. W., Lillo, C., Shu, X., Parapuram, S. K., He, S., Akimoto, M., Wright, A. F., Margolis, B., Williams, D. S. and Swaroop, A. RPGR-ORF15, which is mutated in retinitis pigmentosa, associates with SMC1, SMC3, and microtubule transport proteins J Biol Chem 2005; 280(39) 33580-33587

[74] Ghosh, A. K., Murga-Zamalloa, C. A., Chan, L., Hitchcock, P. F., Swaroop, A. and Khanna, H. Human retinopathy-associated ciliary protein retinitis pigmentosa GTPase regulator mediates cilia-dependent vertebrate development Hum Mol Genet 2010; 19(1) 90-98

[75] Shu, X., Zeng, Z., Gautier, P., Lennon, A., Gakovic, M., Patton, E. E. and Wright, A. F. Zebrafish Rpgr is required for normal retinal development and plays a role in dynein-based retrograde transport processes Hum Mol Genet 2010; 19(4) 657-670

[76] Murga-Zamalloa, C. A., Atkins, S. J., Peranen, J., Swaroop, A. and Khanna, H. Interaction of retinitis pigmentosa GTPase regulator (RPGR) with RAB8A GTPase: implications for cilia dysfunction and photoreceptor degeneration Hum Mol Genet 2010; 19(18) 3591-3598

[77] Bartolini, F., Bhamidipati, A., Thomas, S., Schwahn, U., Lewis, S. A. and Cowan, N. J. Functional overlap between retinitis pigmentosa 2 protein and the tubulin-specific chaperone cofactor C J Biol Chem 2002; 277(17) 14629-14634

[78] Evans, R. J., Hardcastle, A. J. and Cheetham, M. E. Focus on molecules: X-linked Retinitis Pigmentosa 2 protein, RP2 Exp Eye Res 2006; 82(4) 543-544

[79] Kuhnel, K., Veltel, S., Schlichting, I. and Wittinghofer, A. Crystal structure of the human retinitis pigmentosa 2 protein and its interaction with Arl3 Structure 2006; 14(2) 367-378

[80] Veltel, S., Gasper, R., Eisenacher, E. and Wittinghofer, A. The retinitis pigmentosa 2 gene product is a GTPase-activating protein for Arf-like 3 Nat Struct Mol Biol 2008; 15(4) 373-380

[81] Chapple, J. P., Grayson, C., Hardcastle, A. J., Bailey, T. A., Matter, K., Adamson, P., Graham, C. H., Willison, K. R. and Cheetham, M. E. Organization on the plasma membrane of the retinitis pigmentosa protein RP2: investigation of association with detergent-resistant membranes and polarized sorting Biochem J 2003; 372(Pt 2) 427-433

[82] Hurd, T. W., Fan, S. and Margolis, B. L. Localization of retinitis pigmentosa 2 to cilia is regulated by Importin beta2 J Cell Sci 2011; 124(Pt 5) 718-726

[83] den Hollander, A. I., Roepman, R., Koenekoop, R. K. and Cremers, F. P. Leber congenital amaurosis: genes, proteins and disease mechanisms Prog Retin Eye Res 2008; 27(4) 391-419

[84] Murga-Zamalloa, C. A., Ghosh, A. K., Patil, S. B., Reed, N. A., Chan, L. S., Davuluri, S., Peranen, J., Hurd, T. W., Rachel, R. A. and Khanna, H. Accumulation of the Raf-1 kinase

inhibitory protein (Rkip) is associated with Cep290-mediated photoreceptor degeneration in ciliopathies J Biol Chem 2011; 286(32) 28276-28286

[85] Kim, J., Krishnaswami, S. R. and Gleeson, J. G. CEP290 interacts with the centriolar satellite component PCM-1 and is required for Rab8 localization to the primary cilium Hum Mol Genet 2008; 17(23) 3796-3805

[86] Tsang, W. Y., Bossard, C., Khanna, H., Peranen, J., Swaroop, A., Malhotra, V. and Dynlacht, B. D. CP110 suppresses primary cilia formation through its interaction with CEP290, a protein deficient in human ciliary disease Dev Cell 2008; 15(2) 187-197

[87] Rachel, R. A., May-Simera, H. L., Veleri, S., Gotoh, N., Choi, B. Y., Murga-Zamalloa, C., McIntyre, J. C., Marek, J., Lopez, I., Hackett, A. N., Brooks, M., den Hollander, A. I., Beales, P. L., Li, T., Jacobson, S. G., Sood, R., Martens, J. R., Liu, P., Friedman, T. B., Khanna, H., Koenekoop, R. K., Kelley, M. W. and Swaroop, A. Combining Cep290 and Mkks ciliopathy alleles in mice rescues sensory defects and restores ciliogenesis J Clin Invest 2012; 122(4) 1233-1245

[88] Roepman, R., Letteboer, S. J., Arts, H. H., van Beersum, S. E., Lu, X., Krieger, E., Ferreira, P. A. and Cremers, F. P. Interaction of nephrocystin-4 and RPGRIP1 is disrupted by nephronophthisis or Leber congenital amaurosis-associated mutations Proc Natl Acad Sci U S A 2005; 102(51) 18520-18525

[89] Evans RJ, Schwarz N, Nagel-Wolfrum K, Wolfrum U, Hardcastle AJ, Cheetham ME. The retinitis pigmentosa protein RP2 links pericentriolar vesicle transport between the Golgi and the primary cilium. Hum Mol Genet. 2010 Apr 1;19(7):1358-67

Chapter 3

Utilization of Portable Digital Camera for Detecting Cataract

Retno Supriyanti, Hitoshi Habe and Masatsugu Kidode

Additional information is available at the end of the chapter

http://dx.doi.org/10.5772/48428

1. Introduction

Cataract is a kind of eye disease [1]; that is a clouding in the lens of the eye that affects vision. Cataract exhibits a lot of whitish color inside a pupil. The three classes of cataracts are immature, mature and hypermature, which differ in seriousness. In an immature cataract, a whitish color appears inside the pupil but less so than in mature or hypermature cataracts. Usually, the condition is not yet serious. A Hypermature cataract exhibits much whitish color inside the pupil and can cause the lens of the eye to break if surgery is not carried out. This condition is very dangerous. Figure 1 shows examples of the range of serious and non-serious conditions.

The World Health Report published in 2001 estimated that there were 20 million people who are bilaterally blind (i.e., with eyesight of less than 3/60 in the better eye) whose blindness was caused by age related cataracts [2]. That number will have increased to 40 million by the year 2020. Increasing age is associated with an increasing prevalence of cataracts, but in most developing countries, cataracts often occur earlier in life. One of the developing countries that have the highest number of people with cataracts is Indonesia. There are about 6 million people in Indonesia who suffer from cataracts, but Indonesia only has about 1160 ophthalmologists for a population of more than 200 million people (one for every 350.000 people). In addition, ophthalmologists are not evenly distributed. Many ophthalmologists are located in the capital city, yet many people have no access to ophthalmologists because of geographic conditions.

Usually ophthalmologists will use various equipment like slit lamp or ophthalmoscope to determine the type, opacities and the location of the cataract, and to distinguish it from other eye diseases that have symptoms similar to cataracts. Basically, both equipments use a light source to determine the condition of the patient's eye lens. By using these kinds of equipment, lens opacities can be assessed by observing the width of the edge of the iris in a cloudy lens. If the remote location and the large shadow means immature cataracts, if it is a small shadow and close to the pupil occurs in mature cataracts. It is expected with early diagnosis, the cataract can be monitored whether to continue or will cause complications that must be treated to prevent blindness; However, using this equipment have some limitations including expensive price and special training needed. It will be a problem for some developing countries which has a limited number of both ophthalmologists and health facilities like Indonesia, Nepal, and Vietnam, for example. To solve this problem, we developed a method for detecting cataract based on digital image processing techniques. These techniques support the use of low-cost and easy-to-use equipment such as digital camera. We choose to use a digital camera as the main equipment with reference to the working principle of the slit-lamp camera and ophthalmoscope in which this equipment using the light to check the condition of the eye lens, so we adopted the use of the slit-lamp camera or ophthalmoscope light with a flash light on digital camera lenses to represent the condition. The two types of equipment are shown in Figure 2.

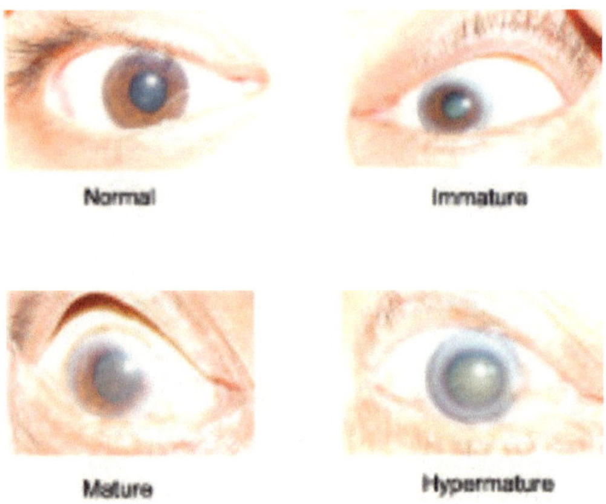

Non Serious Condition

Serious Condition

Figure 1. Example of eye images

In our method, we extracted all information about cataract from pupil area only because all information about cataracts comes from the lens only. This is based on the fact that the opacities as an important sign of cataracts occur in the lens. However, when using a compact digital camera, we found problems such as insufficient image quality and uncontrolled illumination. For example, if we employ intensity value for screening cataract, i.e. higher intensity corresponds to a serious condition; it would fail for a cataract eye image taken under low illumination as shown in Figure 3. It appears that a non-serious condition eye image has an average intensity about 155 inside a pupil while a serious condition eye image only has an average intensity about 55 inside a pupil. In order to develop a robust cataract screening techniques, we proposed to use specular reflection analysis as the core method for cataract screening because specular reflection always brighter than surrounding area and it is not depend on illumination condition. We also were considering texture information as the supporting method.

This chapter will discuss step by step instructions on the use of digital cameras as the main equipment for detecting cataract, complete with an explanation of image processing techniques for the analysis of digital images produced by digital cameras.

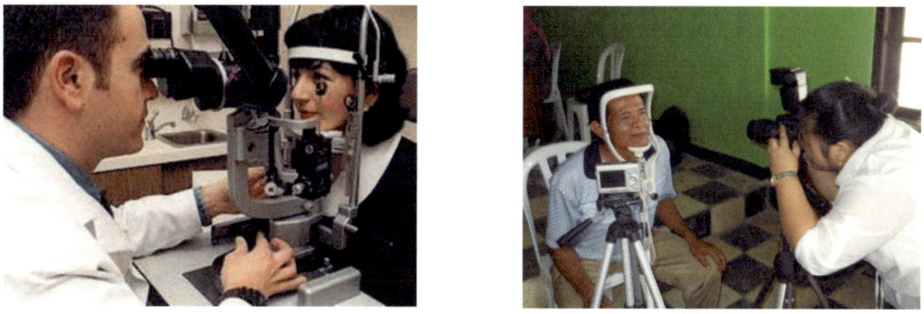

(a) Slit-lamp (b) Digital camera

Source: http://www.mrcopth.com/examinationtechniques
Source: Private documentation

Figure 2. Examination using (a) slit lamp (b) our system

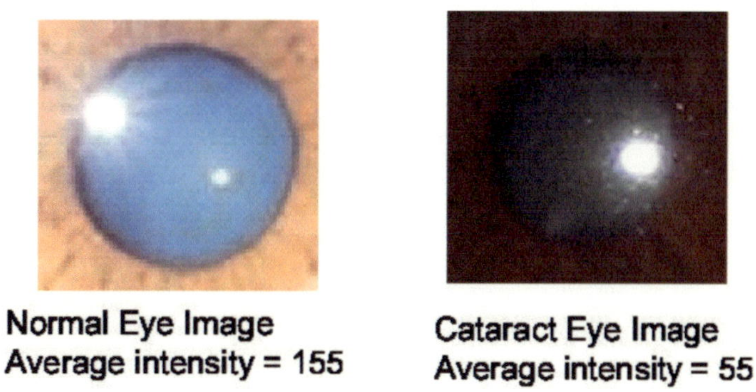

Figure 3. Example of photographs under uncontrolled illumination

2. Images processing analysis

2.1. Definition of pupil

As discussed in Section 1, we extracted all information inside the pupil including specular reflection and texture appearance because all information about cataract is taken from the pupil region only. The pupil of the eye is simply a hole in the iris through which one can peer into the eye. It appears black because of the darkness inside [3][4]. Based on these definitions, we can conclude that the color of the pupil is universal; it does not depend on ethnicity, although the color of the iris is different for different ethnicity, as shown in Figure 4.

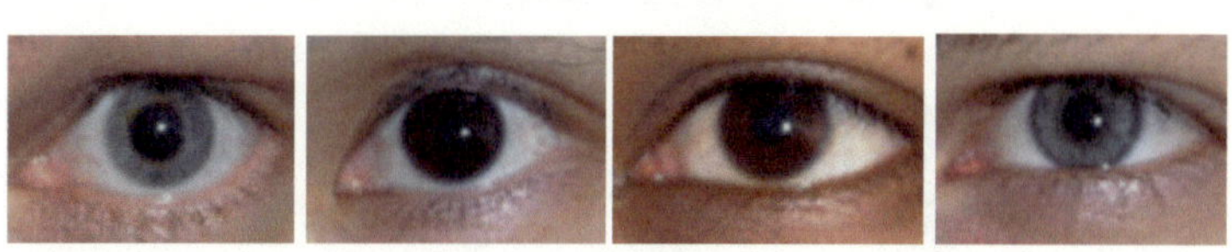

Figure 4. Figure 4. Color of pupil does not depend on ethnicity

The pupil gets wider in the dark but narrower in light. When narrow, the diameter is 3 to 4 millimeters. In the dark it will be the same at first, but will approach the maximum distance for a wide pupil of 5 to 8 mm depending on a person's age [5]. There are some definitions regarding pupil size in Figure 5.

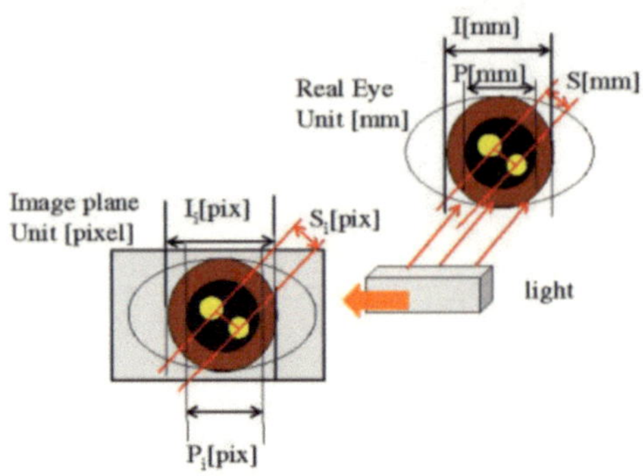

Figure 5. Definitions of pupil

The pupil's size always changes while the iris's size is fixed, therefore, to make pupil size independent in various conditions, in this paper we will use a ratio between pupil and iris as a unit to express size measurement, indicated by the symbol P_r and ex pressing by Equation 1.

$$P_r = \frac{P_i}{I_i} \approx \frac{P}{I} \tag{1}$$

2.2. Pupil localization

In general, the algorithm used in pupil localization is using 3 stages. Before performing these steps, the original image size changed to 50%. This is done to simplify the image processing operations.

1. Masking Step, namely the separation process of facial images based on skin color. How this is done by utilizing the luminance component and Cb and Cr to form the face of the box based on skin color as described in Figure 6.

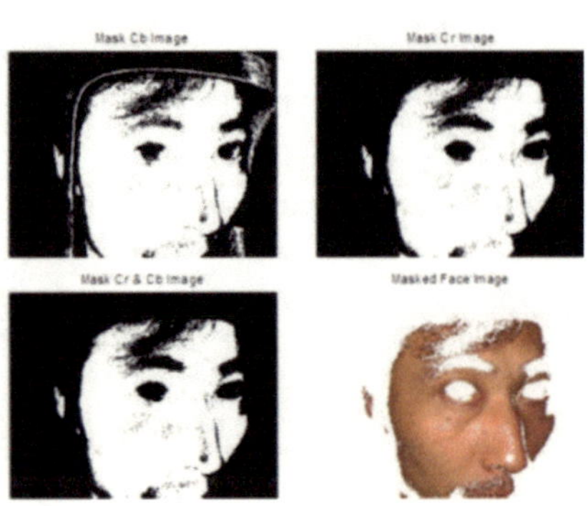

Figure 6. Face masking process

2. Region of eye Step, when it was getting a face image in the box and then take the eye area. Cutting the eye area is based on the normal form has a face that the proportion of 1 / 3 the length of a human face [6] as described in Figure 7.

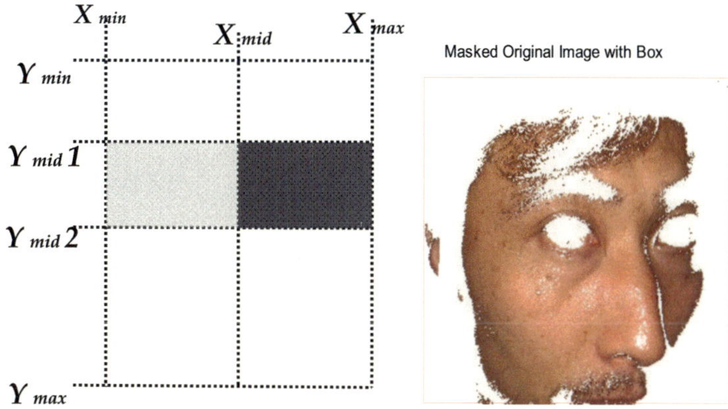

Figure 7. Estimation of eye area

3. Pupils Step, at this stage to use Lab color characteristics to determine the image of the pupil. Then using a fixed radius circle Hough to determine the center point of the circle which is the center point of pupil candidates as described in Figure 8.

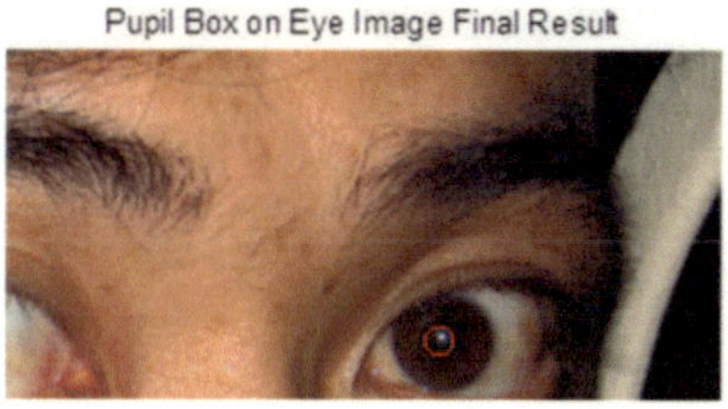

Figure 8. Pupil circle

2.3. Specular reflection analysis

The core of our method is specular reflection analysis. We develop our algorithm refer to the working principles of ophthalmoscope and slit lamp. An ophthalmoscope is an instrument that enables a doctor to examine the inside of a person's eye. The instrument has an angled mirror, various lenses, and a light source. A slit lamp is an instrument that enables a doctor to examine the entire eye under high magnification and that allows measurement of depth. The slit lamp focuses a bright light into the eye. Both equipments have a similarity for diagnosing cataract.

Figure 9 describes the principle work of the specular reflection method. Light hits the frontal surface of the lens and makes a reflection called frontside reflection. But actually light also hits the rear side of the lens. For a non serious condition, there is not a whitish color inside the lens so it will be reflected again, which is called backside reflection. For a serious condition especially, because there is a lot of clouding in the lens, light will not be reflected again. The different characteristics are shown in Figure 10. Based on the reflection theorem, the direction of the normal vector always goes to the center of the pupil, so when we look at the image appearance we can find the relationship of the location between the two reflections and the center of the pupil; they are on a single line

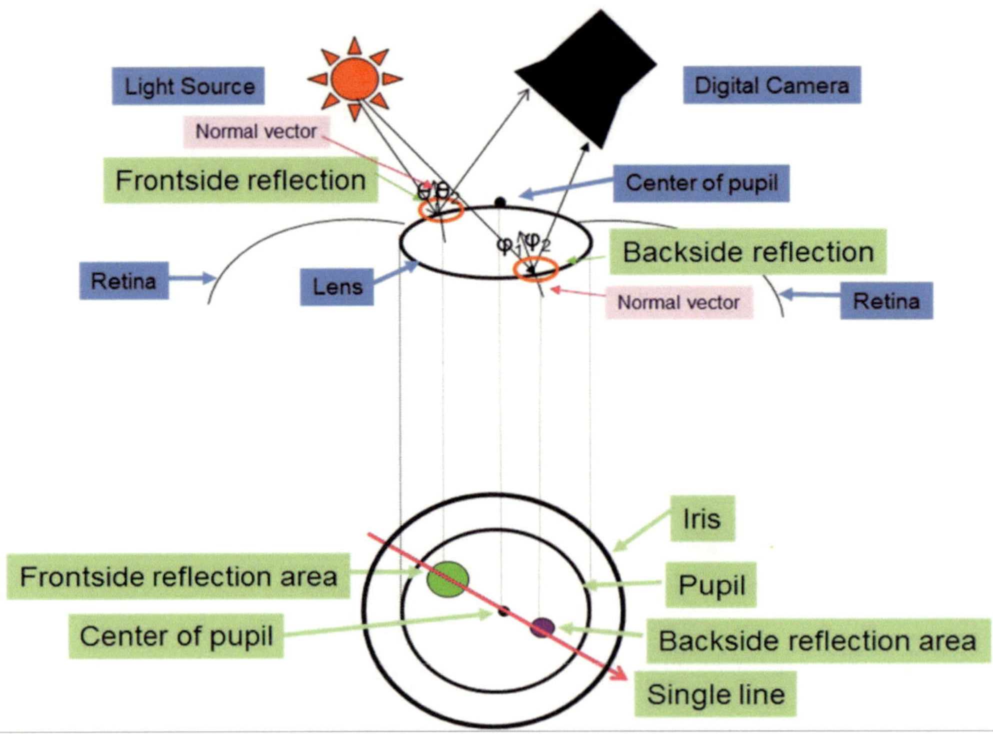

Figure 9. Model of reflection characteristics in eye

Using the relationship between both reflections, we conducted a search to find the backside reflection, as depicted in Figure 11. Using coordinate of the center and the radius of frontside reflection, we then searched for the backside reflection by searching for areas of higher intensity beside frontside reflection compared with their immediately surrounding areas in a line that expressed by Equation 2

$$A = d + r - \delta \tag{2}$$

Where A is the length of backside reflection searching, d is the distance between center of pupil and center of frontside reflection, r is the radius of pupil and δ is the radius of backside reflection.

In fact, the shapes of specular reflections are varied as described in Figure 12. As shown in Figure 12, some variations of the specular reflections shape are circle, cube, rectangular and ellipse, although we used the same flash light during taking photographs. Therefore, during searched for backside reflections area as described in Figure 11, we considered to assume various shapes of specular reflections and did intensity searching based on the shape that we assumed before as shown in Figure 13.

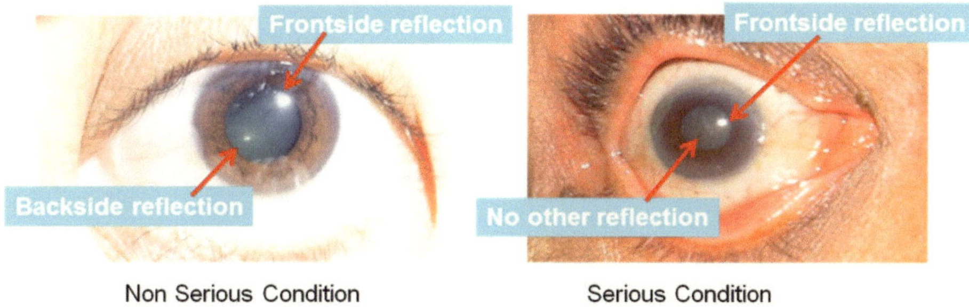

Figure 10. Example of Reflection Appearance

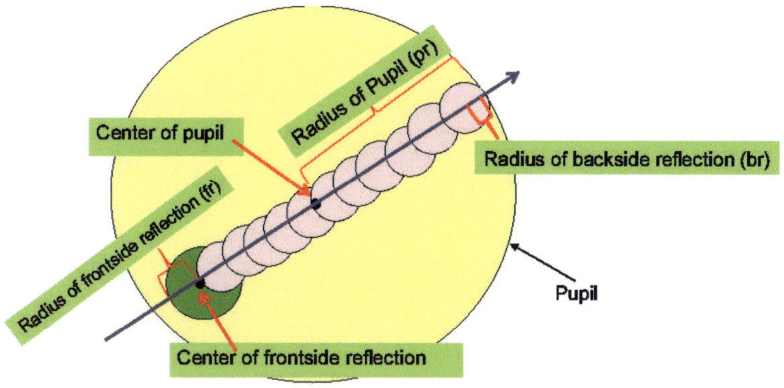

Figure 11. Searching backside reflection area data

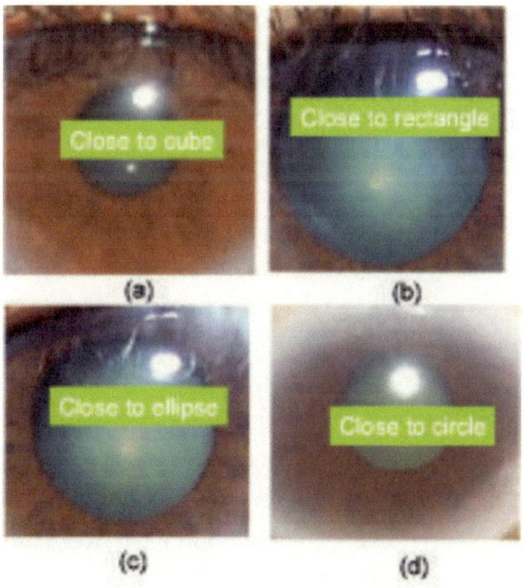

Figure 12. Various shapes of specular reflections inside the pupil

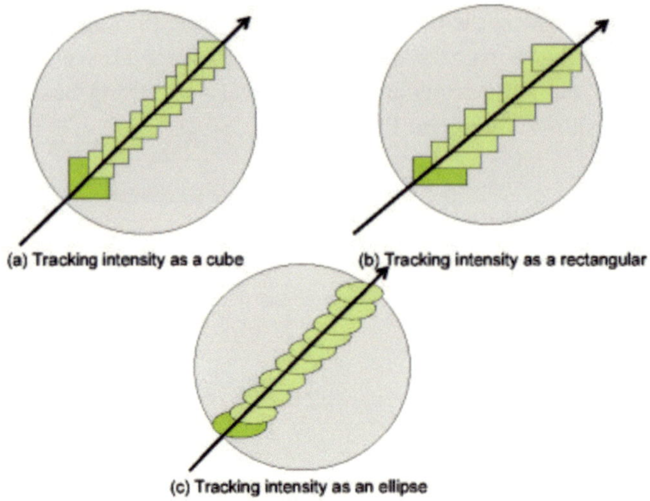

Figure 13. Intensity tracking using various shapes of specular reflections

We apply Eq. 2 which the value of δ is determined by following the assumption of specular reflection as shown in Figure 14.

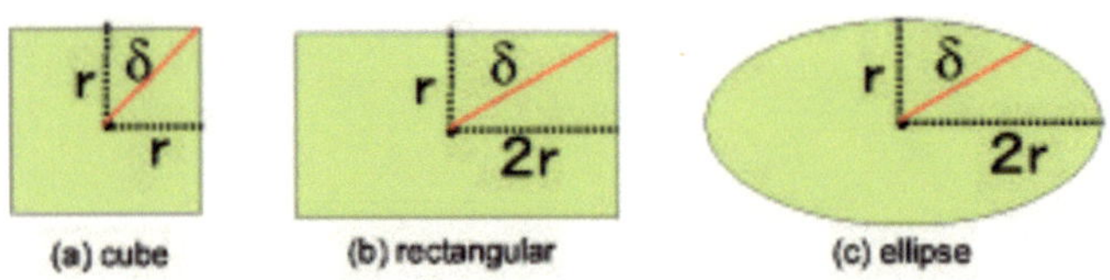

Figure 14. The size using for intensity tracking

Then, we compare the performance of each shapes of specular reflections in order to provide a recommendation on the tendency of specular reflection's shape that can give the best results for cataract screening sistem we apply an Eq.4.

Based on the result of intensity tracking as shown in Figure 11, we implemented a differential function in a discrete system to develop an automatic screening between the serious condition and not serious condition based on intensity tracking result and expressed by Equation 3.

$$D = I(s) - I(s-1)\ldots \tag{3}$$

Where I is intensity and S is a distance between center of frontside reflection and the next circle that will be investigated. During intensity searching, if $D(S) > 0$ it means there is an increasing intensity value. Otherwise if $D(S) < 0$ it means there is a decreasing intensity value. Based on the discussion in above paragraph, that non serious condition always have a great increasing intensity that indicated existence of backside reflection but it doesn't mean that serious condition didn't have increasing intensity during intensity tracking. Because we have variations of the numbers of intensity searching so we define normalized number of increasing value determined by Equation 4.

$$P_n = \frac{P}{n} \tag{4}$$

Where P is the numbers of point that has increasing intensity value and n is the numbers of point along an intensity tracking line. The main characteristic of serious and non-serious conditions depends on the presence of backside reflection in an image that is shown by increasing intensity in an area during intensity searching. Figure 15 shows the examples of the result of intensity tracking for serious and non-serious.

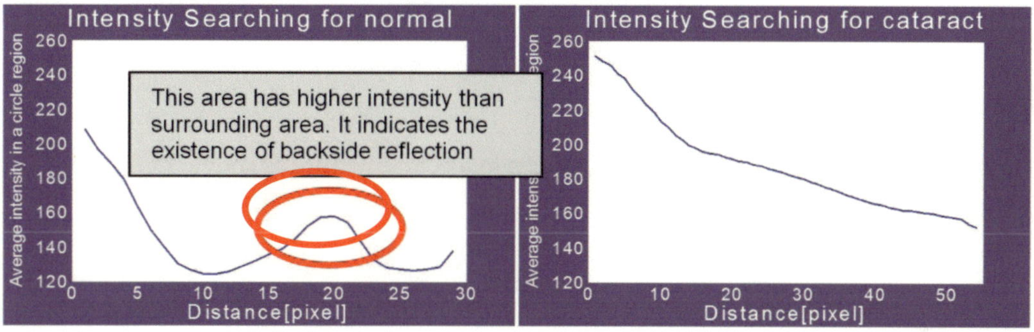

Figure 15. Analyzing backside reflection

2.4. Texture analysis

2.4.1. Uniformity

An important approach to region description is to quantify texture content. In statistical texture analysis, the descriptor measures properties such as smoothness, coarseness and regularity. Basically, there are two kinds of textures inside the pupil; smooth and coarse. This can be calculated by the uniformity value expressed in Eq.5. Where U is the value of uniformity, H is probability histogram of the intensity levels in a region, and N is the number of pixel in an image, Let i = 0, 1, 2, …., , L − 1, be the corresponding histogram, where L is the value of possible intensity. Uniformity will be maximum when all gray levels are equal [7]. Whitish color inside the lens has two kinds' distributions. First, whitish color spread smoothly inside the pupil. In the early stage, this kind of cataract has a thin layer of whitish color and covers the whole lens surface gradually until the whitish color layer becomes thick. Second, whitish color spread uneven inside the lens. It will appear a coarse texture inside the pupil. Almost all non serious conditions have a smooth texture with a high value of uniformity.

$$U = \sum_{i=0}^{L-1} \left(\frac{H(i)}{N}\right)^2 \quad \text{........(5)}$$

For example, in a 3 x 3 region and belongs to a smooth texture as shown in Figure 16 , the uniformity is shown in calculation below:

$$U = \left(\frac{9}{9}\right)^2 = 1$$

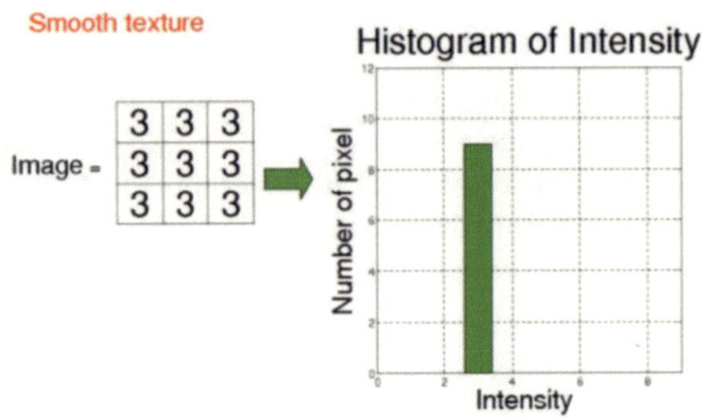

Figure 16. Example of Smooth Texture

Another example, in a 3 x 3 region and belongs to a coarse texture as shown in Figure 17, the uniformity is shown in calculation below:

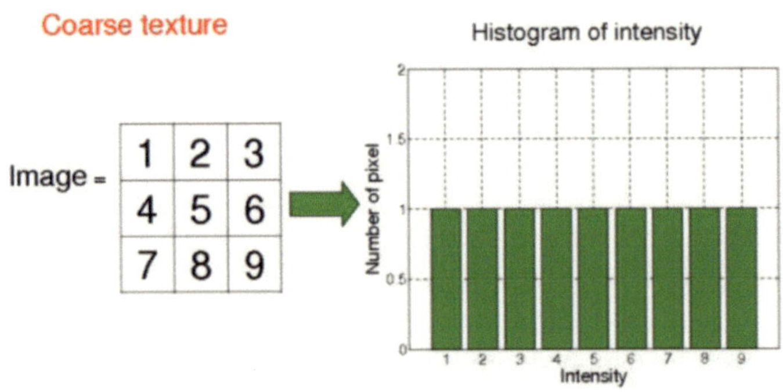

Figure 17. Example of coarse Texture

$$U = \left(\frac{1}{9}\right)^2 + \left(\frac{1}{9}\right)^2 + \left(\frac{1}{9}\right)^2 + \left(\frac{1}{9}\right)^2 + \left(\frac{1}{9}\right)^2 + \left(\frac{1}{9}\right)^2 + \left(\frac{1}{9}\right)^2 + \left(\frac{1}{9}\right)^2 + \left(\frac{1}{9}\right)^2 = 0{,}111$$

Figure 18(a) shows an image of eye in serious condition with a high value of uniformity caused by the whitish color is spreading smoothly inside the pupil. In the early stage, this kind of cataract has a thin layer of whitish color and covers the whole lens surface gradually until the whitish color layer becomes thick. Figure 18(b) shows an image of an eye with a coarse texture because the whitish color is spreading unevenly inside the pupil. Figure 18(c) shows an image of an eye in non-serious condition. Almost all non-serious conditions have a smooth texture with a high value of uniformity.

2.4.2. *Average intensity*

The equation to measure an average intensity expressed in Equation 6, where m is mean (average) of intensity, I is possible intensity, and N is number of pixel in an image [7]. It will be very simple intuition that cataract eyes have brighter intensities than normal eyes.

$$m = \sum_{i=0}^{L-1} \left(\frac{I(i)}{N}\right) \tag{6}$$

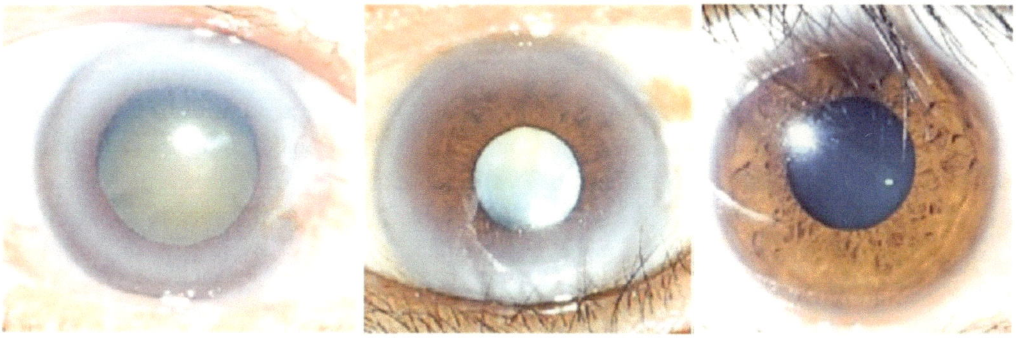

(c) Serious (b) Serious (a) Non- Serious

Figure 18. Example of Texture Appearance

For example, in a 3x3 region as shown in Figure 19 , the average intensity is shown in calculation below :

$$m = \frac{3+3+2+1+2+5+7+1+4}{9} = 3,11111$$

$$\text{Image} = \begin{array}{|c|c|c|} \hline 3 & 3 & 2 \\ \hline 1 & 2 & 5 \\ \hline 7 & 1 & 4 \\ \hline \end{array}$$

Figure 19. An example of average intensity

The whitish color inside a pupil has a corresponding with increasing intensity. Figure 20 shows an eye normal image and a cataract eye image. It appears that a cataract eye image has a higher intensity than a normal eye image. By assuming that a serious condition has a higher intensity than a non-serious condition, we distinguish both conditions.

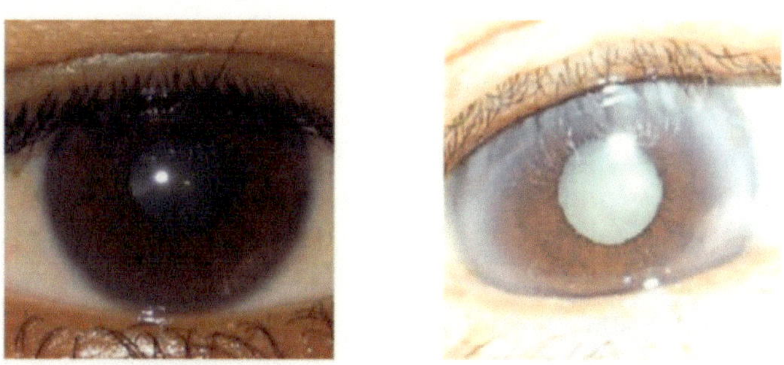

Normal Cataract

Figure 20. Intensity difference between normal and cataract

3. Diagnosing by classification

To build the system, we used Matlab R2007B with image processing toolbox. Also, for building a classifier to classify between serious and non-serious condition, we use SVM toolbox developed by Canu [3]. In order to make a classification for cataract screening we need two kinds of data: training data and testing data. Training data used to train the system to recognize the characteristics of a serious condition and non-serious condition so the system can determine the threshold for distinguishing between two conditions automatically. While testing data used to evaluate system performance refer to the characteristics obtained in the training data.

To test the performance of our system, we use several parameters. The first is True Positive Rate (TPR). TPR determines a classifier or a diagnostic test performance on classifying positive instances correctly among all positive samples available during the test. The second is FPR (False Positive Rate). FPR, on the other hand, defines how many incorrect positive results occur among all negative samples available during the test.

Criterion values for getting TPR and FPR parameters are described in Figure 21.

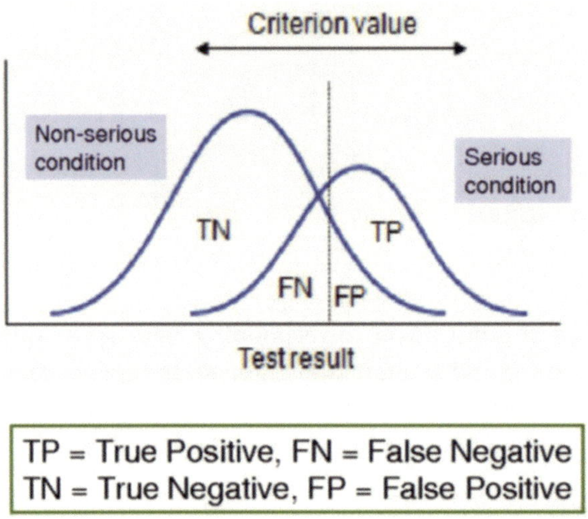

Figure 21. Parameter for measuring performance

To evaluate the overall system performance, we use cross validation techniques in which we did evaluation several times until all data were evaluated.. So that all images produced by various kinds of cameras are grouped into two groups. The first group is the images that show the serious conditions, while the second group is the images that show the non-serious conditions. We did some testing times by taking 90% of data as training data and 10% of data as testing data. Data changed each time, until finally all data used as training data and testing data. Figure 22 shows a summary of performance our algorithm. The result shows that current method has a good performance than other method.

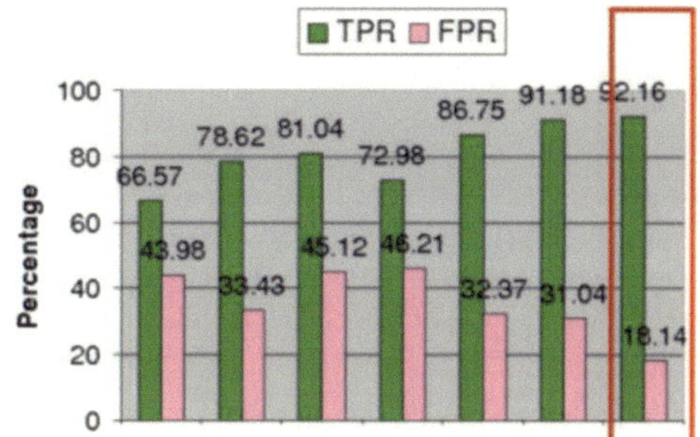

Average instensity	V			V	V		V
Texture uniformity		V		V		V	V
Specular reflection			V		V	V	V

proposed

Figure 22. Performance comparison for each method

4. Practical screening system and data acquisition

As discussed in subsection 2.3, the core of our method is specular reflection analysis. Referring to the reflection theorem, light hits the frontal surface of the lens and makes a reflection called frontside reflection. However, light also hits the rear side of the lens. For a non-serious condition, there is not a whitish color inside the lens, therefore, it will be reflected again, which is called backside reflection. For a serious condition especially, because there is a lot of clouding in the lens, light will not be reflected again. In order to investigate the availability of frontside reflection and backside reflection inside the lens, and also to obtain a minimum distance between two reflections that can be observed by our algorithm, we did a simulation. Refer to the experiments, our algorithm can observe availability of two reflections with minimum ratio between distance and iris of about 0.125. It is an important value because if our algorithm fails to investigate availability of the two reflections, will face problems. First, patient really has a serious condition. Second, it is caused by a wrong position between camera and patient during taking a photograph.

Regarding these problems, we have to make sure that we put camera and patient in an appropriate position. Therefore, a simulation of the angle's position is very important. In our simulation, we assume that a light is attached in camera. The purposes are:

1. Getting an optimal position of angle between camera and lens.
2. Getting an optimal pupil size to get an appropriate distance between two reflections.

The lens has an ellipsoid, biconvex shape. It is typically circa 10 mm in diameter and has an axial length of about 4 mm [5]. An iris is a colored disk inside the eye with diameter of about 12 mm [5]. Figure 23 describes the shape and size of the lens, pupil and iris in our simulation.

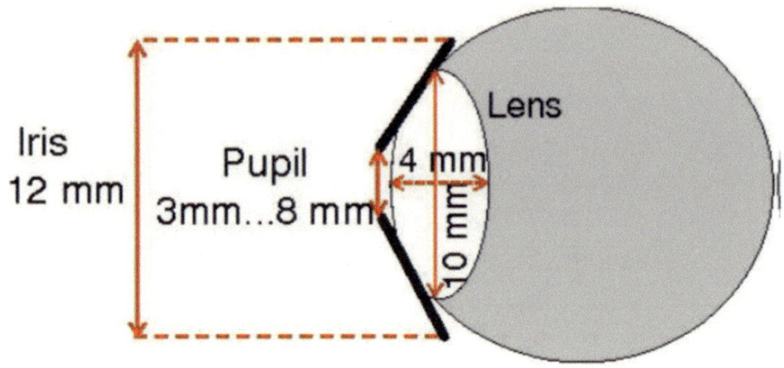

Figure 23. Typical shape and size of pupil

In this part, there are three conditions. First is a condition where the reflection does not occur inside the lens. Second is a condition where only a frontside reflection occurs and can be observed inside the lens. Third is an appropriate condition where a frontside reflection and backside reflection occur and can be observed in an image plane. Figures 24-26 show each condition, respectively.

During simulation, we change the position of the camera with light attached based on angle (φ) between camera and lens. It starts from angle 1° to angle 180°. Figure 24 shows that the position of light cannot reach the lens because light hits the surface of the iris; therefore, there is no reflection in the lens

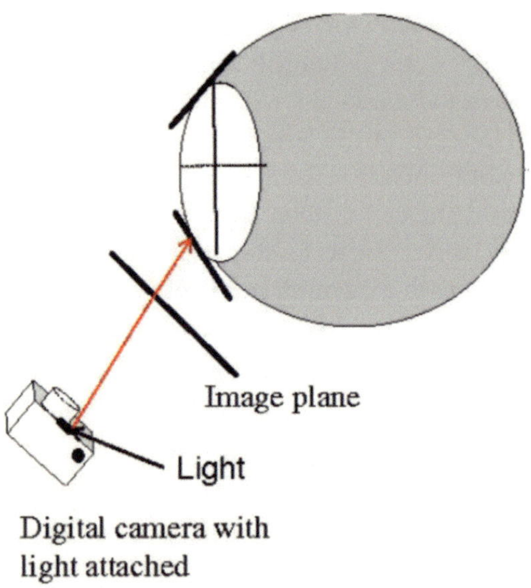

Figure 24. Condition in which no reflection occurs

Figure 25 shows that light hits the frontal surface of the lens therefore, a reflection occurs and is observed. However, when the light hits the rear side of the lens, a reflection occurs but it cannot be observed in the image plane. Therefore, in this condition, only frontside reflection is observed in the image plane. Figure 26 shows an appropriate condition in which both reflections occur and are observed in the image plane. This kind of parameter will be useful for distinguishing between serious and non-serious conditions.

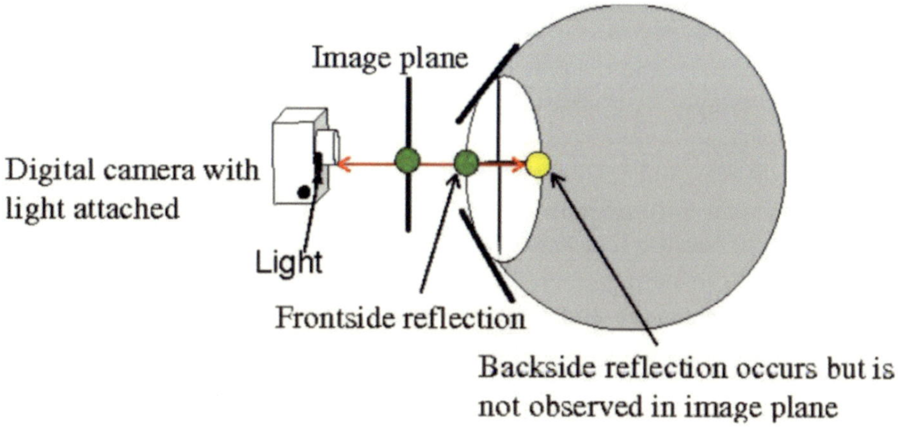

Figure 25. Condition in which only frontside reflection occurs and is observed in an image plane

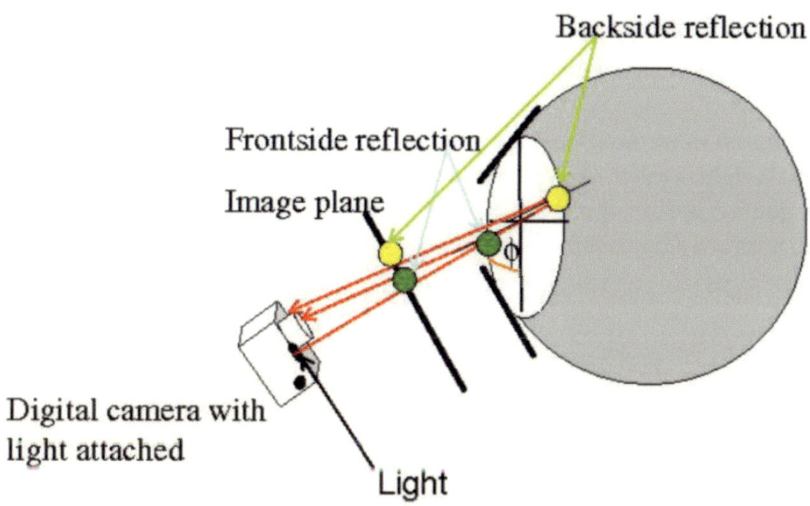

Figure 26. An appropriate condition in which both reflections occur and are observed in an image plane

In the real condition, As already discussed in the section 1, that our system is expected to be used by all people in all places, so that the equipment will be used in our system must also be simple as shown in Figure 28. Brief description about the function of equipment is described in the following paragraph.

3. Chin rest - This is equipment for patient to lean forward and place his or her in the chin rest and forehead against the bar. We use a simple chin rest created manually by using a board that is placed on something that could make it stand upright. The main goal is

to put the patient's chin so that patients feel comfortable during taking a photograph. On the other hand, by using a chin rest so will allow a user to get the right eye image during taking a photograph because the patient does not move his head movement that will result in the patient's eye movement. We should be emphasized here that this tool is not absolutely necessary in our system, if users can take photograph that make an appropriate input image and the patient feel comfortable, not moving their head so that the position of the eyes in a state of permanent, then the use of these tools are not needed.

4. Tripod - Tripods are used for both still and motion photography to prevent camera movement. The main purpose of using a tripod in our system is to make it easier to get good quality photo because the camera will be in a fixed position and not moving so the possibility of blur can be prevented. Another reason is to get more accurate angular position between the camera and the patient because they will affect the existence of specular reflection inside a pupil as be described in above paragraph. It should be noted here that as well as the use of chin rest, the use of a tripod in our system is not an absolute thing. If users able to get an appropriate input image without using a tripod therefore this equipment is not required in our system.
5. Digital Camera - This is the most important equipment in our system because all the input images are taken from a digital camera. In our system, we use all types of digital cameras from various brands available such as Canon and Nikon. We do not consider about the performance of cameras such as the number of pixels, zooming capabilities,and other facilities. Most important for our system is the camera has flash facility as a light source to get specular reflections, has a macro facility to get a good enough quality when taking photographs for the pupil of the eye area. Referring to Figure 2, it can be said that the performance of each camera is almost evenly.

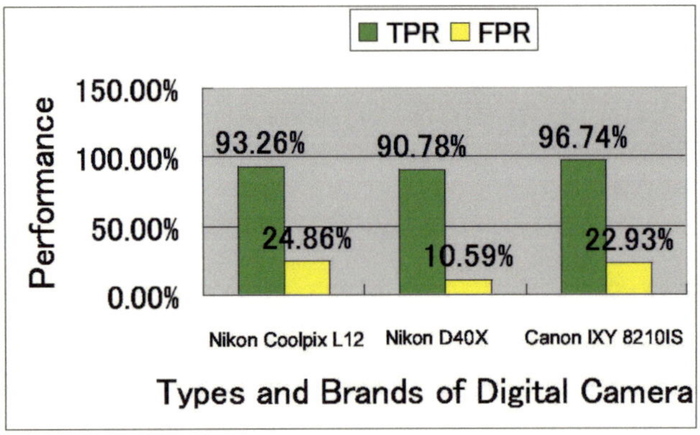

Figure 27. System performance based on types and brands of digital camera

6. Scale - This is equipment to provide guidance angle camera placement. We use a kind of plastic mats that have been marked to measure the angle between the patient and the camera.
7. Personal Computer

The main function is an interface for analyzing of input images that have been obtained in the data acquisition session. Our method written in the form of graphical user interface (GUI) so that user easily uses it just by pressing the command buttons available. Users do not need to analyze the complicated result because our methods give results about the patient's condition which he included in serious or non serious condition.

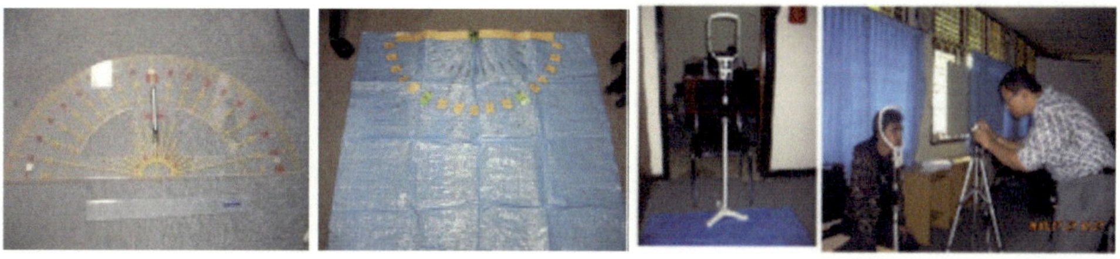

Figure 28. Equipment were used in our system

Figure 29 and Figure 30 describe about the implementation of data acquisition in the real condition.

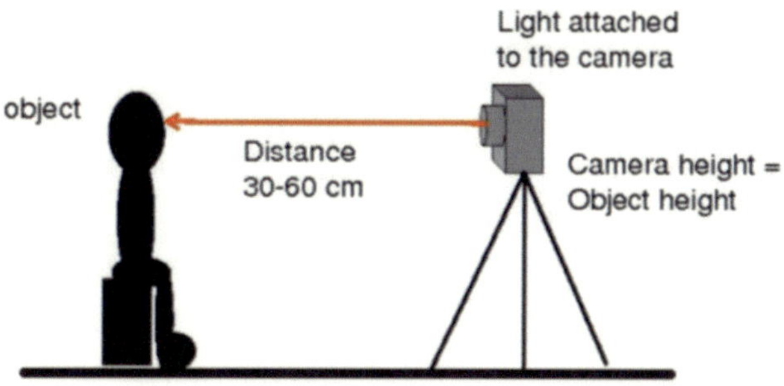

Figure 29. Side view of camera configuration

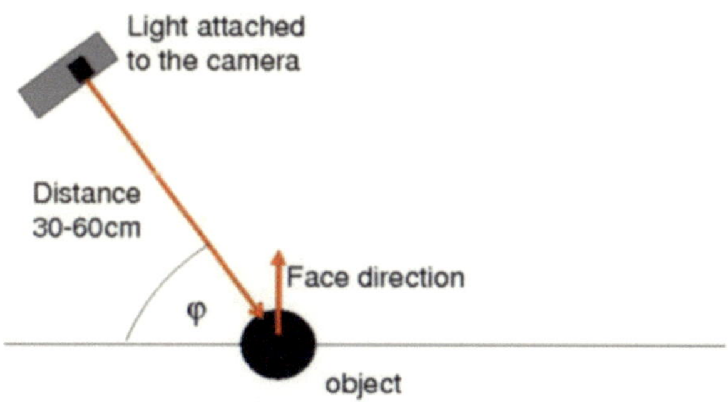

Figure 30. View from above camera configuration

5. Conclusion

Regarding the conditions in developing countries which have limitations both of eye doctors and health facilities, using simple equipment such as digital camera for cataract screening is promising and sufficient. Because digital camera is small and easily carried out, easy to use and inexpensive. Also, the method for supporting digital camera has a good performance for distinguishing between serious and non-serious condition; therefore, it is very useful for determining people who need a surgery as soon as possible.

Author details

Retno Supriyanti
Faculty of Science and Engineering, Jenderal Soedirman University, Indonesia

Hitoshi Habe and Masatsugu Kidode
Graduate School of Information Science, Nara Institute of Science and Technology, Japan

Acknowledgement

We Would like to thank the head and staffs of the Kamandaka Eye Clinic in Purwokerto Indonesia, Students and staffs of Electrical Engineering Dept, Jenderal Soedirman University Indonesia.The staffs of NAIST Japan, all members of the Advanced Intelligence Laboratory at NAIST, and members of the elder peoples house (CHOMEISHO) in Ikoma Japan , for their permission and willingness have photographs taken of cataract and normal patients. Also, this work is partly supported by the Konika Minolta Imaging Science Foundation and the Foundation for NAIST, also DIPA Jenderal Soedirman University through International Research Collaboration Project.

6. References

[1] Ilyas, Sidharta, 2005 "Eye Diseases", Balai Penerbit FKUI, Jakarta.

[2] Brian Gary, Hugh Taylor, 2001, "Cataract Blindness – challenges for 21st century", Bulletin of the World Health Organization.

[3] Medical Encyclopedia. 2007, Pupil. Available : http:// www. nlm. nih. gov/ medlineplus / ency/ article, accessed 2007 july 20.

[4] Eyemakeart. 2009, Anatomi mata. Available: http://eyemakeart.com/anatomi-mata/, accessed 2009 July 20..

[5] Taylor.Karen,2001, "Forensic Art and Illustrations ", CRC Press LLC, Florida.

[6] David B.L. Bong dan Kok Houi Lim, 2009, "Application of Fixed-Radius Hough Transform In Eye Detection". International Journal of Intelligent Information Technology Application, 2(3):121-127.

[7] Gonzales, RC, and R.E. Woods. 2002, "Digital Image Processing. 2nd ed." New Jersey: Prentice Hall, Inc.

[8] Canu. S, Y. Grandvalet, V. Guigue, and A. Rakotomamonjy. 2005, SVM and kernel methods matlab toolbox. Perception Systmes et Information, INSA de Rouen, Rouen, France.

Chapter 4

Clinical Application of Photodisruptors in Ophthalmology

Emina Alimanović Halilović

Additional information is available at the end of the chapter

http://dx.doi.org/10.5772/48625

1. Introduction

In ophthalmology today, laser photodisruptors are used besides laser photocoagulators. Photocoagulators transform light energy into heat energy, causing microcauterisation of tissue. Photodisruptors act non-thermally by controlled cutting of the unwanted tissue, causing microexplosions. The most frequently used photodisruptors are Neodymium YAG, Holmium YAG and Erbium YAG lasers. They differ by type of the active crystal. The laser beam of these lasers is highly coherent, low-divergent, which enables it a high precision. It is used as a microscalpel to cut optical membranes and tissues.

Meyer-Schwickerath was the first to describe the laser beam transmission through optical media. Photodisruptors such as Nd-YAG laser work by principles of the optical "breakdown". Laser beam energy is brought to as small focal point as possible, thus achieving a high energy density with a strong destructive effect. In the focal point there occurs a microexplosion with disruption of electrons from their nuclear orbits. This free floater is known as electronic plasma. The electronic plasma is able to absorb any further energy entering the eye in the same focal point. This significant feature of the protective plasma prevents damage to the eye structures beyond the protective plasma formation, i.e., conduction of the destructive effect outside the focus. Inside the protective plasma, the temperature is 15,000 ºC with a high pressure, so the plasma expands in concentric waves, "shock waves". In about 150ns after the "optical breakdown", it is possible to biomicroscopically see air bubbles as a sign of collapse and pressure equalisation inside the wave with atmospheric pressure. The "shock wave" is accompanied by an acoustic wave that is sometimes audible.

Two methods are used in the Nd-YAG laser beam production: "Q-switched" and "mode-locked". The former compresses energy in a single „nanosecond" pulse, and the latter produces a series of "picosecund" pulses. In the "mode-locked" method, we have a low energy power of single pulsations, while in the "Q-switched" method, pulse energy is higher at the same energy level. The "Q-switched" technology produces chiefly pulses whose main effect is mechanical – buckling. This is photodisruption, i.e., tearing of atoms with energy shocks. The effect of this method is creation of energy in the pipe being let through in short impulses, and during the still interval energy is kept, accumulated and enhanced, so that each impulse has a very high performing power.

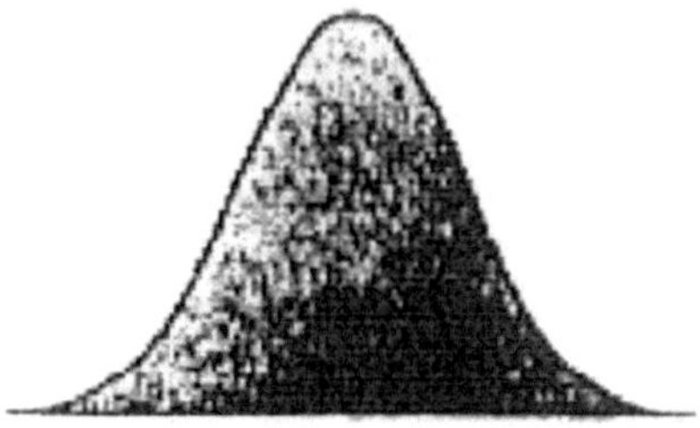

Figure 1. Q-switched pulse;

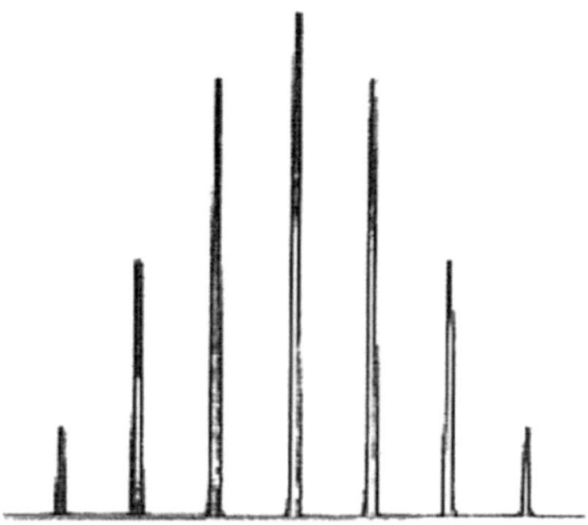

Figure 2. Mode-locked pulse train

The Nd-YAG laser beam causes damage to the tissue in the form of craters in the fields of vaporisation. The crater edges are carbonised, then towards the edges there follows the coagulation necrosis area, and at the far periphery the oedema area.

Erbium-YAG laser has found a broad application in aesthetic plastic microsurgery of eyelids, in blepharochalasis, ectropium, and phthisis. Multifocal Erbium-YAG laser systems have a multiple use in ophthalmology, in the cataract phaco surgery, vitrectomy and sclerectomy.

It is also used in dermatology for dermoabrasion for the skin rejuvenation.

2. Nd-Yag laser in ophthalmology

Modern cataract microsurgery with implantation of intraocular lenses is inseparable from the Nd-YAG laser microsurgery. The microsurgery of glaucoma and problems of the posterior segment also imply the use of Nd-YAG laser. Application of Nd-YAG laser:

with cataract in	anterior capsulotomy
	posterior capsulotomy
	removal of pigment from the anterior surface of IOL
	discission of secondary cataract and membrane
	synechiolysis
	cutting of corneal sutures after the cataract surgery or cheratoplastica
with corneal diseases	dendritic ulcers
	microabscesses
with glaucoma	transscleral cycolophotocoagulation
	iridectomy
	sphinteroctomy
with the vitreous body	anterior vitreoruption
	cutting of intravitreal vitreoretinal tractions and membranes

Table 1. Clinical application of Nd-YAG laser in ophthalmology

2.1. Nd-Yag laser posterior capsulotomy

The most frequent practical application of Nd-YAG laser is in posterior capsulotomy and discission of secondary membranes in aphakic (conditions after the cataract surgery), and pseudophakic (conditions after the cataract surgery with implantation of intraocular lens into the anterior or posterior eye chamber) of the eyes.

The surgical technique of intraocular lens placement is important for the development of posterior capsular opacity. The intraocular lens placement itself, manipulation with the iris, and lens contact with the posterior capsule may be a cause of accumulation of pigment on the lens anterior surface and development of opacity. Also, the lens implant size, its shape and the type of material of which it is made have a significant impact on the development of secondary cataract. Posterior lens capsular opacity develops through the migration of epithelium from the remaining parts of the anterior lens capsule, proliferation of the remaining epithelial cells of the anterior pole of lens and lens fibres. Through their metaplasia, myofibroblasts are developed, forming folds, reticles, uneven membranes which are difficult to see biomicroscopically; they do not significantly affect visual acuity. If epithelial cells accumulate in the form of round, uneven, pearl-shaped opacity - Elschnig's pearls - then such opacity reduces significantly vision. There may be also some other causes of opacity of the posterior lens capsule: remaining parts of the lens cortex intraoperatively and after incomplete aspiration. Masses can incorporate between the implanted lens and posterior capsule. Also, the remaining parts of the lens nucleus, blood cells in hyphema, pigment cells of the iris and ciliary body may accumulate on the lens or posterior capsule. Low-virulent, slow-growing, still bacterial colonies such as Propionibacterium acnes may settle in the posterior capsule field and look like ordinary opacity. If we mistake them for normal capsular opacity and perform the laser capsulotomy, we have opened a path for bacteria into the vitreous body, which can result in the occurrence of endophthalmitis.

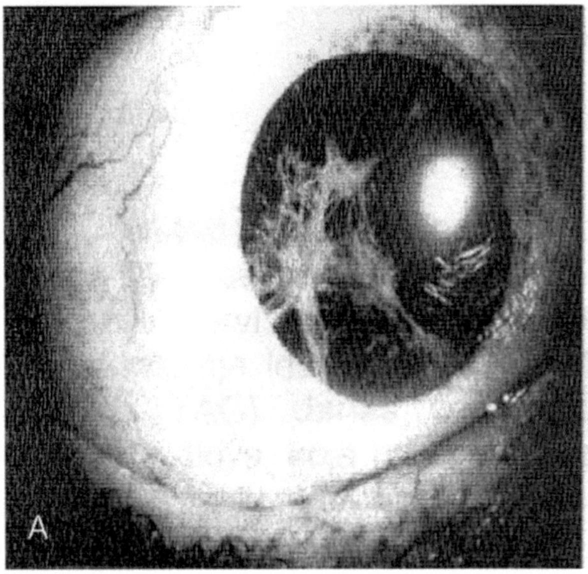

Figure 3. Posterior capsular opacification

Postoperative posterior capsular opacity leads to a fall of visual acuity. Patients complain of blurred images, they see things as if through "gauze or a sieve". In the first postoperative year, opacity occurs in 83% patients and from the second to the fifth years in 50% cases. The Nd-YAG laser posterior capsulotomy is a routine technique with which we resolve the problem. With the laser beam we make the "fenestra" opening on the posterior capsule through which light beams reach the retina without obstruction and form a clear image of an object.

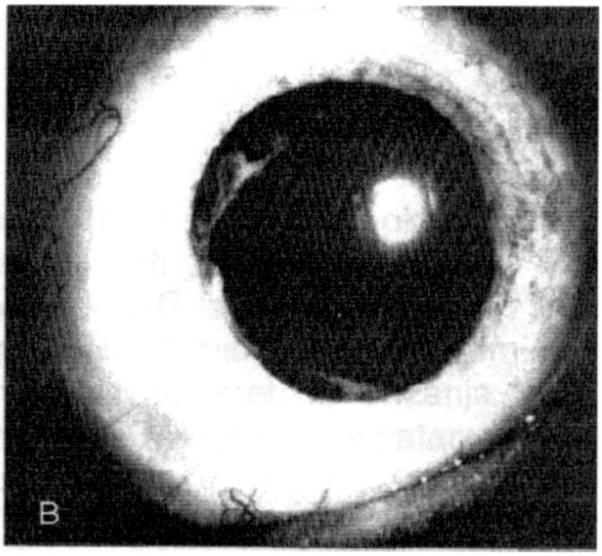

Figure 4. After Nd-YAG capsulotomy

Prior to the intervention itself, it is necessary to examine the patient's visual acuity, take intraocular pressure, examine biomicroscopically capsular opacity, direct and through the procedure of retroillumination of the capsule itself and the retrolental space. Opacity of the posterior lens capsule may be measured echographically, and the quantitative measuring "in vivo" with the Scheimpflug photographic computer system. The intervention is performed on the pupil dilated to the maximum, in the darkroom, with the surgeon's prior adaptation to the dark, with optimal enlargement on the biomicroscope, with the optimal light intensity, on the dilated pupil. The patient has to cooperate with the surgeon, keep still on the apparatus and follow the instructions from the surgeon in moving the eyes. The procedure is performed under local anaesthesia, by means of condensing Abraham or Peyman YAG planconvex contact lens for the posterior capsulotomy. Such lenses concentrate the laser beam to the smallest possible focus. At the same time, they immobilise the eye in restless patients. The angle of the incoming convergent laser beam depends on technical possibilities of the apparatus and it is selected by the surgeon. According to Eisner's discussions, the widest incoming angle, with the smallest focal point (mark), and clear focusing produce the clean beam, with the highest energy concentration in the focus and the smallest energy dispersion in the cornea or retina. The most frequently used capsulotomy techniques are Seaman's, which imply the knowledge of quality and thickness of opacity:

a. the „vertical opening" technique from 12 o'clock position to 6 o'clock position is applied in posterior capsular opacity;
b. the „cross-shaped" technique when horizontal cutting is performed by vertical opening from 9 o'clock position to 6 o'clock position;

c. the „concentric spreading" technique from the periphery to the centre, in abundant secondary;
d. the „fragmentation" technique with the widening of opening edges in fibrous membranes.

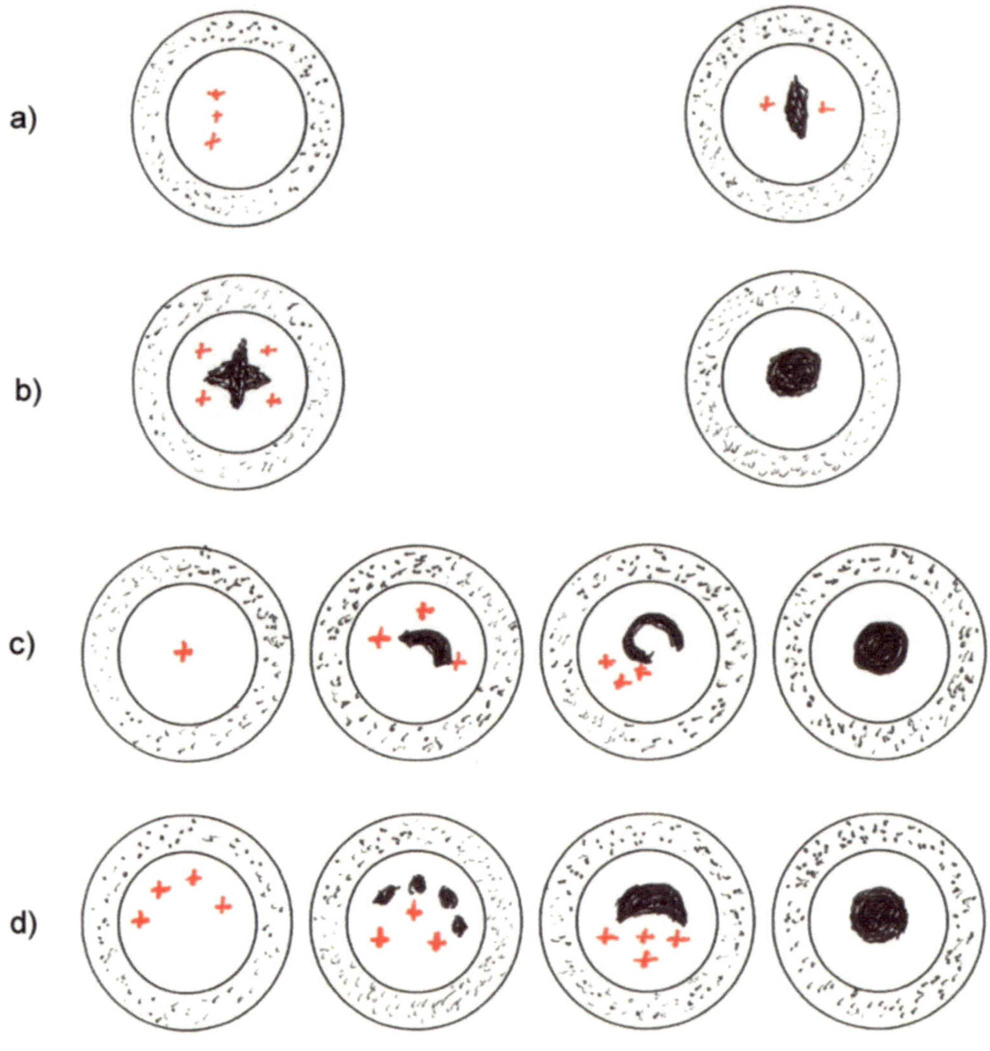

Figure 5. „Seaman's" capsulotomy techniques

Although the Nd-YAG laser capsulotomy is a non-invasive technique, efficient, painless, practical, easily-applicable, cost-effective, with fast recovery, today the method of choice, it is necessary that the laser surgery be performed by a well-trained, educated and experienced ophthalmologist. Only with the expertise and ethics of the laser surgeon can complications be avoided and reduced. All complications are a result of correlation of the laser action, methodological errors in performance and the condition of the eye. Use of the

Nd-YAG laser beam can lead to certain unwanted complications on the anterior and posterior poles of the eye.

On the anterior segment, we usually have: damage to the corneal epithelium, corneal perforation, damage to the intraocular lens, dislocation of the intraocular lens, changes of intraocular pressure, development of iritis, and hemorrhage into the anterior chamber.

On the posterior eye segment, the following complications can develop: rupture of the anterior hyaloid membrane, prolapse of the vitreous body into the anterior chamber, retinal rupture, cystic macular oedema, retinal detachment, retinal bleeding, macular fibrosis, macular rupture, and rarely endophthalmitis.

2.2. A jump of intraocular pressure

We have transient increase in IOP in 50-97% laser-treated patients after the posterior capsulotomy. Numerous investigations have shown that the highest jump takes place in the first four hours, and in the first 24-48 hours it returns to normal, stays increased by 5 mmHg respectively in the first week. In some cases, the increased IOP may stay on for two or three months. The IOP maximal values after the laser capsulotomy are 50-60 mmHg. Transient IOP increase after the Nd-YAG laser posterior capsulotomy is explained by the mechanical obstruction of the trabecular exhaust system with the posterior capsular residual particles, inflammatory cells, and high-molecular soluble proteins of the lens. An increased secretion of the ciliary epithelium is considered to be a cause of extended intraocular hypertension as a consequence of the "shock" wave effect. Also, according to Terry AC's opinion, there is a significant effect of prostglandins on the blood-aqueous barrier, which results in increased production of ocular water. The IOP jump is more frequent in the aphakic eye than in the pseudophakic eye. A higher IOP jump was proved in the lens implant into the anterior chamber compared to the eyes with the lens in the posterior chamber, or fixed to the iris. Glaucoma patients have a higher IOP jump compared to non-glaucoma patients.

2.3. Corneal damage

The laser beam, going through the cornea, may cause corneal oedema or perforation, usually unintentionally, due to the bad focusing or use of too much energy. The cornea absorbs 6% Nd-YAG laser energy, lens 15%, the vitreous body 36%. Capsulotomy causes a loss of endothelial cells of the cornea from 0 to 7%, but this loss does not decompensate the cornea.

Corneal damages are a consequence of the mechanical destruction and a heat effect of the linearly and non-linearly absorbed laser energy. Corneal epithelisation is completed in the first 24 hours. Corneal oedema may occur as secondary due to the increased IOP, or may be caused by exacerbation of inflammatory processes of the anterior segment after the YAG laser.

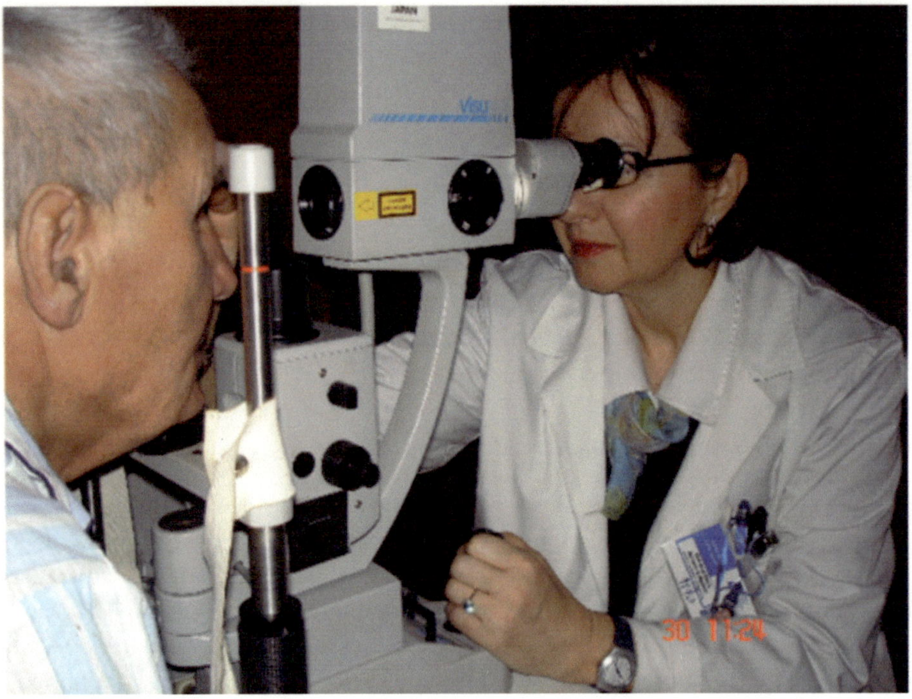

Figure 6. The Nd YAG laser procedure

2.4. Iris haemorrhage

As a consequence of damage to the delicate iris blood vessel by the laser beam during posterior capsulotomy, we can have bleeding in the anterior chamber with a slight pain. Incidence of this complication ranges from 1% to 3%. A slight pressure of the contact lens onto the cornea usually stops bleeding.

2.5. Damage to the intraocular lens

During posterior laser capsulotomy, damage to the intraocular lens may occur in 5% to 40% cases. They are usually recesses, fissures, cracks, lattice, and bursts of stellar shape. These damages affect visual acuity, especially if centrally located. They produce various visual effects, usually in the form of blinding glare, which affects the normal vision. The lens damage depends on individually and totally used energy, impulse duration, number of impulses, and the kind of the IOL material. Polymethylmethacrylat (PMMA) lenses may endure bigger energy without damages, and they are crater-shaped. Silicon lenses have damages in the form of smooth stratification.

2.6. Dislocation of the intraocular lens

Upon the Nd-YAG laser posterior capsulotomy, the IOL shifts to the vitreous body. The implanted lens shifting is monitored by measuring the depth of the anterior chamber with ultrasound biometry. It is a dislocation of 25μm (from 9 to 55 μm) with SD 13. It is difficult to prove the effect of dislocation on visual acuity as capsulotomy is followed by improvement of visual acuity.

2.7. Rupture of the anterior hyaloid membrane

Rupture of the anterior hyaloids membrane occurs as a complication after the Nd-YAG laser capsulotomy in 19% cases, which enables a prolapse of the vitreous body into the anterior chamber.

2.8. Prolapse of the vitreous body into the anterior chamber

We usually notice this complication three weeks after capsulotomy within the scope from 1.5% to 16%. Herniation of the vitreous body may cause an increased intraocular pressure. There are reports by the authors who, within a four-year period after intervention, do not find an increased IOP. Shifting of the vitreous body forward increases a danger of occurrence of macular oedema, retinal ruptures, and retinal detachment.

2.9. Retinal ruptures

After the laser posterior retinal capsulotomy, the number of retinal ruptures increases. The number, type and location of retinal ruptures are characteristic. They are asymptomatic, round, atrophic retinal ruptures observable usually a month upon capsulotomy, with incidence of 2.3%. The possibility of rupture occurrence is twice as big in laser-treated compared to non-laser treated eyes. Atrophic round retinal ruptures are more numerous than u-shaped ones. They occur in all meridians, including the macula, too. They may be isolated or within peripheral degenerations. They are chiefly localised in the upper temporal and nasal quadrants.

2.10. Retinal detachment

Occurrence of retinal detachment and retinal ruptures is statistically significantly more frequent in the eyes on which laser posterior capsulotomy was performed. Retinal detachment incidence after laser capsulotomy varies from 0.08% to 3.6% or 13% respectively, depending on the sample. Multiple studies have shown that post-laser retinal detachments occur more frequently in younger males. Risk factors, such as myopia, lattice degeneration, anamnesis of existence of retinal detachment on the other eye, and complicated surgeries, demonstrably increase the number of retinal detachments after capsulotomy. Retinal ablation development is influenced by tissue ionization and formation of gaseous "plasma", which then expands accompanied with the "shock and acoustic" wave. After the laser incision of tissue, we have a condition of a latent stress which further disintegrates the structures. All the three mechanisms act simultaneously, and the extent of destruction of the tissue around the optimal "breakdown" area depends on the laser pulse total energy, time of occurrence, and duration of electronic plasma, and the "shock" wave action. It is believed that the passage of the laser beam through the vitreous body and its "shock" and "acoustic" wave cause significant biochemical changes in the vitreous body. Animal experiments prove penetration of the physiological barrier, processes of depolymerisation of hyaluronic acid, liquefaction and separation of the vitreous body, and all this activates processes of vitreoretinal proliferation; as a consequence we have the occurrence of retinal ruptures and retinal detachment.

2.11. Cystoid macular oedema

Cystoid macular oedema incidence after the Nd-YAG laser capsulotomy varies in different authors from 0.5% to 4.9%. Oedema develops in first six months after the laser capsulotomy. Occurrence of cystoid macular oedema is related to the hyaloid membrane rupture, intraocular lens damage and a short time interval between the cataract surgery and laser intervention. Diagnosis is usually established on the basis of ophthalmoscopic finding and an unexpected fall of vision. Fluorescein angiography shows the flow of the contrast into the macular area. Fine and Brucker proved that cystoid macular oedema is a liquid which from perifoveolar capillaries pours via the damaged endothelium and accumulates in the plexiform, Henle's layer. The laser beam passing through optical tissues releases prostaglandin and leukotriene from the iris, which triggers a change of permeability of parafoveolar capillaries.

2.12. Macular rupture

After the Nd-YAG laser capsulotomy, we can have macular ruptures as a consequence. They are observable as early as 24 hours upon capsulotomy, and in the period from 10 to 21 days. They occur unilaterally more frequently, but there have been reports about bilateral occurrence as well. Macular rupture is almost always associated with other complications such as: a jump of intraocular pressure, prolapse of the vitreous body into the anterior chamber, macular haemorrhage, and occurrence of cystoid macular oedema. It manifests with a sudden fall of vision, appearance of central black spots and paracentral scotoma. They may create difficulties with recognition of colours.

Post-capsulotomy macular rupture occurs as a consequence of several mechanisms: thermal damages, mechanical disruptions, "optical breakdown" which leads to blood vessel bursts of the retina and chorioidea, thus causing subretinal, intraretinal, and vitreal bleeding. The third mechanism is the "shock wave" responsible for the occurrence of a series of changes in the vitreous body leading to the separation and ablation of the vitreous body. As a secondary effect, there occurs contraction of the perifoveolar vitreous body creating tangent tractions. They are considered to be a cause of macular rupture occurrence.

In most cases the macular rupture closes spontaneously within a period from three weeks to six months, and visual acuity improves significantly. Recently third-degree Gass macular ruptures are resolved surgically by vitrectomy with interior tamponade. After vitrectomy the macular rupture closes and visual acuity improves.

2.13. Macular fibrosis

After the Nd-YAG laser capsulotomy, macula bleeding may follow. Blood resorption is accompanied with formation of preretinal and retinal fibrogliosis bands and membranes which can be filled with abnormal blood vessels. Occurrence of macular fibrosis, after the Nd-YAG laser capsulotomy, is statistically significant. Macular fibrosis significantly reduces visual acuity and it is followed with metamorphopsia. It is confirmed by ophthalmological examination, fluorescein angiography, and fundus microphotography. Histologically, macular fibrosis is made up of: cells of retinal pigment epithelium 51%, astocytes 29%, fibrocytes 14%, and myofibroblasts 7%. With the epiretinal peeling technique within vitrectomy, preretinal membranes are removed. This technique requires the surgeon's enormous experience, and it gives significant results in the sphere of central visual functions.

2.14. Other photomacular damages

After the Nd-YAG laser capsulotomy, photomacular damages have incidence from 7% to 20%. Most photomacular damages appear asymptomatically or with a minimal symptomatology due to their frequent extrafoveolar location. They may manifest as macular haemorrhage, subretinal, intraretinal, and preretinal bleeding, or as semi-ruptures. Sometimes bleeding may occur in the vitreous body, which significantly reduces vision transiently. Despite big, visible, semi-ruptured macular changes, the condition may be almost fully repaired after the Nd-YAG laser capsulotomy.

2.15. Endophthalmitis

After the Nd-YAG laser capsulotomy, there may develop endophthalmitis. It develops from the fifth day to the sixth week after intervention. Proved causative agents are Propionibacterium acnes and Staphylococcus epidermis all-present, saprophyte bacteria with a low degree of pathogenicity. They are found in the normal conjunctival flora. Propionibacterium acnes is gram-positive, anaerobic, producing lipolytic enzyme which serves as a trigger of inflammatory processes. During the extra-capsular cataract extraction with lens implantation, bacteria are brought into the eye. The Nd-YAG laser capsulotomy is an activating factor, a trigger for the development of the anterior uveitis, which then spreads into panuveitis, endophthalmitis respectively. Formation of the fenestra on the posterior capsule, often on the anterior hyloid membrane as well, opens the path for bacteria from the anterior to the posterior ocular chamber, i.e., into the middle and posterior parts of the vitreous body. Diagnosis is confirmed by the characteristic ophthalmological picture, i.e., positive cultures of ocular water and vitreous body. The ocular water culture grows in nine days, while the vitreous body culture is earlier and more frequently positive.

Research has shown that the most common complication is a jump of ocular pressure, then damage to the intraocular lens, anterior hyaloid membrane rupture, bleeding in the anterior chamber, retinal rupture, and macular fibrosis.

Development of complications is significantly affected by a total of applied energy, number of pulsations, individual pulse energy, and opening diameter made during capsulotomy.

To prevent complications, the suggested optimal pulse energy is up to 2.0 mJ, total applied energy of 200-300 mJ. The optimal size of the opening made on the posterior capsule is 4 mm.

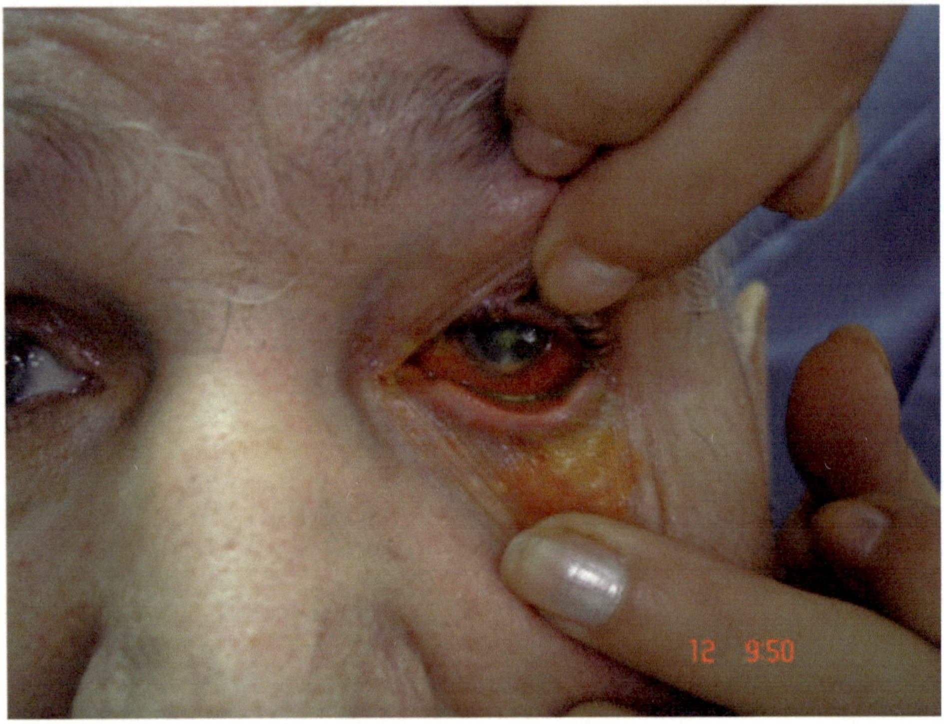

Figure 7. Endophthalmitis after Nd-YAG laser capsulotomy

3. Neodymium Yag laser iridectomy

Nd-YAG laser is used as an alternative treatment to the classic iridectomy in primary glaucoma of the closed angle, puppilary block, and secondary glaucoma of various mechanisms of origin.

Intervention is performed under local anaesthesia, in artificial myosis provoked by 2-4% pilocarpine. Abraham or Goldmann lenses are used. A total to be applied is from 1 to 12 mJ, usually from 3 to 5 mJ through 1-10 applications. The most common location is the central part of the iris on the basis of the iris crypts in the upper nasal quadrant in the 10:30 meridian, or the upper temporal quadrant in the 1:30 meridian. Studies carried out on a larger sample point to a successful iridectomy in 99% cases. After 1-2 hours intraocular pressure falls. The use of corticosteroid drops is suggested in the postoperative period. Upon the Nd-YAG laser iridectomy, there may occur complications described earlier in the chapter on posterior capsulotomy.

4. Nd-Yag laser on the posterior segment

Within diabetic retinopathy, the Valsalva retinopathy, or a sudden rupture of arterial retinal aneurysm, premacular haemorrhage may develop with a sudden loss of vision. According to the accepted opinions, such condition could be observed, waiting for spontaneous haemorrhage resorption. Vitrectomy with premacular haemorrhage aspiration is certainly a more effective method. Today membranectomy with the double-frequency Nd-YAG laser is offered a as an alternative therapy.

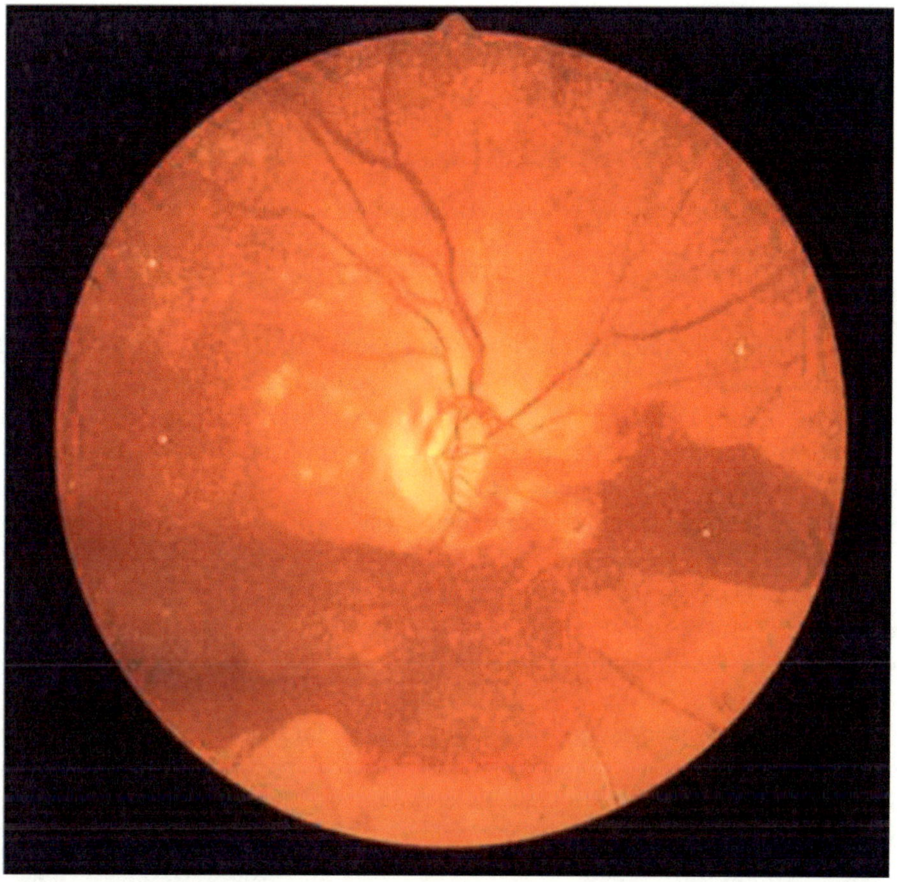

Figure 8. Preretinal haemorrhage

By this intervention, we drain haemorrhage and speed up blood resorption. Immediately upon the laser intervention, vision improves significantly. So today the Nd-YAG laser membranectomy, in premacular haemorrhage, occurs as a non-invasive alternative method to vitrectomy, due to the good results it achieves. Within proliferative diabetic retinopathy with vitreoretinal proliferation, Neodymium-YAG laser may be used to cut adhesions located in the central and posterior vitreous. Prior to that, bases of such proliferations may be ensured by placing argon laser barriers. We can have adhesions in the anterior vitreous body as well; we see them after cataract operations complicated with the vitreous body prolapse and development of iridicyclitis. In these interventions, special Peyman lenses are used for the middle and posterior vitreous.

5. Erbium-Yag laser

Erbium-YAG laser has also found its application in ophthalmology in phaco surgeries. Micropulse laser waves break up blurred lenses, which is followed with aspiration of the broken up and fragmented masses. The laser beam, in this surgery, is an alternative to the ultrasound wave. Erbium-YAG laser, which is introduced by means of special endo-probes into the bulbus, is used in sclerectomy and vitrectomy.

Author details

Emina Alimanović Halilović
University Clinical Center Sarajevo, Sarajevo, Bosnia and Herzegovina

6. References

Alimanović-Halilović E. Complications after Neodymium-YAG laser capsulotomy in Phakic and Pseudophakic Eyes : PhD thesis. Sarajevo: Faculty of Medicine, 2001:5-20;78-105.

Alward WLM. Laser Iridotomy. In: Weingeist TA. Laser Surgery in Ophthalmology Practical Applications. San Mateo California USA: Appleton & Lange, 1992:139-147.

Aron-Rose DS et al. Rhegmtogenous retinal Detachment After Neodymium-YAG. Laser capsulotomy in Phakic and Pseudophakic Eyes. In Richard R et al. Use of apulsed picosecond Nd-YAG laser. Am J of Ophthalmology 1986;(101):81-9.

Blacharski AP, Newsome AD. Bilateral macular holes after Nd-YAG laser posterior capsulotomy. American Journal of Ophthalmology 1988:417-8.

Carstocea B, Pascu RA. Yttrium Aluminium Garnet Crystal (I).Oftalmologia 2005;49(3): 3-9.

Cinal A. Intraocular lens position after capsulotomy. J Cataract Refract Surg 2000;26:5-6.

Collins JF, Donnenfeld ED. Opthalmic Desk Reference. New York: Raven Press, 1991: 456-7.

Farvadin M, Mehryar M, Maghaddasi H, Farvadin M. Neodymium-YAG laser treatment for macular hemorrhages. Arch Indian Med 2005; 8(1):8-13.

Georg E. Learning to be a YAG Surgeon. In: March FW. Ophthalmic Laser. 1990; 119-29.

Glacet-Bernard, Brahim R, Mokhtari et al. Retinal detachment following Nd-YAG capsulotomy. A retrospective study of 144 capsulotomies. J Fr Ophthalmol 1993;16(2):87-94.

Holweger R, Marefat B. Intraocular pressure change after neodymium-YAG capsulotomy. Journal of Cataract & Refractive Surgery 1997; 23(7):1095-102.

Hal DB, Wayne FM, James HL. Use of the YAG Laser in Posterior Capsulotomies. In: Wayne FM. Ophthalmic Laser 1990:131-9.

Hayashi K, Hayashi H, Nakao F, Hayash F. In vivo quantitative measurement of posterior capsule opacification after extracapsular catarac surgery. Am J of Ophthalmology 1998;125:837-43.

Isola V, Spinelli G, Misefari W. Transpupillary retinopexy of chorioretinal lesions predisposing to retinal detachment with the use of diode (810 nm) microlaser. Retina 2001;21(5):453-9.

Javitt et.al In: Ninn-Pedersen K, Bauer B. Cataract patients in a defined Swedish population 1986-1990. Nd-YAG laser capsulotomies in relation to preoperative and surgical conditions. Act Ophthal Scandinavica 1996;114:382-86

Lerman S, Thrasher B, Moran M. Vitreus changes after Neodymium-YAG laser irradiation of the posterior lens capsule or midvitreus. Am J of Ophthalmology 1997;470-5.

Mackool JR. Antiinflammatory regimen for cystoid macular edem after cataract surgery. J Cataract Refract Surg 2000;26:474.

Meisler et al. In: Tetz MR, Apple JD et al. A newly described complication of Nd-YAG laser capsulotomy: Exacerbation of an intraocular infection. Arch Ophthalmology 1987;105:1324 5.

Ranta P, Kivela T. Retinal detachement in pseudophakic eyes with and without Nd-YAG laser posterior capsulotomy. Ophthalmology 1998;105(11):2127-33.

Rennie CA, Newman DK, Snead MP, Flanagan DW. Nd:YAG laser treatment for premacular subhyaloid haemorrhage. Eye 2001;15(Pt 4):519-24.

Rakofsky S, Koch D. et al. Levobunolol 0,5% and Timolol 0,5% to prevent intraocular pressure elevation after Neodymium-YAG laser posterior capsulotomy. J of Cataract & Refractive Surgery 1997;23(7):1075-80.

Sefić S, Firdus H, Alimanović E, Ljaljević S, Sefić M. Oštećenja oka kod pomraèenja sunca. Med Arch 2000;54(1):41-4.

Sefić M. Bolesnik sa kataraktom pita: Da li se može poboljšati vid laserom? Sarajevo: KCU, 1999: 10.

Smith RT, Moscoso WE, Trokel S, Auran J. The barrier function in Neodymium-YAG laser capsulotomy. Arch Ophthalmol 1995;113:645-52.

Stilma JS, Boen-Tan TN. Timolol and intraocular pressure elevation following Neodymium-YAG laser surgery. Documenta Ophthalmologica 1986; 64:59-67.

Sheidow T, Gonder RJ, Merchea MM. Macular hole following Nd-YAG capsulotomy. Br J of Ophthalmology 1999;83(6):755.

Thach AB, Lopez PF, Snady-Mc Coy LC. et al. Accidental Nd-YAG laser injuries to the macula. Am J of Ophthalmology 1995; 119(6):767-773.

Zeyen P, Zeyen T. The long term effect of YAG laser posterior capsulotomy on intraocular pressure after combined glaucoma and cataract surgery. Belge d Ophthalmologie 1999; 271:99-103.

Bhargava R, Kumar P, Prakash A, Chaudhary KP. Estimation of mean ND: Yag laser capsulotomy energy levels for membranous and fibrous posterior capsular opacification. Nepal J Ophthalmol. 2012;4(7):108-13.

Larrañaga-Osuna G, Garza-Cantú D. Intraocular pressure in patients undergoing capsulotomy Nd: YAG laser Rev Med Inst Mex Seguro Soc. 2011;49(3):259-66.

Giocanti-Aurégan A, Tilleul J, Rohart C, Touati-Lefloc'h M, Grenet T, Fajnkuchen F, Chaîne G. OCT measurement of the impact of Nd:YAG laser capsulotomy on foveal thickness. J Fr Ophtalmol. 2011;34(9):641-6.

Chapter 5

Hydrogel Contact Lenses Surface Roughness and Bacterial Adhesion

Maria Jesus Giraldez and Eva Yebra-Pimentel

Additional information is available at the end of the chapter

http://dx.doi.org/10.5772/48436

1. Introduction

Contact lenses are a safe and effective mode of vision correction and today's industry offers wearers the choice of continuous wear, overnight orthokeratology, frequent-replacement or daily-disposable lenses among others. However, despite these options, including different care and maintenance systems, there are still features of contact lenses that could be improved such as possible microbial contamination (Weisbarth et al., 2007).

Microbial keratitis (MK) is a serious complication of contact lens (CL) wear that can lead to vision impairment (Buehler et al., 1992; Catalonotti et al., 2005; Leitch et al., 1998; Mah-Sadorra et al., 2005; Keay et al., 2009). Although the incidence of CL-related MK is only 0.02–0.5% (Cheng et al., 1999; Holden et al., 2005), the use of CL is so wide-spread that the problem may affect several millions of people and must therefore be considered a major health threat.

The CL surface is a suitable substrate for bacterial adhesion and biofilm formation, and can sustain the growth of microorganisms in prolonged contact with the cornea (Elder et al., 1995). In addition, CL wear may impair the immune response of the cornea by distorting its epithelial barrier function, and thus promote MK (Liesegang, 2002). To improve the corneal/CL interface, new soft hydrogel lens materials incorporate several co-polymers, including silicone polymers for increased oxygen permeability and phosphoryl-choline to increase biocompatibility. Further, the new modalities of wear, such as daily disposable (DD) hydrogel CL, avoid the need for regular cleaning and storage, which are known to be an important cause of microbial contamination (Laughlin-Borlace et al., 1998). However, several studies have surprisingly shown that users of DD and silicone hydrogel CL do not show a reduced risk of MK (Dart et al., 2008; Stapleton et al., 2008; Willcox et al., 2010). In effect, in the paper by Dart et al., differences in soft CL design and/or the composing polymer rather than the mode of wear were found to determine susceptibility to MK (Dart et al., 2008).

The process of initial adhesion of bacteria to the CL surface has been extensively examined in terms of the physical and chemical properties of both the bacterial cell and CL surface, such as hydrophobicity and roughness. Thus, the results of several *in vivo* studies suggest that a rougher CL surface is prone to more extensive bacterial adhesion (Bruinsma et al., 2002; Bruinsma et al., 2003) since imperfections in the lens surface is where deposits are likely to form (Hosaka et al., 1983). Also, depending on the surface thermodynamics, hydrophilic strains seem to preferentially adhere to hydrophilic surfaces, while more hydrophobic strains have a preference for hydrophobic surfaces (Bos et al., 1999; Bruinsma et al., 2001). Apart from lens surface factors, adhesion is also conditioned by features of the bacterial surface including flagella and fimbriae (Fletcher et al., 1993a; Fletcher et al., 1993b; Gupta et al., 1994; Gupta et al., 1996; Willcox et al., 2001; Donlan, 2002; Donlan, 2002; Kogure et al., 1998; Morisaki et al., 1999) or the presence or release of extracellular substances such as polysaccharides, proteins and biosurfactants (Mack et al., 1999; Mack et al., 1996; Mack et al., 1994).

Occasionally, a contact lens wearer will suffer an adverse response to a lens. These problems are frequently caused by bacterial contamination of the contact lens surface, and MK is one of the most feared complications (Patel and Hammersmith, 2008; Stapleton et al., 2008). Contact lenses absorb tear film proteins and lipids and this induces lens contamination and deterioration. Moreover, the build-up of tear film components on contact lenses can cause discomfort and inflammatory complications such as giant papillary conjunctivitis (GPC) (Skotnitsky et al., 2002; Skotnitsky et al., 2006), and this may occur with any type of daily or extended wear lenses (Donshik PC, 2003). This adsorption depends mainly on the contact lens material, and varies according to the tear secretion rate and certain pathological conditions. Research on conventional poly-HEMA-based lens materials has shown that the deposition of lysozyme and albumin depends upon the polymer's composition (Bohnert et al., 1988), charge (Garrett et al., 2000; Soltys-Robitaille et al., 2001) and water content (Garrett et al., 1999). Silicone-hydrogel materials give rise to different deposition profiles to those associated with the use of conventional poly-HEMA hydrogel lenses in that they induce less protein deposition and more lipid deposition (Jones et al., 2003; Subbaraman et al., 2006; Carney et al., 2008). Surface roughness also need to be considered since deposits are more likely to form on imperfections of the lens surface (Hosaka et al., 1983). It was also previously demonstrated that as surface roughness increases, the biofilm deposited on the lens also increases (Baguet et al., 1995) and that bacterial transfer from a contact lens is determined by the roughness and hydrophobicity of the surface receiving the bacteria (Vermeltfoort et al., 2004).

Further, a smooth surface is essential for the optical quality of a contact lens since reduced scattered light improves the performance of an optical system (Bennett, 1992). Developments in soft contact lens materials continue to be an important issue, since the performance and comfort of a contact lens will depend on the material, its surface architecture and the quality of the lens manufacturing process (Lorentz et al., 2007; Riley et al., 2006; Guillon and Maissa, 2007). In addition, the performance of contact lenses does not remain constant over time and lens surface changes induced by wear will affect their performance and determine a need to replace the lens.

The aim of this chapter was to qualitatively and quantitatively characterize the surfaces of unworn hydrogel contact lenses using Atomic Force Microscopy (AFM) and White Light Optical Profiling (WLOP), and to analyze how these surface characteristics affect on bacterial adhesion.

2. Contact lens surface roughness

2.1. Roughness parameters

The actual geometry of a surface is very complex (Gadelmawla et al., 2002). Even areas considered "very smooth" show a complex mix of geometric features. Surface roughness is becoming increasingly important for applications in many fields (Bennett, 1992). Among other factors, surface roughness of devices in direct contact with living systems will influence their biological reactivity. How a surface is finished is an important factor for a good operation of many types of products, which include optical products (Bennett, 1992), related to engineering (Blunt, 2006), food (Sheen et al., 2008; Wang et al., 2009) and biomedical products (Hooton et al., 2004; Hooton et al., 2006; Linneweber et al., 2007; Lee et al., 2009). The surface of any body or object is the part which interacts with the surrounding environment. Roughness is a biological factor that affects in a molecular scale, the manner in which bacteria adhere to surfaces, above all for initial adhesion. (Mitik-Dineva et al., 2008; Mitik-Dineva et al., 2009). The real geometry of a surface is so complex that only by increasing the number of parameters used can a more accurate description be obtained (Gadelmawla et al., 2002). Surface parameters can be considered as height and shape parameters:

2.1.1. Height parameters

The parameters generally used to quantify roughness include height parameters such as average roughness (R_a), mean-square-roughness (R_{ms}) and Maximum Roughness (R_{max}) (Baguet et al., 1993; Guryca et al., 2007; Bhatia et al., 1997; Hinojosa Rivera and Reyes Melo, 2001; Lira et al., 2008; Gonzalez-Meijome et al., 2009; Giraldez et al., 2010a; Giraldez et al., 2010c; Gonzalez-Meijome et al., 2006a). R_a is the average deviation or arithmetic mean of the profile from the mean line; it is universally accepted and is the most used international parameter of roughness. R_{ms} is the standard deviation from the mean surface plane. Although R_a and R_{ms} seem to be the most informative and consistent parameters used to define the surface topography of contact lenses (Gonzalez-Meijome et al., 2006a), they both show a dependency on sample length (Hinojosa Rivera and Reyes Melo, 2001; Kiely and Bonnell, 1997; Kitching et al., 1999). Degree of their variation with sample length could be representative of how homogeneous a surface is in its irregularities distribution. R_{max} is the maximum peak-to-valley height identified within the observed area. It could be affected by local imperfections or sample contamination leading to higher values than expected, so material characterization based on this parameter could be unreliable.

2.1.2. *Shape parameters*

Two statistical parameters of roughness, not generally used to analyze contact lens surfaces, are kurtosis (R_{ku}) and skewness (R_{sk}). R_{ku} is a measure of the sharpness of the profile about the mean line that provides information on the distribution of spikes above and below the mean line. Thus, spiky surfaces will have a high kurtosis value ($R_{ku} > 3$) and bumpy surfaces a low value ($R_{ku} < 3$). R_{sk} is a measure of the symmetry of the profile about the mean line, giving information on asymmetrical profiles for surfaces with the same values of R_a and R_{ms}. Negative values of R_{sk} indicate a predominance of troughs, while positive ones are observed for surfaces with peaks. The use of both shape parameters, R_{ku} and R_{sk}, which serve to distinguish between two profiles with the same R_a and/or R_{ms}, (Gadelmawla et al., 2002) has been reported in several biomedical fields (Hansson, 2000; Olefjord and Hansson, 1993; Yang et al., 2007; Linde et al., 1989; Zyrianov, 2005; Raulio et al., 2008; Szmukler-Moncler et al., 2004; Cehreli et al., 2008). Figure 1 shows the amplitude distributions/shape profiles of two surfaces with a similar R_a but different values of R_{sk} or R_{ku} (Gadelmawla et al., 2002).

The clinical applications of R_{ku} and R_{sk} in the contact lens field could be to provide a measure of the susceptibility of a contact lens surface to deposit formation or colonization by microorganisms. Also, different shapes could determine a greater specific surface area, and thus more available active sites for thermodynamic reactions. As two surfaces with similar Ra or R_{ms} could differ in shape (Figure 1), they may also differ in their performance.

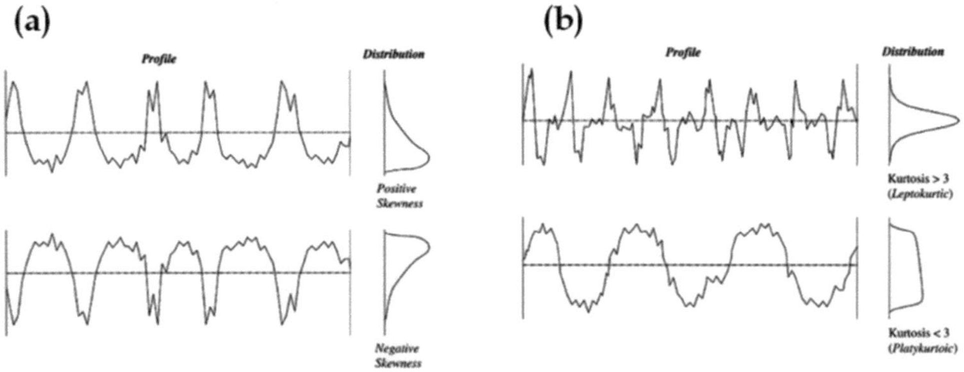

Figure 1. Amplitude distribution curve about the mean line for two surfaces showing similar R_a values but different values of R_{sk} (a) or R_{ku} (b).

2.2. Surface roughness measurement

A wide variety of methods are available for measuring surface roughness and the light scattering the roughness produces. As commented previously, the apparent surface roughness depends upon the size of the sample area, so in order to provide a better description of the surface roughness, measurements must be acquired for a variety of sample sizes (Kiely and Bonnell, 1997; Kitching et al., 1999); with roughness parameters being calculated for areas with different location and size.

2.2.1. Atomic force microscopy

Atomic force microscopy (AFM) provides detailed information on the surface characteristics of contact lenses (Bhatia et al., 1997; Baguet et al., 1993; Baguet et al., 1995; Bruinsma et al., 2003; Lira et al., 2008; Guryca et al., 2007; Gonzalez-Meijome et al., 2006a; Gonzalez-Meijome et al., 2009; Teichroeb et al., 2008; Maldonado-Codina and Efron, 2005) and is a powerful tool for the high resolution examination of the structure of the hydrated contact lens surface. The method has the advantages that it avoids artefacts due to dehydration and coating (Bhatia et al., 1997; Kim et al., 2002), and allows for non-destructive surface topography and roughness measurements. AFM consists of a microscale cantilever with a sharp tip (probe) that is used to scan the specimen surface. The cantilever is typically made of silicon or silicon nitride with a tip radius of curvature of the order of nanometers. When the tip is brought into the proximity of a sample surface, forces between the tip and the sample cause the cantilever to deflect according to Hooke's law. (Lira et al., 2008) The advantage of AFM over conventional microscopy or scanning electron microscopy (SEM) is the high level resolution offered in three dimensions and that topographic information can be obtained in aqueous, nonaqueous or dry conditions, eliminating the need for sample preparation (e.g., dehydration, freezing or coating). In effect, AFM has proved useful for characterizing tear deposits on worn soft contact lens surfaces (Baguet et al., 1995; Rebeix et al., 2000) or characterizing the rigid gas permeable contact lens surface (Bruinsma et al., 2003). In fact, detailed information about the surface quality of CL has been studied previously by Atomic Force Microscopy (AFM) (Bhatia et al., 1997; Baguet et al., 1993; Baguet et al., 1995; Bruinsma et al., 2003; Gonzalez-Meijome et al., 2006a; Gonzalez-Meijome et al., 2009; Giraldez et al., 2010c) and Cryo-SEM (Gonzalez-Meijome et al., 2006b; Guryca et al., 2007). AFM is a very powerful tool for high resolution examination of hydrated CL surface structure. The method avoids artifacts due to dehydration and coating (Bhatia et al., 1997; Kim et al., 2002). However, when using AFM to analyse CL surface the area of measurement is very small, so it may be answered how representative of the total lens are R_a and R_{ms} obtained by AFM. Cryo-SEM, a modification of the Scanning Electron Microscopy (SEM), requires that the material be frozen in nitrogen before examination (Serp et al., 2002). In hydrogels, this usually means the destruction of the material, which is the main disadvantage of this technique.

2.2.2. White Light Optical Perfilometer

White Light Optical Perfilometer (WLOP) is one of the preferred methods of precision surface characterization in many fields (Caber, 1993; Windecker and Tiziani, 1999; Bennett, 1992; O'Mahony et al., 2003). WLOP is a topographic technique, that as well as AFM, enables the analysis of surface topography and roughness by means of a nondestructively methodology. It is a powerful and well-established technique for non-contact measurement of surface topography for quickly determining three-dimensional surface shape over larger areas at high vertical and moderate lateral resolution (Bennett, 1992; O'Mahony et al., 2003; Novak et al., 2003). Two modes of operation are generally available for the optical profilers. For smooth surfaces the phase-shifting integrating bucket technique (PSI) is generally used since it gives sub-nanometer height resolution capability. For rougher surfaces, a vertical scanning coherence sensing technique can be used to give a nanometer height resolution over several hundred microns of surface height. WLOP allows analyze larger areas than techniques used before in contact lenses, so the values and statistics could be more representative of roughness distribution over the lens surface. Topographic information can be obtained from the surface in aqueous conditions.

2.3. Contact lens surface roughness characteristics

Surface topography and roughness parameters showed different characteristics depending on the type of contact lens (material, water content, manufacture system, replacement frequency). Moreover roughness varies with magnification, so the size of the measured area must be considered when comparing the results of different studies (Kiely and Bonnell, 1997; Kitching et al., 1999). R_a is the arithmetic mean of the departures of the profile from the mean line (Hinojosa Rivera and Reyes Melo, 2001). Thus, it should not vary with magnification for a surface with homogeneously distributed irregularities, regardless of how smooth or rough the surface is. However, the irregularities of most surfaces are not perfectly homogeneously distributed, and effectively differences in contact lens surface roughness values have been observed at different magnifications, with higher roughness scores obtained for larger areas more enlarged areas (Gonzalez-Meijome et al., 2006a). Hence, the amount of variation could reflect how homogeneous a surface is.

Contact lens surface characteristics determined by AFM and by WLOP are presented in the next sections.

2.3.1. CL surface roughness by AFM

Contact lens surfaces roughness and topography can be determined by AFM (Veeco, multimode-nanoscope V) in tapping mode™. (Giraldez et al., 2010c) Although the method used is the same as for dry conditions, a special cell could be necessary so measurements could be made on the lenses in their original shipping fluid (physiological saline) to keep CL hydrated during microscopy observation. All procedures and examinations must be conducted in the same room kept at 21ºC and approximately 50% relative humidity. Then images have to be processed, for example, using the Vision®32 and Nanoscope v7.20 software packages.

Table 1 and table 2 shows height (R_a and R_{ms}) and shape (R_{ku} and R_{sk}) parameters of 6 hydrogel CL. The specific characteristics of these CL are provided in Table 3. They were all manufactured by cast-molding and had no surface treatment. Although all the lenses are suitable for daily wear, manufacturers recommend a different replacement frequency (Table 1). Senofilcon A and comfilcon A are silicone-hydrogel contact lenses, while hioxifilcon (Osmo 2®), omafilcon A and ocufilcon B are hydroxyethylmethacrylate (HEMA) copolymers and nefilcon A is a polyvinyl alcohol (PVA). The main monomers of the material used to manufacture Osmo 2 contact lenses are those that comprise hioxifilcon (2-HEMA GMA; GMA, glycerylmethacrylate) plus MA (methacrylic acid).

Contact lens	25 μm²		196 μm²	
	R_a (nm)	R_q (nm)	R_a (nm)	R_q (nm)
Hioxifilcon-based	4.31 ± 0.59	5.50 ± 0.58	5.91 ± 0.65	7.90 ± 0.89
Omafilcon A	1.90 ± 0.39	2.78 ± 0.45	4.66 ± 2.05	6.80 ± 2.74
Nefilcon A	11.25 ± 0.38	15.41 ± 1.26	12.99 ± 0.05	18.34 ± 0.25
Ocufilcon B	11.01 ± 1.79	14.38 ± 2.13	11.45 ± 2.56	23.11 ± 4.49
Senofilcon A	3.33 ± 0.28	4.06 ± 0.38	3.76 ± 0.05	4.70 ± 0.005
Comfilcon A	1.56 ± 0.37	2.34 ± 0.69	2.76 ± 0.80	4.21 ± 0.44

Table 1. Mean roughness parameters recorded for the hydrogel contact lenses using AFM on surface areas of 25 μm² and 196 μm²

	Hioxifilcon-based	**Omafilcon A**	**Nefilcon A**	**Oculfincon B**	**Senofilcon A**	**Comfilcon A**
R_{ku}	3.71± 0.94	23.54 ± 14.81	5.86 ± 2.03	5.45 ± 1.95	3.74 ± 1.63	31.09 ± 0.95
R_{sk}	-0.22 ± 0.17	2.04 ± 1.07	1.43 ± 0.32	0.98 ± 0.17	0.74 ± 0.41	2.93 ± 0.82

Table 2. Mean R_{ku} and R_{sk} values recorded for the hydrogel contact lenses using AFM on a 25 μm² surface area

Brand name	Material Generic name	Charge	Water content (%)	Type of hydrogel	Replacement Frequency*
Osmo 2	Hioxifilcon-based	Non ionic	72	HEMA copolymer	Three months
Proclear	Omafilcon A	Non ionic	62	HEMA copolymer	One month
Focus Dailies	Nefilcon A	Non ionic	69	Polyvinylalcohol	One day
Frequency 1 day	Ocufilcon B	Ionic	52	HEMA copolymer	One day
Acuvue Oasys	Senofilcon A	Non ionic	38	Silicone hydrogel	Two weeks
Biofinity	Comfilcon A	Non ionic	48	Silicone hydrogel	One month

* Manufacturer's recommendation

Table 3. Specifications of the contact lenses analyzed by AFM.

The corresponding 3-D image of the lenses with the lowest (comfilcon A and omafilcon A) and highest (nefilcon A and ocufilcon B) roughness scores are shown in figure 2. Figure 3 and 4 show the corresponding image for senofilcon A and hioxifilcon CL respectively.

A different surface roughness in a new lens can be the result of the manufacturing method and the material's properties. The spin casting method generates contact lenses with the smoothest surfaces, followed by cast-molding and then lathe-cut lenses (Guryca et al., 2007; Grobe, 1996). All the lenses presented here were cast-molded, and their roughness parameters were similar to the ranges reported for other non surface-treated cast-molded lenses (Guryca et al., 2007). Thus, the roughness differences between lenses cannot be attributed only to the manufacturing procedure. Besides the mode of elaboration, other authors have linked the presence of methacrylic acid (MA) (Baguet et al., 1993) or a reduced water content (Guryca et al., 2007; Vermeltfoort et al., 2004) to a greater lens surface roughness.

Daily replacement hydrophilic contact lenses (nefilcon A and ocufilcon B), showed the highest roughness values for both surface areas analyzed. In contrast, comfilcon A showed the smoothest, or flattest surface (R_a = 1.56 nm), followed closely by omafilcon A (R_a = 1.90 nm). Similar roughness values were observed for the hioxifilcon-based material and senofilcon A, yet their surface appearance was different (figures 3 and 4). Although the hioxifilcon-based contact lens contains MA, which should determine a greater surface roughness, its similar R_a to senofilcon A could be attributed to its high water content. As may be observed in Figure 3, senofilcon A shows a granulated surface structure, which is similar to that previously reported for the AFM observation of senofilcon A (Teichroeb et al., 2008), of galyficon A (Lira et al., 2008) and for the cryogenic SEM visualization of the latter. (Gonzalez-Meijome et al., 2006b) Galyfilcon A is a non surface-treated silicone hydrogel contact lens that contains PVP as an internal wetting agent.

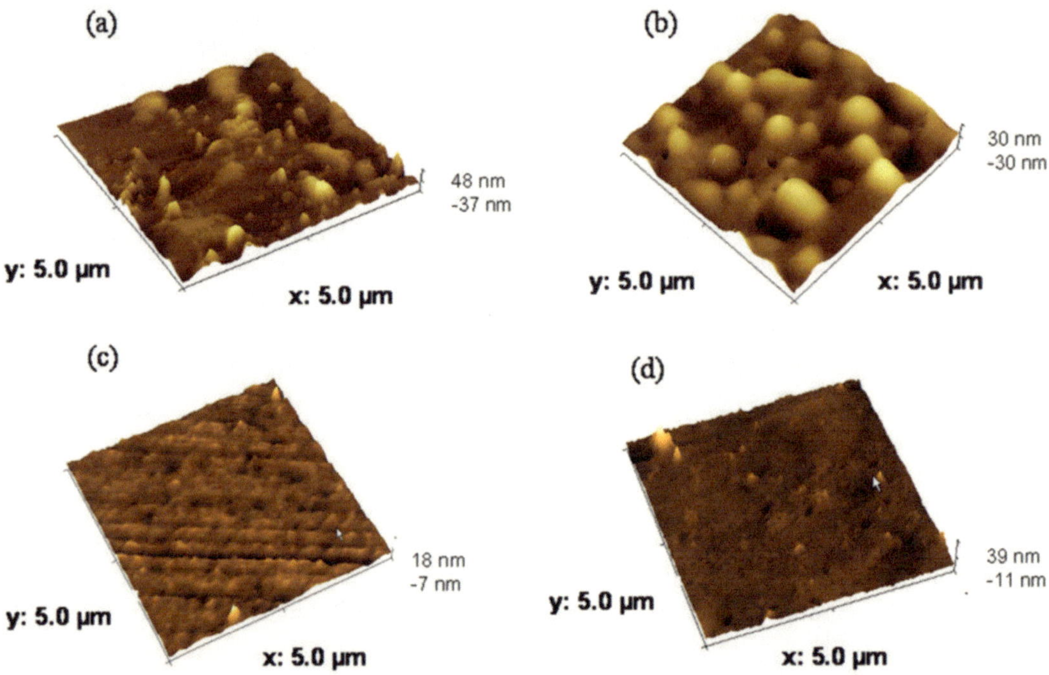

Figure 2. Three-dimensional images generated by the AFM analysis of a 25 µm² area of nefilcon A (a), ocufilcon B (b), comfilcon A (c) and omafilcon A (d).

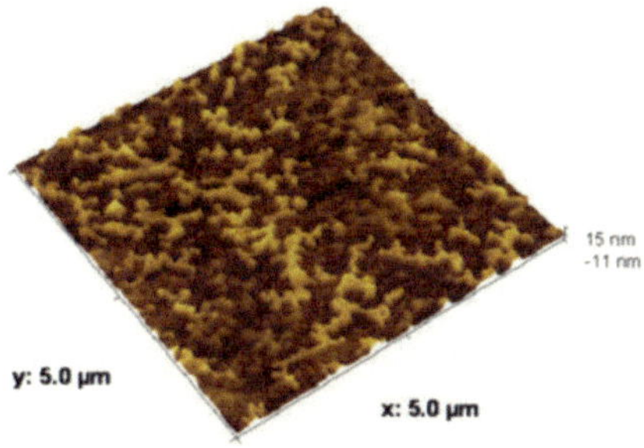

Figure 3. Three-dimensional image generated by the AFM analysis of senofilcon A over a 25 μm^2 area.

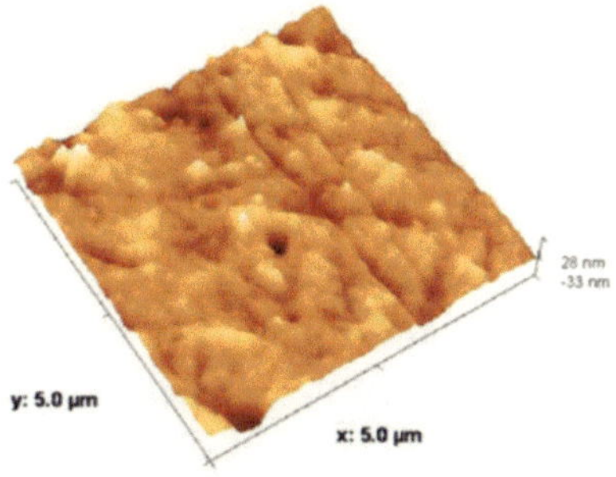

Figure 4. Three-dimensional image generated by the AFM analysis of hioxifilcon over a 25 µm2 area..

Silicone-hydrogel contact lenses exhibit different surface characteristics depending on their chemical composition and surface treatments (Nicolson PC, 2003). Surface treatments are targeted at obtaining wettable surfaces (Jones L and Dumbleton K, 2002), although the surfaces of the silicone-hydrogel contact lenses presented here were untreated. Thus, senofilcon A incorporates an internal wetting agent (polyvinyl pyrrolidone) that apparently leaches to the lens surface, and the Aquaform™ technology used in comfilcon A minimizes lens dehydration by forming hydrogen bonds with water molecules, creating a naturally hydrophilic contact lens that retains water inside the lens (Szczotka-Flynn L, 2007; Whittaker G, 2008). The roughness parameters obtained for these lenses were similar to those observed previously in silicone-hydrogel contact lenses lacking surface treatment, such as galyfilcon A and comfilcon A (Lira et al., 2008; Gonzalez-Meijome et al., 2009), but lower than those reported for surface-treated designs (Gonzalez-Meijome et al., 2006a; Guryca et al., 2007). Despite the similar surface appearance of silicone hydrogels included here and those examined by others, (Teichroeb et al., 2008; Gonzalez-Meijome et al., 2009) Teichroeb et al. observed higher roughness parameters for senofilcon A than Comfilcon A when measuring a 25 μm^2 area. These differences could be related to the fact that the lenses were analysed after drying in ambient conditions for 15 minutes.

2.3.2. CL surface roughness by WLOP

The issue of measurement area is an important point to be considered in all surface roughness measurements (Bennett, 1992; Blunt, 2006; Hinojosa and Reyes, 2001; kiely and

Bonnell, 1997; Kitching et al., 1999). WLOP allows analysing larger areas than other techniques used before in CL. In this regard, the maximum Hydrogel CL area studied by AFM was 400 μm² (Gonzalez-Meijome et al., 2006a), which means that for a 14.00 mm diameter CL, only about $2.6x10^{-4}$ % of the entire CL surface area would be analyzed. When using WLOP we were able to determine roughness parameters in areas as large as 67646μm², which is almost 170 higher than the greatest area evaluated by AFM, so values and statistics are suppose to be more representative of the total CL surface (Giraldez et al., 2010a).

WLOP measurements can be obtained with the interference microscopy Wyko®-NT1100, a tool that combines a microscopy and an interferometer into the same instrument and which was previously used for hydrogel CL surface analysis. (Giraldez et al., 2010a)

Table 4, 5 and 6 shows values for R_a, R_{ms} and R_{max} parameters of 4 hydrogel CL obtained from WLOP analysis for 625 μm², 2500 μm², 10829 μm² and 67646 μm² areas. The specific characteristics of these CL are provided in Table 7. All these CL were manufactured by cast-moulding and had no surface treatment. Although all lenses are indicated for daily wear, different replacement frequency is recommended by manufacturer (table 1). According with material, hioxifilcon, omafilcon A and ocufilcon B are hydroxyethylmethacrylate (HEMA) copolymers and nefilcon A is a polyvinylalcohol (PVA). Osmo 2 contact lens material is based in hioxifilcon, as their main monomers are those from hioxifilcon (2-HEMA GMA; GMA, glycerylmethacrylate) and MA (methacrylic acid). Lenses were obtained in the original containers filled with a physiological saline solution. As an example, surface appearance of hydrogel contact lenses at different magnification is shown in figure 5.

	625 μm²	**2500 μm²**	**10829 μm²**	**67646 μm²**
Hioxifilcon-based	31,04 ± 1,75	32,88 ± 2,18	42,26 ± 7,92	47,89 ± 3,97
Omafilcon A	17,62 ± 2,50	22,18 ± 0,55	49,84 ± 9,83	67,12 ± 12,59
Ocufilcon B	31,11 ± 3.03	35,68 ± 2,50	30,70 ± 4,50	173,11 ± 95,55
Nefilcon A	25,04 ± 5.04	54,73 ± 17,31	114,93 ± 7,29	323,77 ± 16,11

Table 4. Average Roughness (R_a) of hydrogel contact lenses determined by WLOP for 625 μm², 2500 μm², 10829 μm² and 67646 μm² areas. Mean and Standard Deviation are shown. Values are in nanometers (nm).

	625 μm²	**2500 μm²**	**10829 μm²**	**67646 μm²**
Hioxifilcon-based	40,07 ± 2,24	44,94 ± 4,25	61,54 ± 13,32	63,25 ± 4,22
Omafilcon A	22,41 ± 3,22	28,20 ± 0,88	65,99 ± 16,08	89,37 ± 17,87
Ocufilcon B	46,04 ± 3,74	52,92 ± 2,28	53,07 ± 5,80	307,61 ± 178,88
Nefilcon A	39,08 ± 12,71	97,89 ± 30,97	175,03 ± 5,40	508,47 ± 49,04

Table 5. Root-Mean-Square (Rms) of hydrogel contact lenses determined by WLOP for 625 μm², 2500 μm², 10829 μm² and 67646 μm² areas. Mean and Standard Deviation are shown. Values are in nanometers (nm).

	625 μm²	2500 μm²	10829 μm²	67646 μm²
Hioxifilcon-based	433,98 ± 27,40	869,04 ± 117,33	1996,67 ± 426,18	2306,67 ± 1259,61
Omafilcon A	280,67 ± 59,22	353,57 ± 35,63	1303,86 ± 528,49	2646,67 ± 2019,53
Ocufilcon B	583,65 ± 103,34	854,75 ± 43,99	1401,80 ± 352,84	18196,67± 10208,47
Nefilcon A	620,39 ± 94,48	1800,00 ± 612,20	2723,33 ± 583,12	22970,00 ± 4690,00

Table 6. Maximum Roughness (R_{max}) of hydrogel contact lenses determined by WLOP for 625 μm², 2500 μm², 10829 μm² and 67646 μm² areas. Mean and Standard Deviation are shown. Values are in nanometers (nm).

Brand	Manufacturer	Material (USAN)	Charge	Water content (%)	Principal monomers	Replacement Frequency*
Osmo 2	MarkEnnovy	Hioxifilcon-based	Non ionic	72	2-HEMA GMA MA	Three months
Proclear	Cooper Vision	Omafilcon A	Non ionic	62	HEMA, PC	One month
Frequency 1 day	Cooper Vision	Ocufilcon B	Ionic	52	2-HEMA EGDMA	One day
Focus Dailies+	Ciba Vision	Nefilcon A	Non ionic	69	PVP NAAADA	One day

* Manufacturer recommendation

+All Day Comfort (with enhanced lubricating agents)

Table 7. Specifications of the contact lenses analyzed by WLOP.

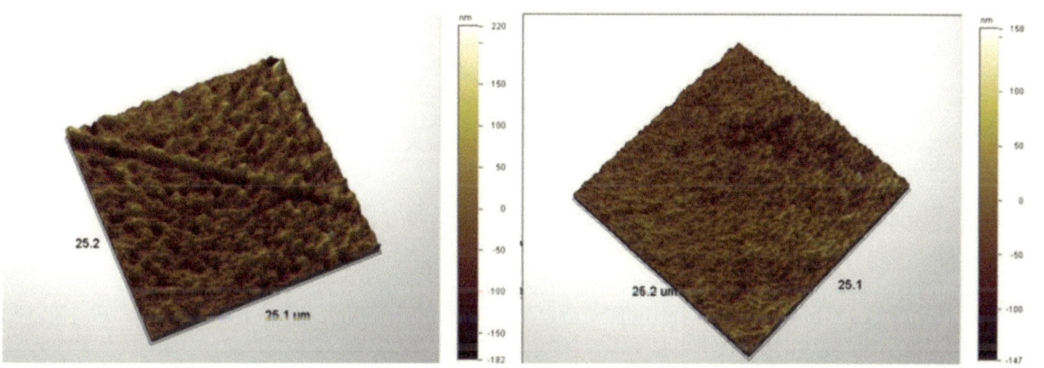

Figure 5. Surface topography of hioxifilcon and omafilcon A contact lenses (surface area: 625 μm²) obtained by WLOP.

According with the 625 μm² and 2500 μm² area, ocufilcon B and hioxifilcon based CL showed statistical rougher surface scores than those obtainded by omafilcon A, although differences between lenses were not large enough to be clinically relevant. However, when higher areas were considered, it could be observed that daily CL showed an important increase in their roughness values, which is not observed in hioxifilcon based and Omafilcon A lenses (Figures 6 and 7). According to this, analyzing higher areas could assist to detect differences between lenses surface characteristics, which may be not so obvious if smaller areas are studied.

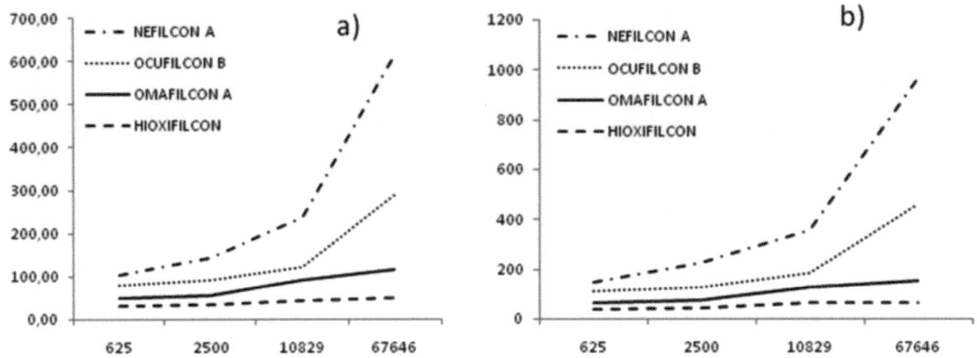

Figure 6. Variation of R_a (a) and R_{ms} (b) parameters for different scanning surface areas. Y-values represent nanometers (nm). X-values represent μm^2.

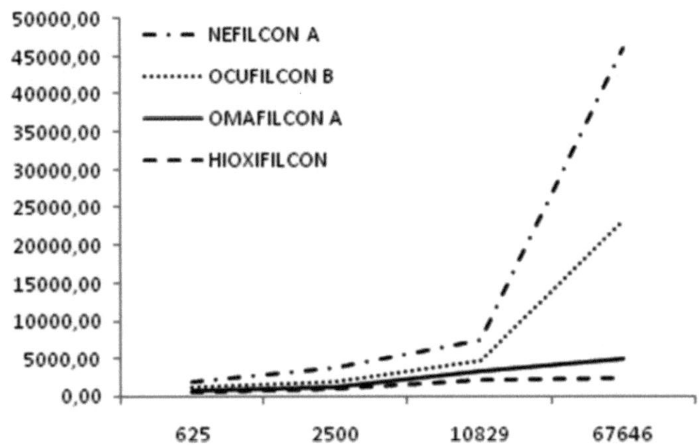

Figure 7. Variation of Maximum Roughness (R_{max}) for different scanning surface areas. Y-values represent nanometers (nm). X-values represent μm^2.

As can be observed, roughness analysis varies with the magnification. R_a is the arithmetic mean of the departures of the profile from the mean line. So, when a surface presents irregularities homogeneously distributed, R_a should not vary with magnification, irrespective of its roughness degree. However, this is not the usual situation, as most of surfaces are not perfectly homogeneous in their irregularities distribution. In fact, there has been reported differences in CL surface roughness values at different magnifications using AFM technique, showing higher roughness scores in higher areas (Gonzalez-Meijome et al., 2006a; Giraldez et al., 2010c). Degree of variation of roughness parameters when increasing size of the measured area could be representative of how homogeneous a surface is. From the data presented here, hioxifilcon based CL has the most homogeneous surface, showing the lower R_a and R_{ms} variation when comparing values from different areas (Figure 6 and 7). Conversely, Nefilcon A showed the highest increase in roughness, displaying the less homogeneous surface of the study.

Local imperfections or sample contamination could affect R_a, R_{ms} and R_{max} values. However, their effect on R_a and R_{ms} is supposed to be lower than that on R_{max}, since R_a and R_{ms} are average values that should be less affected by local imperfections when higher areas are considered. On the other hand, R_{max} might show higher values than expected when imperfections are present, as it indicate maximum peak to valley distance in a measured area, independently of its size. When comparing CL presented here, R_{max} variation with area size had a similar pattern than that observed in R_a and R_{ms} for all CL. This can be easily observed when comparing figures 6 and 7. This finding could indicate that the higher R_{max} values observed in larger areas, especially in daily CL, would not be due to local imperfections or sample contamination, but rather due to the actual surface roughness of the CL.

Roughness parameters values obtained by WLOP are significantly higher than those previously observed in other hydrogel CL by AFM. This difference between techniques could be related to the effect of the measured area size on the R_a and R_{ms} values, as they tend to be higher when the analyzed area increases (Hinojosa and Reyes, 2001; kiely and Bonnell, 1997; Kitching et al., 1999).

CL surface roughness degree is an important issue as imperfections in the lens surface is where deposits are likely to form (Hosaka et al., 1983). It was also previously demonstrated that the surface roughness increase, the biofilm deposited on the lens increase (Baguet et al., 1995), and that bacterial transfer from a CL is determined by the roughness and hydrophobicity of the surface receiving the bacteria (Vermeltfoort et al., 2004). Daily replacement CL in present study are suppose to acquire more deposits during wear as they had the highest increase in roughness values when higher areas are considered. So, strict replacement regime must be follow in nefilcon A and ocufilcon B CL wear. By gaining a better understanding of the surface roughness of different types of CL, practitioners will be better placed to prescribe the most suitable lens for any given patient and to interpret the clinical performance of lenses they prescribe in relation to patient symptoms and ocular surface signs.

3. Bacterial adhesion to contact lenses

The process of initial adhesion of bacteria to the CL surface has been extensively examined in terms of the physical and chemical properties of both the bacterial cell and CL surface such as hydrophobicity and roughness. Thus, depending on the surface thermodynamics, hydrophilic strains seem to preferentially adhere to hydrophilic surfaces, while more hydrophobic strains have a preference for hydrophobic surfaces. (Bos et al., 1999; Bruinsma et al., 2001)Also, the results of several *in vivo* studies suggest that a rougher CL surface will be prone to more extensive bacterial adhesion (Bruinsma et al., 2002; Bruinsma et al., 2003) since imperfections in the lens surface is where deposits are likely to form. (Hosaka et al., 1983)

Microbial colonization can be quantified by enumerating colony-forming units (CFU) using different bacterial strains, as the *P. aeruginosa* strain CECT 110 or *S. epidermidis* strain CECT 4184 (both from the Spanish Type Culture Collection). Adhesion can be determined by immersing each CL, convex side up, in 1 ml of a cell suspension of *P. aeruginosa* or *S. epidermidis* whose concentration of 1.2 x 10^9 CFU/ml (adjusted to McFarland scale No.4) is determined by dilution in sterile saline solution (SS) and spreading on Tryptic Soy Agar (TSA) plates. Following incubation of the bacterial suspension for 2 h at 37ºC with continuous shaking (15 rpm), each CL has to be carefully removed and washed 3 times in sterile SS. Next each lens is placed in 2 ml of sterile SS and sonicated using a Bronson Sonifier 250 for 1 min. The suspensions then spread on TSA-1 plates and CFU enumerated after 24 h of incubation at 37ºC.

3.1. Microbial keratitis on contact lens wear

The adhesion of bacteria to contact lenses (CL), notably that of *Pseudomonas aeruginosa* and *Staphylococcus epidermidis,* is considered a primary risk factor of serious corneal problems (Buehler PO et al., 1992; Catalonotti P et al., 2005; Leitch EC et al., 1998). The CL surface is a suitable substrate for bacterial adhesion and biofilm formation, and can sustain the growth of an inoculum of organisms in prolonged contact with the cornea (Elder Mj et al., 1995). In addition, corneal interaction with the CL can override the protective mechanisms of the cornea, augmenting the capacity of microbial cells to adhere to the cornea and progress to microbial keratitis (MK). To improve the corneal/CL interface, several co-polymers have been incorporated into soft hydrogel lens materials, including silicone polymers for increased oxygen permeability and phosphoryl-choline to increase biocompatibility. Further, the new modalities of wear, such as daily disposable (DD) hydrogel CL, avoid the need for regular cleaning and storage, which are known to be an important cause of microbial contamination (Laughlin-Borlace et al., 1998). Notwithstanding, studies have shown that users of DD and silicone hydrogel CL do not show a reduced risk of MK (Dart et al., 2008; Stapleton et al., 2008). In the paper by Dart et al., differences in soft CL design and/or the composing polymer rather than the mode of wear were found to determine susceptibility to MK (Dart et al., 2008).

Several microbial strains have been isolated from clinical samples of MK. Approximately two thirds of these strains are Gram-negative bacterial strains, most notably *Pseudomonas aeruginosa* but also some *Serratia* species, while one third comprises Gram-positive cocci, including *Staphylococcus aureus* and *Staphylococcus epidermidis* (Catalonotti P et al., 2005; Leitch EC et al., 1998; Seal et al., 1999). *S epidermidis* is one of the microorganisms most frequently isolated from the normal microbiota of the human eye surface (Ayoub M et al., 1994; Doyle A et al., 1995; Hara J et al., 1997). Despite this, this bacterium has been held responsible for infections such as chronic blepharitis, conjunctivitis and keratitis, especially in immunocompromised hosts (Pinna A et al., 1999), and may account for 45 per cent of all cases of bacterial keratitis (Nayak et al., 2007; Nayak and Satpathy, 2000). In CL wearers, *S. epidermidis* finds itself in a privileged position to act as an opportunistic pathogen, colonizing the lens surface from the eye and surrounding areas. The microorganism also shows an adhesion preference for foreign materials and has the capacity to produce an extracellular substance comprised of polysaccharides (slime) (Perilli et al., 2000).

Pseudomonas aeruginosa is a common Gram-negative bacillus that acts as an opportunistic pathogen under several circumstances (Lyczak et al., 2000). As a Gram-negative bacterium, the lipopolysaccharides (LPS) composing its outer membrane act as key virulence factor, promoting infection by interfering with the host immune response (Wilkinson, 1983; Cryz, Jr. et al., 1984). Other virulence factors encoded by *P. aeruginosa* could help bacterial survival on the ocular surface. These factors are those needed for strategies such as biofilm formation, resistance against killing, communication between bacteria (e.g., quorum sensing), invading epithelial cells and surviving within them, destroying tear components, breaking down cell-to cell junctions and extracellular matrices, and injecting toxins into cells (Alarcon et al., 2009; Angus et al., 2008; Evans et al., 2007; Fleiszig et al., 1994; Fleiszig, 2006; Hauser, 2009; Lyczak et al., 2000; Wagner and Iglewski, 2008; Willcox, 2007; Zolfaghar et al., 2003; Zolfaghar et al., 2005; Zolfaghar et al., 2006). *Pseudomonas aeruginosa* also possesses factors that are highly immunogenic (initiate inflammation) while being able to evade the immune responses they initiate (Choy et al., 2008; Evans et al., 2007; Hazlett, 2007; Lyczak et al., 2000). Interestingly, *P. aeruginosa* virulence factors can also confer resistance to contact lens disinfectants (Lakkis and Fleiszig, 2001).

3.2. Effect of hydrophobicity and surface roughness

Bacterial adhesion to a biomaterial is thought to depend on the hydrophobicity of the biomaterial, such that adhesion decreases with the water content of the CL (Ahanotu et al., 2001; Kodjikian et al., 2004; Magnusson, 1982). The effect of surface roughness on bacterial adhesion to a CL is still far from being well understood. According to prior work, it seems clear that surface roughness is related to deposit formation and microorganism colonization of the surface (Baguet et al., 1995; Vermeltfoort et al., 2004). Greater surface roughness determines a greater specific surface area, thus creating more available active sites for thermodynamic reactions. Bacterial adhesion initiates on surface irregularities that serve as microenvironments where bacteria are sheltered from unfavorable environmental factors and then promote their survival (Shellenberger and Logan, 2002; Chae et al., 2006; Jones and Velegol, 2006). The effects of surface roughness have been examined over a wide range of physical scales (Bruinsma et al., 2001; Li and Logan, 2004; Li and Logan, 2005; Emerson et al., 2006; Mitik-Dineva et al., 2008; Park et al., 2008) and previous studies suggest that nanoscale surface roughness may greatly influence bacterial adhesion (Mitik-Dineva et al., 2008).

3.2.1. *Staphylococcus epidermidis*

Initial adhesion of *S. epidermidis* to unworn or worn conventional hydrogel CL has been reported to be strain and substrate related, the hydrophilic nature of the lens being a key factor (George et al., 2003; Henriques et al., 2005). The incorporation of silicone in a hydrogel polymer achieves high oxygen permeability but on the other hand reduces hydrophilicity (Tighe B, 2009). According with previous studies (Giraldez et al., 2010b), unworn silicone hydrogel CL (more hydrophobic) show a greater susceptibility to *S. epidermidis* adhesion than the conventional hydrogel CL (Figure 6). This observation is consistent with the established relationship between microbial adhesion and lens surface hydrophobicity. Notwithstanding, Santos et al. (Santos et al., 2008) were unable to detect any difference in microbial adhesion when comparing unworn silicone hydrogel and conventional hydrogel CL. This discrepancy could be explained by the different extents of microbial colonization observed for different *S. epidermidis* strains, and/or the different methodologies employed (Henriques et al., 2005; Kodjikian et al., 2007). In both hydrophobic and hydrophilic groups, the lenses showing the lowest R_a values (omafilcon A and comfilcon A) also returned the lowest numbers of *S. epidermidis* CFU, despite their high R_{ku} and R_{sk} values. Roughness values corresponding to these lenses are shown in tables 1 and 2.

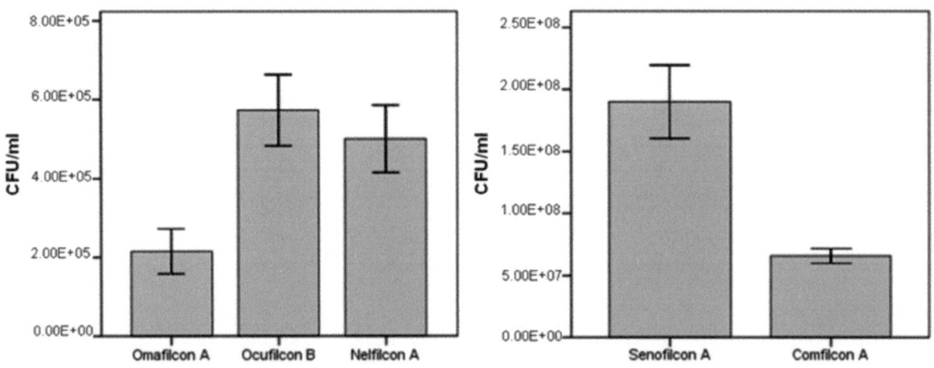

Figure 8. Adhesion of *S. epidermidis* CECT 4184 to hydrophilic (a) and hydrophobic (b) hydrogel contact lenses.

3.2.2. Pseudomona aeruginosa

Figure 7 provides the quantities, in CFU, of *P. aeruginosa* that adhered to six unworn CL (4 silicone hydrogel and 2 conventional hydrogel CL). In these lenses, it can be observed no substantial preference of *P. aeruginosa* to adhere to unworn hydrophilic or hydrophobic CL. Although this is consistent with other studies for other bacterial strains (Borazjani et al., 2004; Santos et al., 2008), it challenges the established relationship between microbial adhesion and lens surface hydrophobicity (Pritchard et al., 1999; Doyle, 2000; Young et al., 2002; van Oss, 2003; Giraldez et al., 2010b). This discrepancy could be explained by the different extents of microbial colonization observed for different bacterial strains, and/or the different methodologies employed (Henriques et al., 2005; Kodjikian et al., 2007). In fact, most *P. aeruginosa* strains have a more hydrophilic surface than *S. epidermidis* or other bacteria (Gottenbos et al., 2001; Mitik-Dineva et al., 2009). This could explain the scarce difference observed between *P. aeruginosa* adhesion to hydrophilic and hydrophobic contact lenses relative to previously observed *S. epidermidis* adhesion patterns (Bos et al., 1999; Bakker et al., 2002; Giraldez et al., 2010b).

In relation with roughness effect, the lenses showing the highest R_a values accompanied by low R_{ku} and R_{sk} values (for a 25 μm^2 area, ocufilcon B: R_a=11.01 ± 1.79 nm, R_{ku}=5.45 ± 1.95 and R_{sk}= 0.98 ± 0.17; and lotrafilcon B: R_a=26,97 ± 3,91nm, R_{ku}=4,11 ± 1,28 and R_{sk}= -0,34 ±

0,07) also returned the lowest numbers of *P. aeruginosa* CFU. Nanomaterials are those with constituent dimensions smaller than 100 nm in at least one direction and have numerous biomedical applications (Park et al., 2008). Nanophase materials have greater surface areas, more surface defects, increased surface electron delocalization and greater numbers of surface grain boundaries. Since they show a higher percentage of atoms at their surfaces compared to conventional materials, the surface properties of nanophase materials differ and this results in higher surface reactivity to cell responses (Park et al., 2008; Mitik-Dineva et al., 2008). Although changes in metabolic responses have not been clearly defined, research has shown altered attachment rates for certain bacteria on nanophase surfaces, which could translate to enhanced or reduced adhesion (Park et al., 2008; Mitik-Dineva et al., 2008; Mitik-Dineva et al., 2009). Thus, while nanophase materials show reduced *Staphylcoccus epidermidis* colonization compared to conventional materials (Colon et al., 2006; Giraldez et al., 2010b) they nevertheless show improved *P. aeruginosa* colonization (Mitik-Dineva et al., 2009; Webster et al., 2005).

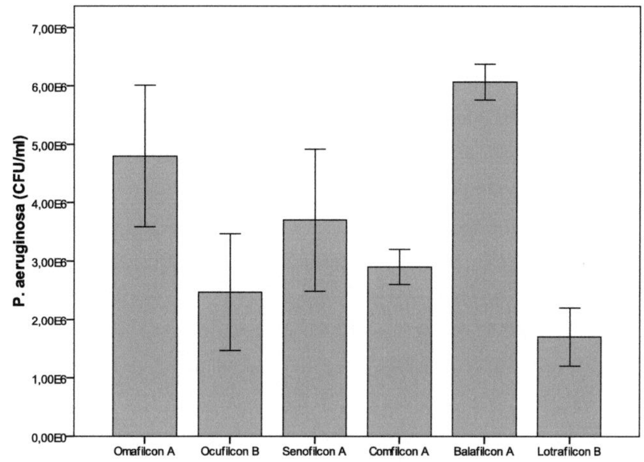

Figure 9. Adhesion of *P. aeruginosa* to both hydrophilic (omafilcon A and ocufilcon B) and hydrophobic (senofilcon A, comfilcon A, balafilcon A and lotrafilcon B) contact lenses.

4. Conclusion

Surface hydrophobicity and roughness are critical factors for bacterial adhesion; the surface of any body or object is the part which interacts with the surrounding environment. Hydrophobicity effect on bacterial adhesion to contact lenses is different in depending on bacterial strains; it seems to have a higher influence in *S epidermidis* than in *P aeruginosa* adhesion. Moreover, roughness is a biological factor that affects the manner in which bacteria adhere to surfaces, above all for initial adhesion; so by gaining a better understanding of the surface roughness of different types of CL, practitioners will be better placed to prescribe the most suitable lens for any given patient and to interpret the clinical performance of lenses they prescribe in relation to patient symptoms and ocular surface signs.

Author details

Maria Jesus Giraldez and Eva Yebra-Pimentel
Santiago de Compostela University, Spain

5. References

Ahanotu, E. N., Hyatt, M. D., Graham, M. J. and Ahearn, D. G. (2001) Comparative radiolabel and ATP analyses of adhesion of Pseudomonas aeruginosa and Staphylococcus epidermidis to hydrogel lenses. *CLAO J* 27, 89-93.

Alarcon, I., Kwan, L., Yu, C., Evans, D. J. and Fleiszig, S. M. (2009) Role of the corneal epithelial basement membrane in ocular defense against Pseudomonas aeruginosa. *Infect.Immun.* 77, 3264-71.

Angus, A. A., Lee, A. A., Augustin, D. K., Lee, E. J., Evans, D. J. and Fleiszig, S. M. (2008) Pseudomonas aeruginosa induces membrane blebs in epithelial cells, which are utilized as a niche for intracellular replication and motility. *Infect.Immun.* 76, 1992-2001.

Ayoub M, Badr A and Elian S. (1994) A study of the effect of antibiotics on the normal flora of the eye. *Med J Cairo Univ* 62, 121-8.

Baguet, J., Sommer, F., Claudon-Eyl, V. and Duc, T. M. (1995) Characterization of lacrymal component accumulation on worn soft contact lens surfaces by atomic force microscopy. *Biomaterials* 16, 3-9.

Baguet, J., Sommer, F. and Duc, T. M. (1993) Imaging surfaces of hydrophilic contact lenses with the atomic force microscope. *Biomaterials* 14, 279-84.

Bakker, D. P., Busscher, H. J. and van der Mei, H. C. (2002) Bacterial deposition in a parallel plate and a stagnation point flow chamber: microbial adhesion mechanisms depend on the mass transport conditions. *Microbiology* 148, 597-603.

Bennett, J. M. (1992) Recent developments in surface roughenss characterization. *Meas Sci Technol* 3, 1119-27.

Bhatia, S., Goldberg, E. P. and Enns, J. B. (1997) Examination of contact lens surfaces by Atomic Force Microscope (AFM). *CLAO J.* 23, 264-9.

Blunt, R. T. (2006). *White light interferometry- a production worthy technique for measuring surface roughness on semiconductor wafers. CS Mantched Conference. Proceedings of the CS Mantched Conferences.*

Bohnert JL, Horbett TA, Ratner BD and Royce FH. (1988) Adsorption of proteins form artificial tear solutions to contact lens materials. *Ophthalmol Vis Sci* 29, 362-73.

Borazjani, R. N., Levy, B. and Ahearn, D. G. (2004) Relative primary adhesion of Pseudomonas aeruginosa, Serratia marcescens and Staphylococcus aureus to HEMA-type contact lenses and an extended wear silicone hydrogel contact lens of high oxygen permeability. *Cont Lens Anterior Eye* 27, 3-8.

Bos, R., van der Mei, H. C. and Busscher, H. J. (1999) Physico-chemistry of initial microbial adhesive interactions--its mechanisms and methods for study. *FEMS Microbiol Rev* 23, 179-230.

Bruinsma, G. M., Rustema-Abbing, M., de Vries J, Busscher, H. J., van der Linden, M. L., Hooymans, J. M. and van der Mei, H. C. (2003) Multiple surface properties of worn RGP lenses and adhesion of Pseudomonas aeruginosa. *Biomaterials* 24, 1663-70.

Bruinsma, G. M., Rustema-Abbing, M., de, V. J., Stegenga, B., van der Mei, H. C., van der Linden, M. L., Hooymans, J. M. and Busscher, H. J. (2002) Influence of wear and overwear on surface properties of etafilcon A contact lenses and adhesion of Pseudomonas aeruginosa. *Invest Ophthalmol.Vis.Sci.* 43, 3646-53.

Bruinsma, G. M., Rustema-Abbing, M., van der Mei, H. C. and Busscher, H. J. (2001) Effects of cell surface damage on surface properties and adhesion of Pseudomonas aeruginosa. *J.Microbiol.Methods* 45, 95-101.

Buehler PO, Schein OD, Stamler JF, Verier DD and Karz J. (1992) The increased risk of ulcerative keratitis among disposable soft contact lens users. *Arch Ophthalmol* 110, 1555-8.

Caber, P. (1993) Interferometric profiler for rough surfaces. *Appl Opt* 32, 3438-41.

Carney, F. P., Nash, W. L. and Sentell, K. B. (2008) The Adsorption of Major Tear Film Lipids In Vitro to Various Silicone Hydrogels over Time. *Invest Ophthalmol.Vis.Sci.* 49, 120-4.

Catalonotti P, Lanza M, Del Prete A, Lucido M, Catania MR, Calle F, Boggia D, Perfetto B and Rossano F. (2005) Slime-producing Staphylococcus epidermidis and S. aureus in acute bacterial conjunctivitis in soft contact lens wearers. *New Microbiol* 28, 345-54.

Cehreli, Z. C., Lakshmipathy, M. and Yazici, R. (2008) Effect of different splint removal techniques on the surface roughness of human enamel: a three-dimensional optical profilometry analysis. *Dental Traumatology* 24, 177-82.

Chae, M. S., Schraft, H., Truelstrup, H. L. and Mackereth, R. (2006) Effects of physicochemical surface characteristics of Listeria monocytogenes strains on attachment to glass. *Food Microbiol.* 23, 250-9.

Cheng, K. H., Leung, S. L., Hoekman, H. W., Beekhuis, W. H., Mulder, P. G., Geerards, A. J. and Kijlstra, A. (1999) Incidence of contact-lens-associated microbial keratitis and its related morbidity. *Lancet* 354, 181-5.

Choy, M. H., Stapleton, F., Willcox, M. D. and Zhu, H. (2008) Comparison of virulence factors in Pseudomonas aeruginosa strains isolated from contact lens- and non-contact lens-related keratitis. *J.Med.Microbiol.* 57, 1539-46.

Colon, G., Ward, B. C. and Webster, T. J. (2006) Increased osteoblast and decreased Staphylococcus epidermidis functions on nanophase ZnO and TiO2. *J.Biomed.Mater.Res.A* 78, 595-604.

Cryz, S. J., Jr., Pitt, T. L., Furer, E. and Germanier, R. (1984) Role of lipopolysaccharide in virulence of Pseudomonas aeruginosa. *Infect.Immun.* 44, 508-13.

Dart, J. K., Radford, C. F., Minassian, D., Verma, S. and Stapleton, F. (2008) Risk factors for microbial keratitis with contemporary contact lenses: a case-control study. *Ophthalmology* 115, 1647-54, 1654.

Donlan, R. M. (2002) Biofilms: microbial life on surfaces. *Emerg.Infect.Dis.* 8, 881-90.

Donshik PC. (2003) Contact lens chemistry and giant papillary conjunctivitis. *Eye Contact Lens* 29, S37-S39.

Doyle A, Belgi B, Early A, Blake A, Eustace P and Hone R. (1995) Adherence of bacteria to intraocular lenses: a propective study. *Br J Ophthalmol* 79, 347-9.

Doyle, R. J. (2000) Contribution of the hydrophobic effect to microbial infection. *Microbes.Infect.* 2, 391-400.

Elder Mj, Stapleton F, Evans E and Dart JK. (1995) Biofilm-related infections in ophthalomology. *Eye* 9, 102-9.

Emerson, R. J., Bergstrom, T. S., Liu, Y., Soto, E. R., Brown, C. A., McGimpsey, W. G. and Camesano, T. A. (2006) Microscale correlation between surface chemistry, texture, and the adhesive strength of Staphylococcus epidermidis. *Langmuir* 22, 11311-21.

Evans, D. J., McNamara, N. A. and Fleiszig, S. M. (2007) Life at the front: dissecting bacterial-host interactions at the ocular surface. *Ocul.Surf.* 5, 213-27.

Fleiszig, S. M. (2006) The Glenn A. Fry award lecture 2005. The pathogenesis of contact lens-related keratitis. *Optom.Vis.Sci.* 83, 866-73.

Fleiszig, S. M., Zaidi, T. S., Fletcher, E. L., Preston, M. J. and Pier, G. B. (1994) Pseudomonas aeruginosa invades corneal epithelial cells during experimental infection. *Infect.Immun.* 62, 3485-93.

Fletcher, E. L., Fleiszig, S. M. and Brennan, N. A. (1993a) Lipopolysaccharide in adherence of Pseudomonas aeruginosa to the cornea and contact lenses. *Invest Ophthalmol Vis Sci* 34, 1930-6.

Fletcher, E. L., Weissman, B. A., Efron, N., Fleiszig, S. M., Curcio, A. J. and Brennan, N. A. (1993b) The role of pili in the attachment of Pseudomonas aeruginosa to unworn hydrogel contact lenses. *Curr.Eye Res.* 12, 1067-71.

Gadelmawla, E. S., Koura, M. M., Maksoud, T. M. A., Elewa, I. M. and Soliman, H. H. (2002) Roughness parameters. *Journal of Materials Processing Technology* 123, 133-45.

Garrett Q, Garrett RW and Milthorpe BK. (1999) Lysozime sorption in hydrogel contact lenses. *Invest Ophthalmol.Vis.Sci.* 40, 897-903.

Garrett Q, Laycock B and Garrett RW. (2000) Hydrogel lens monover constituents modulate protein sorption. *Invest Ophthalmol.Vis.Sci.* 41, 1678-95.

George, M., Ahearn, D., Pierce, G. and Gabriel, M. (2003) Interactions of Pseudomonas aeruginosa and Staphylococcus epidermidis in adhesion to a hydrogel. *Eye Contact Lens* 29, S105-S109.

Giraldez, M. J., Garcia-Resua, C., Lira, M., Real Oliveira, M. E. and Yebra-Pimentel, E. (2010a) White light interferometry to characterize the hydrogel contact lens surface. *Ophthalmic Physiol Opt.* 30, 289-97.

Giraldez, M. J., Resua, C. G., Lira, M., Oliveira, M. E., Magarinos, B., Toranzo, A. E. and Yebra-Pimentel, E. (2010b) Contact lens hydrophobicity and roughness effects on bacterial adhesion. *Optom.Vis.Sci.* 87, E426-E431.

Giraldez, M. J., Serra, C., Lira, M., Real Oliveira, M. E. and Yebra-Pimentel, E. (2010c) Soft contact lens surface profile by atomic force microscopy. *Optom.Vis.Sci.* 87, E475-E481.

Gonzalez-Meijome, J. M., Lopez-Alemany, A., Almeida, J. B. and Parafita, M. A. (2009) Surface AFM microscopy of unworn and worn samples of silicone hydrogel contact lenses. *J Biomed Mater Res.B Appl Biomater.* 88, 75-82.

Gonzalez-Meijome, J. M., Lopez-Alemany, A., Almeida, J. B., Parafita, M. A. and Refojo, M. F. (2006a) Microscopic observation of unworn siloxane-hydrogel soft contact lenses by atomic force microscopy. *J.Biomed.Mater.Res.B Appl.Biomater.* 76, 412-8.

Gonzalez-Meijome, J. M., Lopez-Alemany, A., Almeida, J. B., Parafita, M. A. and Refojo, M. F. (2006b) Microscopic observations of superficial ultrastructure of unworn siloxane-hydrogel contact lenses by cryo-scanning electron microscopy. *J.Biomed.Mater.Res.B Appl.Biomater.* 76, 419-23.

Gottenbos, B., Grijpma, D. W., van der Mei, H. C., Feijen, J. and Busscher, H. J. (2001) Antimicrobial effects of positively charged surfaces on adhering Gram-positive and Gram-negative bacteria. *J.Antimicrob.Chemother.* 48, 7-13.

Grobe G. (1996) Surface chemical structure for soft contact lenses as a funciton of polymer processing. *J.Biomed.Mater.Res.* 32, 45-54.

Guillon, M. and Maissa, C. (2007) Use of silicone hydrogel material for daily wear. *Cont.Lens Anterior.Eye* 30, 5-10.

Gupta, S. K., Berk, R. S., Masinick, S. and Hazlett, L. D. (1994) Pili and lipopolysaccharide of Pseudomonas aeruginosa bind to the glycolipid asialo GM1. *Infect.Immun.* 62, 4572-9.

Gupta, S. K., Masinick, S. A., Hobden, J. A., Berk, R. S. and Hazlett, L. D. (1996) Bacterial proteases and adherence of Pseudomonas aeruginosa to mouse cornea. *Exp Eye Res.* 62, 641-50.

Guryca, V., Hobzova, R., Pradny, M., Sirc, J. and Michalek, J. (2007) Surface morphology of contact lenses probed with microscopy techniques. *Cont.Lens Anterior.Eye* 30, 215-22.

Hansson, S. (2000) Surface roughness parameters as predictors of anchorage strength in bone: a critical analysis. *J Biomech.* 33, 1297-303.

Hara J, Yasuda F and Higashitsutsumi M. (1997) Preoperative desinfection of the conjunctival sac in cataract surgery. *Ophthalmologica* 211, 62-7.

Hauser, A. R. (2009) The type III secretion system of Pseudomonas aeruginosa: infection by injection. *Nat.Rev.Microbiol.* 7, 654-65.

Hazlett, L. D. (2007) Bacterial infections of the cornea (Pseudomonas aeruginosa). *Chem.Immunol.Allergy* 92, 185-94.

Henriques, M., Sousa, C., Lira, M., Elisabete, M., Oliveira, R., Oliveira, R. and Azeredo, J. (2005) Adhesion of Pseudomonas aeruginosa and Staphylococcus epidermidis to silicone-hydrogel contact lenses. *Optom Vis Sci* 82, 446-50.

Hinojosa Rivera M and Reyes Melo ME. (2001) La rugosidad de las superficies: topometría. *Ingenierias* 4, 27-33.

Holden, B. A., Sankaridurg, P. R., Sweeney, D. F., Stretton, S., Naduvilath, T. J. and Rao, G. N. (2005) Microbial keratitis in prospective studies of extended wear with disposable hydrogel contact lenses. *Cornea* 24, 156-61.

Hooton, J. C., German, C. S., Allen, S., Davies, M. C., Roberts, C. J., Tendler, S. J. and Williams, P. M. (2004) An atomic force microscopy study of the effect of nanoscale contact geometry and surface chemistry on the adhesion of pharmaceutical particles. *Pharm.Res.* 21, 953-61.

Hooton, J. C., German, C. S., Davies, M. C. and Roberts, C. J. (2006) A comparison of morphology and surface energy characteristics of sulfathiazole polymorphs based upon single particle studies. *Eur.J Pharm.Sci* 28, 315-24.

Hosaka, S., Ozawa, H., Tanzawa, H., Ishida, H., Yoshimura, K., Momose, T., Magatani, H. and Nakajima, A. (1983) Analysis of deposits on high water content contact lenses. *J.Biomed.Mater.Res.* 17, 261-74.

Jones L and Dumbleton K. (2002) Silicone hydrgels contact lenses, Part 1. Evolution and current status. *Optometry Today* 20, 26-32.

Jones L, Senchyna M, Glasier MA, Schickler J, Forbe I, Louie D and May C. (2003) Lysozyme and lipid deposition on silicone hydrogel contact lens materials. *Eye Contact Lens* 29, S75-S79.

Jones, J. F. and Velegol, D. (2006) Laser trap studies of end-on E. coli adhesion to glass. *Colloids Surf.B Biointerfaces.* 50, 66-71.

Keay, L., Edwards, K. and Stapleton, F. (2009) Signs, symptoms, and comorbidities in contact lens-related microbial keratitis. *Optom.Vis.Sci.* 86, 803-9.

Kiely JD and Bonnell DA. (1997) Quantification of topographic structure by scanning probe microscopy. *J Vac Sci Technol B* 15, 1483-93.

Kim, S. H., Opdahl, A., Marmo, C. and Somorjai, G. A. (2002) AFM and SFG studies of pHEMA-based hydrogel contact lens surfaces in saline solution: adhesion, friction, and the presence of non-crosslinked polymer chains at the surface. *Biomaterials* 23, 1657-66.

Kitching S, Williams PM, Roberts CJ, Davies MC and Tendler SJB. (1999) Quantifying surface topography and scannig probe image reconstruction. *J Vac Sci Technol B* 17, 273-9.

Kodjikian, L., Burillon, C., Roques, C., Pellon, G., Renaud, F. N., Hartmann, D. and Freney, J. (2004) Intraocular lenses, bacterial adhesion and endophthalmitis prevention: a review. *Biomed Mater Eng* 14, 395-409.

Kodjikian, L., Casoli-Bergeron, E., Malet, F., Janin-Manificat, H., Freney, J., Burillon, C., Colin, J. and Steghens, J. P. (2007) Bacterial adhesion to conventional hydrogel and new silicone-hydrogel contact lens materials. *Graefes Arch.Clin.Exp.Ophthalmol.*

Kogure, K., Ikemoto, E. and Morisaki, H. (1998) Attachment of Vibrio alginolyticus to glass surfaces is dependent on swimming speed. *J Bacteriol.* 180, 932-7.

Lakkis, C. and Fleiszig, S. M. (2001) Resistance of Pseudomonas aeruginosa isolates to hydrogel contact lens disinfection correlates with cytotoxic activity. *J Clin Microbiol.* 39, 1477-86.

Laughlin-Borlace, L., Stapleton, F., Matheson, M. and Dart, J. K. (1998) Bacterial biofilm on contact lenses and lens storage cases in wearers with microbial keratitis. *J Appl Microbiol* 84, 827-38.

Lee, S. P., Lee, S. J., Lim, B. S. and Ahn, S. J. (2009) Surface characteristics of orthodontic materials and their effects on adhesion of mutans streptococci. *Angle Orthod.* 79, 353-60.

Leitch EC, Harmis NY, Corrigan KM and Willcox MD. (1998) Identification and enumeration of staphylococci form the eye during soft contact lens wear. *Optom Vis Sci* 75, 258-65.

Li, B. and Logan, B. E. (2004) Bacterial adhesion to glass and metal-oxide surfaces. *Colloids Surf.B Biointerfaces.* 36, 81-90.

Li, B. and Logan, B. E. (2005) The impact of ultraviolet light on bacterial adhesion to glass and metal oxide-coated surface. *Colloids Surf.B Biointerfaces.* 41, 153-61.

Liesegang, T. J. (2002) Physiologic changes of the cornea with contact lens wear. *CLAO J.* 28, 12-27.

Linde, Y. W., Bengtsson, A. and Loden, M. (1989) 'Dry' skin in atopic dermatitis. II. A surface profilometry study. *Acta Derm.Venereol.* 69, 315-9.

Linneweber, J., Dohmen, P. M., Kertzscher, U., Affeld, K., Nose, Y. and Konertz, W. (2007) The effect of surface roughness on activation of the coagulation system and platelet adhesion in rotary blood pumps. *Artif.Organs* 31, 345-51.

Lira, M., Santos, L., Azeredo, J., Yebra-Pimentel, E. and Oliveira, M. E. (2008) Comparative study of silicone-hydrogel contact lenses surfaces before and after wear using atomic force microscopy. *J.Biomed.Mater.Res.B Appl.Biomater.* 85, 361-7.

Lorentz, H., Rogers, R. and Jones, L. (2007) The impact of lipid on contact angle wettability. *Optom.Vis.Sci.* 84, 946-53.

Lyczak, J. B., Cannon, C. L. and Pier, G. B. (2000) Establishment of Pseudomonas aeruginosa infection: lessons from a versatile opportunist. *Microbes.Infect.* 2, 1051-60.

Mack, D., Haeder, M., Siemssen, N. and Laufs, R. (1996) Association of biofilm production of coagulase-negative staphylococci with expression of a specific polysaccharide intercellular adhesin. *J Infect.Dis.* 174, 881-4.

Mack, D., Nedelmann, M., Krokotsch, A., Schwarzkopf, A., Heesemann, J. and Laufs, R. (1994) Characterization of transposon mutants of biofilm-producing Staphylococcus epidermidis impaired in the accumulative phase of biofilm production: genetic identification of a hexosamine-containing polysaccharide intercellular adhesin. *Infect.Immun.* 62, 3244-53.

Mack, D., Riedewald, J., Rohde, H., Magnus, T., Feucht, H. H., Elsner, H. A., Laufs, R. and Rupp, M. E. (1999) Essential functional role of the polysaccharide intercellular adhesin of Staphylococcus epidermidis in hemagglutination. *Infect.Immun.* 67, 1004-8.

Magnusson, K. E. (1982) Hydrophobic interaction--a mechanism of bacterial binding. *Scand.J Infect.Dis.Suppl* 33, 32-6.

Mah-Sadorra, J. H., Yavuz, S. G., Najjar, D. M., Laibson, P. R., Rapuano, C. J. and Cohen, E. J. (2005) Trends in contact lens-related corneal ulcers. *Cornea* 24, 51-8.

Maldonado-Codina, C. and Efron, N. (2005) Impact of manufacturing technology and material composition on the surface characteristics of hydrogel contact lenses. *Clin Exp Optom* 88, 396-404.

Mitik-Dineva, N., Wang, J., Mocanasu, R. C., Stoddart, P. R., Crawford, R. J. and Ivanova, E. P. (2008) Impact of nano-topography on bacterial attachment. *Biotechnol.J.* 3, 536-44.

Mitik-Dineva, N., Wang, J., Truong, V. K., Stoddart, P., Malherbe, F., Crawford, R. J. and Ivanova, E. P. (2009) Escherichia coli, Pseudomonas aeruginosa, and Staphylococcus aureus Attachment Patterns on Glass Surfaces with Nanoscale Roughness. *Current Microbiology* 58, 268-73.

Morisaki, H., Nagai, S., Ohshima, H., Ikemoto, E. and Kogure, K. (1999) The effect of motility and cell-surface polymers on bacterial attachment. *Microbiology* 145 (Pt 10), 2797-802.

Nayak, N., Nag, T. C., Satpathy, G. and Ray, S. B. (2007) Ultrastructural analysis of slime positive & slime negative Staphylococcus epidermidis isolates in infectious keratitis. *Indian J Med Res.* 125, 767-71.

Nayak, N. and Satpathy, G. (2000) Slime production as a virulence factor in Staphylococcus epidermidis isolated from bacterial keratitis. *Indian J Med Res.* 111, 6-10.

Nicolson PC. (2003) Continuous wear contact lens surface chemistry and wearability. *Eye Contact Lens* 29, S30-S32.

Novak, E., Pasop, F., and Browne, T. (2003). *Production metrology for MEMS characterization. Proceedings of the 2003 Desing, Test, Integration & Packaging of MEMS/MOEMS.* Cannes-Mandelieu

O'Mahony, C., Hill, M., Brunet, M., Duane, R. and Mathewson, A. (2003) Characterization fo micromechanical structures using white-light interferometry. *Meas Sci Technol* 14, 1807-14.

Olefjord, I. and Hansson, S. (1993) Surface analysis of four dental implant systems. *Int J Oral Maxillofac.Implants.* 8, 32-40.

Park, M. R., Banks, M. K., Applegate, B. and Webster, T. J. (2008) Influence of nanophase titania topography on bacterial attachment and metabolism. *Int.J.Nanomedicine.* 3, 497-504.

Patel, A. and Hammersmith, K. (2008) Contact lens-related microbial keratitis: recent outbreaks. *Curr.Opin.Ophthalmol* 19, 302-6.

Perilli, R., Marziano, M. L., Formisano, G., Caiazza, S., Scorcia, G. and Baldassarri, L. (2000) Alteration of organized structure of biofilm formed by Staphylococcus epidermidis on soft contact lenses. *J Biomed Mater Res.* 49, 53-7.

Pinna A, Zabettu S, Sotgiu M, Sechi LA, Fadda G and Carta F. (1999) Identification and antibiotic susceptibility of coagulase negative staphylococi isolated in corneal /external infections. *Br J Ophthalmol* 83, 771-3.

Pritchard, N., Fonn, D. and Brazeau, D. (1999) Discontinuation of contact lens wear: a survey. *Int Contact Lens Clin* 26, 157-62.

Raulio, M., Jarn, M., Ahola, J., Peltonen, J., Rosenholm, J. B., Tervakangas, S., Kolehmainen, J., Ruokolainen, T., Narko, P. and Salkinoja-Salonen, M. (2008) Microbe repelling coated stainless steel analysed by field emission scanning electron microscopy and physicochemical methods. *J Ind.Microbiol Biotechnol* 35, 751-60.

Rebeix, V., Sommer, F., Marchin, B., Baude, D. and Tran, M. D. (2000) Artificial tear adsorption on soft contact lenses: methods to test surfactant efficacy. *Biomaterials* 21, 1197-205.

Riley, C., Young, G. and Chalmers, R. (2006) Prevalence of ocular surface symptoms, signs, and uncomfortable hours of wear in contact lens wearers: the effect of refitting with daily-wear silicone hydrogel lenses (senofilcon a). *Eye Contact Lens* 32, 281-6.

Santos, L., Rodrigues, D., Lira, M., Real Oliveira, M. E., Oliveira, R., Vilar, E. Y. and Azeredo, J. (2008) Bacterial adhesion to worn silicone hydrogel contact lenses. *Optom Vis Sci* 85, 520-5.

Seal, D. V., Kirkness, C. M., Bennett, H. G. and Peterson, M. (1999) Population-based cohort study of microbial keratitis in Scotland: incidence and features. *Cont.Lens Anterior.Eye* 22, 49-57.

Serp, D., Mueller, M., Von Stockar, U. and Marison, I. W. (2002) Low-temperature electron microscopy for the study of polysaccharide ultraestructures in hydrogels.I. Theoretical and technical considerations. *Biotechnol Bioeng* 79, 243-52.

Sheen, S., Bao, G. and Cooke, P. (2008) Food surface texture measurement using reflective confocal laser scanning microscopy. *J Food Sci* 73, E227-E234.

Shellenberger, K. and Logan, B. E. (2002) Effect of molecular scale roughness of glass beads on colloidal and bacterial deposition. *Environ.Sci Technol* 36, 184-9.

Skotnitsky C, Naduvilath TJ, Sweeney DF and Sankaridurg PR. (2006) Two presentations of contact lens-induced papillary conjunctivitis (CLPC) in hydrogel lens wear: local and general. *Optom Vis Sci* 83, 27-36.

Skotnitsky C, Sankaridurg PR, Sweeney DF and Holden BA. (2002) General and local contact lens induced papillary conjunctivitis (CLPC). *Clin Exp Optom* 85, 193-7.

Soltys-Robitaille CE, Ammon DM jr, Valint PL jr and Grobe G. (2001) The relationship between contact lens surface charge and in-vitro protein deposition levels. *Biomaterials* 22, 3257-60.

Stapleton, F., Keay, L., Edwards, K., Naduvilath, T., Dart, J. K., Franzco, G. B. and Holden, B. (2008) The Incidence of Contact Lens-Related Microbial Keratitis in Australia. *Ophthalmology*

Subbaraman LN, Bayer S, Gepr S, Glasier MA, Lorentz H, Senchyna M and Jones L. (2006) Rewetting drops containing surface active agents improve the clinical performance of silicone hydrogel contact lenses. *Optom Vis Sci* 83, 143-51.

Szczotka-Flynn L. (2007) Lens distinctions. *http://www.clspectrum.com/*

Szmukler-Moncler, S., Testori, T. and Bernard, J. P. (2004) Etched implants: a comparative surface analysis of four implant systems. *J Biomed Mater Res.B Appl Biomater.* 69, 46-57.

Teichroeb, J. H., Forrest, J. A., Ngai, V., Martin, J. W., Jones, L. and Medley, J. (2008) Imaging protein deposits on contact lens materials. *Optom Vis Sci* 85, 1151-64.

Tighe B. (2009) Silicone hydrogels: what are they and how should they be used in everyday practice? *Optician* 218, 31-2.

van Oss, C. J. (2003) Long-range and short-range mechanisms of hydrophobic attraction and hydrophilic repulsion in specific and aspecific interactions. *J Mol.Recognit.* 16, 177-90.

Vermeltfoort, P. B., van der Mei, H. C., Busscher, H. J., Hooymans, J. M. and Bruinsma, G. M. (2004) Physicochemical factors influencing bacterial transfer from contact lenses to surfaces with different roughness and wettability. *J Biomed Mater Res.B Appl.Biomater.* 71, 336-42.

Wagner, V. E. and Iglewski, B. H. (2008) P. aeruginosa Biofilms in CF Infection. *Clin.Rev.Allergy Immunol.* 35, 124-34.

Wang, H., Feng, H., Liang, W., Luo, Y. and Malyarchuk, V. (2009) Effect of surface roughness on retention and removal of Escherichia coli O157:H7 on surfaces of selected fruits. *J Food Sci* 74, E8-E15.

Webster, T. J., Tong, Z., Liu, J. and Katherine, B. M. (2005) Adhesion of Pseudomonas fluorescens onto nanophase materials. *Nanotechnology* 16, S449-S457.

Weisbarth, R. E., Gabriel, M. M., George, M., Rappon, J., Miller, M., Chalmers, R. and Winterton, L. (2007) Creating antimicrobial surfaces and materials for contact lenses and lens cases. *Eye Contact Lens* 33, 426-9.

Whittaker G. (2008) Biofinity silicone hydrogels. *www.opticianonline.net* 19-20.

Wilkinson, S. G. (1983) Composition and structure of lipopolysaccharides from Pseudomonas aeruginosa. *Rev.Infect.Dis.* 5 Suppl 5, S941-S949.

Willcox, M. D. (2007) Pseudomonas aeruginosa infection and inflammation during contact lens wear: a review. *Optom.Vis.Sci.* 84, 273-8.

Willcox, M. D., Harmis, N., Cowell, Williams, T. and Holden. (2001) Bacterial interactions with contact lenses; effects of lens material, lens wear and microbial physiology. *Biomaterials* 22, 3235-47.

Willcox, M. D., Naduvilath, T. J., Vaddavalli, P. K., Holden, B. A., Ozkan, J. and Zhu, H. (2010) Corneal erosions, bacterial contamination of contact lenses, and microbial keratitis. *Eye Contact Lens* 36, 340-5.

Windecker, R. and Tiziani, H. J. (1999) Optical roughness measurements using extended white-light interferometry. *Opt Eng* 38, 1081-7.

Yang, S., Zhang, H. and Hsu, S. M. (2007) Correction of random surface roughness on colloidal probes in measuring adhesion. *Langmuir* 23, 1195-202.

Young, G., Veys, J., Pritchard, N. and Coleman, S. (2002) A multi-centre study of lapsed contact lens wearers. *Ophthalmic Physiol Opt* 22, 516-27.

Zolfaghar, I., Angus, A. A., Kang, P. J., To, A., Evans, D. J. and Fleiszig, S. M. (2005) Mutation of retS, encoding a putative hybrid two-component regulatory protein in Pseudomonas aeruginosa, attenuates multiple virulence mechanisms. *Microbes.Infect.* 7, 1305-16.

Zolfaghar, I., Evans, D. J. and Fleiszig, S. M. (2003) Twitching motility contributes to the role of pili in corneal infection caused by Pseudomonas aeruginosa. *Infect.Immun.* 71, 5389-93.

Zolfaghar, I., Evans, D. J., Ronaghi, R. and Fleiszig, S. M. (2006) Type III secretion-dependent modulation of innate immunity as one of multiple factors regulated by Pseudomonas aeruginosa RetS. *Infect.Immun.* 74, 3880-9.

Zyrianov, Y. (2005) Distribution-based descriptors of the molecular shape. *J Chem.Inf.Model.* 45, 657-72.

Chapter 6

New Biomarkers in the Retina and RPE Under Oxidative Stress

Wan Jin Jahng

Additional information is available at the end of the chapter

http://dx.doi.org/10.5772/ 48785

1. Introduction

Age-related macular degeneration (AMD) involves progressive cell death of post-mitotic retinal pigment epithelial (RPE) cells, which adversely affects rod and cone survival. RPE cells are exposed to chronic oxidative stress, including constant exposure to intense light and increased reactive oxygen species (ROS) from mitochondria due to high levels of oxygen consumption. However, understanding how oxidative stress causes phosphoproteomic alterations that initiate death signals in the RPE is elusive. Lack of such knowledge is an important problem, because, without it, acquiring the ability to modulate cellular protection is highly unlikely.

The RPE, located between photoreceptors and choroid, is in a unique position to mediate the transport of nutrients, oxygen, and retinoid from blood to photoreceptors. For continued vision, the RPE is required for retinoid recycling and phagocytosis, which initiates accumulation of retinoid byproducts that eventually leads to apoptosis. Continuous exposure to light causes the RPE to consume a large amount of oxygen in order to complete the complex processes of nutrient transport, phagocytosis, and the visual cycle. It is still not known why the initial retinal degeneration occurs and how the degenerative processes progress as a result of oxidative stress. Adaptation to changes in oxidative environment is critical for the survival of retina and RPE cells. Clinical trials demonstrated a significant reduction toward retinal degeneration upon intake of antioxidants that include lutein, zeaxanthin, zinc, vitamin C, and vitamin E. Oxidation of polyunsaturated fatty acids (PFA) and photosensitizers in the RPE induces reactive oxygen species (ROS) production upon exposure to visible light. Hydrogen peroxide (H_2O_2) is generated in the RPE during phagocytosis of the photoreceptor outer segment, and it has been used as a direct oxidative-inducing reagent to initiate cellular oxidative stress. Understanding of molecular mechanisms that mediate oxidative stress-induced proteome changes in the RPE may provide insight into the pathogenesis of retinal degeneration. In our study, comparative and differential proteomics have been applied to investigate global changes in the RPE and retina proteome due to oxidative stress induced by light or H_2O_2.

2. Phosphorylation signaling in the RPE

We have focused on understanding the cell death mechanism of the retina and RPE under oxidative stress [Chung et al., 2009; Lee et al., 2010a; Lee et al., 2010b; Zhang et al., 2010; Lee et al., 2011; Arnouk et al., 2011; Sripathi et al., 2011]. Our studies demonstrated that oxidative stress may trigger induction of anti-apoptotic erythropoietin, JAK2, and BCL-xL, as well as pro-apoptotic caspases. Oxidative stress also influences mitochondrial-nuclear communication by shuttling mitochondrial prohibitin. We examined whether phosphorylations of cytoskeletal and anti-apoptotic proteins, including vimentin, PP2A, and crystalline, regulate the initial protecting mechanism. The cytoskeletal network formed by filamentous proteins determines how retinal and RPE cells respond to their extracellular environmental stimuli that include oxidative stress.

Site-specific phosphorylations of crystalline and vimentin regulate protein interactions through positive or negative feedback mechanisms. The significance of proteomic studies is that they are providing a detailed apoptotic mechanism and new potential AMD-related biomarkers. The global phosphoproteome changes in RPE cells under oxidative stress will help to identify key elements of phosphorylation signaling that serve as a framework of biochemical pathways of AMD progression.

It is a critical question to understand the maintenance mechanism of appropriate phosphorylation signaling under chronic stress conditions. Oxidative stress may influence the expression of genetic risk factors, including complement factor H (CFH). Although the potential importance of protein phosphorylation/dephosphorylation as a therapeutic target has been appreciated, no detailed approach to date has been made targeting biomarkers in phosphoproteome to treat ocular diseases. For example, abnormalities in vimentin phosphorylation have been linked to neurodegenerative diseases, including AMD and Alzheimer's disease [Madigan et al., 1994; Yen et al, 1983; Yu et al., 1994], but the phosphorylation network mechanism in RPE cells under oxidative stress remains largely elusive.

Regulation of the phosphate on/off switch is a central tool for RPE cells to survive under stress conditions. Unbiased approach to determine phosphorylation sites and kinetics will help to understand the complex apoptotic network and epigenetic controlling mechanism of RPE death. A general proteomic approach that includes protein identification by mass spectrometry has been used routinely for the last decade, however, RPE phosphoproteomics remains challenging due to the complexity, substoichiometry (less than 50% phosphorylated), and kinetics (short vs. long time frame). Understanding phosphorylation in AMD is not clear, because protein phosphorylation is a very dynamic process, while the aging process is slow. Recent animal models exhibiting some of the features of human AMD are available, but most of these models do not represent the full spectrum of pathological changes observed in human AMD. Animal models that mimic the complex and progressive characteristics of AMD are extremely valuable for studying the pathogenesis of AMD and testing different treatment modalities.

Phosphoproteins have been studied using chemical and affinity-based methods [Zhou et al., 2008; Tao et al., 2005]. However, the rapid and dynamic nature of the underlying changes and the low abundance of phosphoproteins reflecting their substoichiometry present challenges to the quantitative study of the phosphoproteome. Thus, the isolation of the phosphoproteome or phosphopeptidome represents a potentially advanced step in this analysis. We introduced a system-wide, unbiased, and high-throughput approach to investigate global phosphoproteome of oxidative stress-induced or aged RPE and retinal cells using phosphoproteome enrichment and labeling method. Phosphoprotein-enriched extracts from human RPE cells under stress were separated by two-dimensional (2D) electrophoresis. Serine, threonine, and tyrosine phosphorylation were visualized by 2D phospho-Western blotting and specific phosphorylation sites were analyzed by tandem mass spectrometry. We examined phosphoproteome changes under oxidative stress *in vitro* and aging-induced phosphoproteome *in vivo*.

Our results suggest a positive correlation between early biomarkers of phosphoproteome under oxidative stress and RPE proteins from AMD patients. The outcome of the current work is the initial delineation of the underlying physiology of oxidative stress-mediated phosphorylation signaling in RPE apoptosis. In addition, our study suggests a stimulus for understanding oxidative stress-induced cytoskeletal changes and the aggregate formation mechanism by phosphorylations. As a consequence, an effective therapeutic approach and animal model based on the modulation of phosphorylations are expected to result.

Recently, pioneering proteomic profiling studies revealed protein expression changes in human RPE, drusen, and lipofuscin [West et al., 2001; Crabb et al., 2002; Schütt et al., 2007]. Other studies compared native differentiated to cultured dedifferentiated RPE cells [Alge et al., 2003; Alge et al., 2006]. Proteomics proved to be a useful tool in delineating changes in RPE with the progressive stages of AMD [Nordgaard et al., 2006; An et al., 2006; Norgaard et al., 2008], and diabetes [Decanini et al., 2007]. Also, proteomic tools were used to study changes in the vitreous humor associated with diabetic retinopathy [Kim et al., 2007] and retinal proteins in glaucoma model [Tezel et al., 2005]. Since oxidative stress is implicated in the etiology of several RPE diseases that include AMD, identification of molecular mediators and early signaling events under chronic stress is a crucial step for understanding cell death mechanism and retinal degeneration. However, limitations of proteomic approach, including minor proteins with low concentration, hydrophobic membrane proteins, reproducibility, and time and labor demanding processes, exist as huddles to get comprehensive details on the molecular mechanism. Moreover, there is no comprehensive database that could support the analysis of protein phosphorylation in human RPE from the standpoint of spatial and temporal changes.

Phosphorylation of specific amino acids, including serine, threonine, and tyrosine, is a significant modulator of protein function that regulates subcellular localization, protein–protein interaction, conformational change, and signal transduction. Charge changes by phosphorylation creates a protein switch mechanism, allowing reversible phosphorylation to modify intracellular signaling in response to specific microenvironmental and genetic conditions and thereby act as a basic survival tool. However, the rapid and dynamic nature of the underlying changes and the low abundance of phosphoproteins reflecting their substoichiometry present challenges to the quantitative study of the phosphoproteome. The isolation of phosphoproteome or phosphopeptidome represents a potential challenge. Our data and other evidence suggest that phosphorylations are involved in apoptotic or protecting signaling under oxidative stress [Chung et al., 2009; Zhang et al., 2010; Arnouk et al., 2011; Lee et al., 2011; Sripathi et al., 2011].

Proteomic study provides direct evidence and a molecular basis for phosphorylation signaling, cytoskeletal reorganization, and apoptotic mechanisms of AMD [Nordgaard et al., 2006; Crabb et al., 2002; Ethen et al., 2006; An et al., 2006; Warburton et al., 2007]. A detailed proteome analysis of AMD supports our hypothesis that there is a positive correlation between RPE biomarkers under stress and AMD as shown in **Table 1**.

To address the issue of phosphorylation in cytoskeletal reorganization, we examined morphologic and cytoskeletal changes of RPE cells under oxidative stress *in vitro*. The apoptotic cell surface changes initiate the protrusion, develop bubble-like blebs on their surface, and continue phagocytic alteration shown as the membrane disruption. In the middle stage, cells showed apical, basal and surface changes such as dense projection of microvilli. In later stage, cells broke into small, membrane-wrapped fragments.

To examine potential markers corresponding cytoskeletal reorganization under oxidative stress, we examined vimentin, an intermediate filament protein shown in both control and AMD drusen [Crabb et al., 2002]. ARPE-19 contains retinal G-protein receptor (RGR) and peropsin as light detecting chromophore. Previous observation of vimentin in RPE cells derived from human choroidal neovascular membranes in AMD, as well as in drusen and melanolipofuscin, supporting our choice of phosphoproteome biomarkers in RPE cells under stress [Schlunck et al., 2002; Crabb et al., 2002; Warburton et al., 2007]. Previously, proteomic analysis of the retina revealed that the expression levels of vimentin and PP2A are significantly increased when C3HeB/FeJ mice (rd1 allele, 12 weeks, photoreceptor degenerated) are exposed under continuous light for 7 days compared to a condition of 12h light/dark cycling exposure [Zhang et al., 2010]. When melatonin is administered to animals while they are exposed to continuous light, the increased levels of vimentin and PP2A return to a normal level. Further, vimentin has been shown to be a target of PP2A that directly binds vimentin and dephosphorylates it. Vimentin is present in all mesenchymal cells, and often used as a differentiation marker. Like other intermediate filaments, vimentin acts to maintain cellular integrity; however, vimentin may play a role in RPE survival by phosphorylation.

AMD RPE proteome [1]	**AMD drusen** [2]	**RPE blebs** [3]	***RPE proteome under OS in vitro*** *[4]*	***RPE proteome under light in vitro*** *[5]*
ATP synthase β CRABP1 CRALBP Crystallin αA Elf4H GST π HSC 70 HSP 60 HSP 70 Mt HSP 75 Pyruvate kinase VDAC 1	Annexin 5 Clusterin Complement component 9 Crystallin αB Crystallin βA3 Histone H2A2 Serum albumin TIMP3 Vimentin Vitronectin	Annexin 5 Cytoskeleton-associated protein 4 Desmin EF 1 GST GTPase Rab 14 HSP 70 9B Keratin 7, 18 Lamin A/C MMP-14 Peroxiredoxin 5 Thioredoxin reductase 1 Tubulin VDAC3	*Annexin 5* *BUB3* *EF2* *GST π* *Guanine binding protein* *HSP 90 α* *HSP β1* *Lamin A/C* *Peroxiredoxin 1, 2* *Phosphomevalonate kinase* *Plasminogen activator-inhibitor 1* *Prohibitin* *Pyruvate kinase* *Retinol binding protein* *RPE65* *Thioredoxin-dependent-peroxide reductase 3* *VDAC2*	*Actin* *ATP synthase* *CRALBP* *Creatine kinase* *Crystallin αA* *Crystallin αB* *Crystallin βB* *Crystallin γ* *G binding protein β1* *HSP 70* *HSP 90* *HSP β1* *IRBP* *Plasminogen* *Protein kinase 4* *Pyruvate kinase* *RPE65* *Tubulin α1B* *Tubulin β2*
AMD retina proteome [6]	**RPE secretome** [7]	**AMD RPE secretome** [7]	**Melanolipofuscin** [8]	***Retina proteome in vitro under OS*** *[9, 10]*
CRABP Crystallin αA Crystallin αB HSP 60 HSP70 Tubulin α VDAC1	Annexin 5 Caspase 5 CFB CFH Complement C HSP 47 Laminin MMP2 Prasminogen activator inhibitor 1	CFB CFH Collagen α Complement C Custerin Galectin 3 BP MMP2	Annexin 5 ATP synthase Crystallin αB G binding protein HSP 60 HSP 70 Prohibitin RBP 3 RDH 11 RDH 5 RGR RPE65 Tubulin α Tubulin β VDAC 1, 2, 3 Vimentin	*Bcl-xL* *Caspase-3* *c-FOS* *Crystallin αB* *Crstallin βB* *Crystallin βS* *Crystallin γB* *Crystallin γF* *EPO* *EPOR* *G binding protein* *Jak2* *Peroxiredoxin 2* *Peroxiredoxin 6* *PP2A* *Tubulin β* *Vimentin*

[1] Nordgaard et al., 2006 [2] Crabb et al., 2002 [3] Alcazar et al., 2009 [4] Arnouk et al., 2011, [5] Lee et al., 2011, [6] Ethen et al., 2006 [7] An et al., 2006 [8] Warburton et al., 2007 [9] Chung et al., 2009 [10] Zhang et al., 2010

Table 1. Comparison of AMD proteome vs. retina/RPE proteome changes under oxidative stress. Early biomarkers from our studies are in Italics.

Vimentin is a major component of intermediate filament that spread throughout the cell and serve as signal transducer conveying mechanical and molecular information from cell surface to nucleus and intracellular compartments. Modifications of vimentin are essential reactions of filament dynamics. Changes of vimentin phosphorylation are directed to reorganization of the intermediate filament network and altered function of RPE cells. Hyperphosphorylation of vimentin can disassemble intermediate filament into soluble monomeric form. Our results suggest that vimentin is critically involved in the process of light-induced damage in RPE cells. By reducing the light-induced post-translational modification of vimentin, PP2A may assist to maintain the proper filament network in RPE cells.

Next we tested the hypothesis that oxidative stress may induce protein phosphorylation, including vimentin. Vimentin phosphorylation at S38 is downregulated under stress and is a potential PP2A specific site for dephosphorylation. Phosphorylation at S38 suggests a potential antiapoptotic role when considering increased Bak under oxidative stress. Phosphorylation at S55 under stress condition is upregulated compared to β-actin control. We examined whether normal light- induced phosphoproteome was altered in RPE cells. To investigate RPE phosphoproteome, we used 2D electrophoresis to separate proteins from cells incubated under light (7000 lux) or dark conditions for 1 hour. RPE proteins induced by light were visualized using mass spectrometry-compatible silver staining. MALDI-TOF-TOF mass spectrometry analysis revealed that a large proportion of the proteins up-regulated first and foremost by light in the RPE belong to the crystallin family. Our data demonstrated that crystallins were upregulated under oxidative stress in bovine primary RPE cells. Serine phosphorylation of crystallin was markedly increased in light exposure, as shown by pSer-specific Western blotting. Notably, opposite effects on serine and tyrosine phosphorylation may yield positive or negative regulation with the same stimulus [Taniguchi et al., 2006]. Enzymes associated with phosphorylation or energy metabolism, including Ser/Thr protein kinase 4 (STE20) and ATP synthase, were downregulated under intense light. The most abundant light-induced upregulated phosphoproteins were crystallins, including αA and αB crystallins. Our results may suggest that phosphorylation of crystallin is critical to maintain a chaperone function in RPE cells. Phosphorylations at serine residues were next to proline or near proline. The results of phosphoproteome enrichment experiment were confirmed using an affinity-based phosphopeptide-enrichment strategy. In this experiment, in-solution trypsin digested peptides were concentrated using a metal (Ga^{+3}) based column and analyzed by tandem mass analysis.

Phosphorylation-dependent signaling might differ between tissues, and might reflect the microenvironmental diversity among different tissues, including differences in stress stimuli. Phosphoproteome change is an indication of an early signaling event under oxidative stress conditions in RPE. Increased phosphorylation of crystallins, in particular, might suggest a stress-response role for these proteins in the RPE. Accordingly, crystallin phosphorylation may provide an anti-apoptotic signal to attenuate oxidative stress-induced degenerative pathway as early signaling event. However, accumulated phoshprylated crystallins may lead to pathological mechanism [den Engelsman et al., 2005]. In this context, stress-induced up- or down-regulation of crystallins is known to occur in various diseases or age-related conditions [Nordgaard et al., 2006; Ethen et al., 2006]. The functional relationship between heat-shock proteins and cytoskeletal proteins, such as intermediate filaments, vimentin and actin, is well documented [Clark et al., 2000; Xi et al., 2003]. N-terminal phosphorylation of heat-shock proteins is correlated with the stabilization of cytoskeletal elements.

Our studies support the hypothesis that a progressive accumulation of oxidative damage is a fundamental mechanism involved in RPE cell death. Oxidative stress occurs when free radicals produced in RPE cells are not completely modulated by the appropriate endogenous defense systems. Phospholipids are a major component that can be targeted by excess oxidative stress. Lipid peroxidation plays an important role in initiating and mediating phosphorylation and cell death signaling. Establishing the involvement of lipid changes in phosphorylation signaling has not been an easy task. The lipids of cellular membranes serve roles in controlling the structure and fluidity of the membrane, and as signaling molecules that modifies protein functions. The lipid binding assay demonstrated subcellular communication between mitochondria and the nucleus under oxidative stress. The changes in the expression and localization of p-crystallin and p-vimentin triggered by reactive oxygen species are crucial for RPE integrity.

Recently, crystallin location and function in the retina and RPE have been described [Sakaguchi et al., 2003; Organisciak et al., 2011; Zigler et al., 2011; Sreekumar et al., 2010; Gangalum et al., 2011]. αA- and αB-crystallin are located in the ganglion cell layer and photoreceptor layer, whereas β-crystallin is detected in all nuclear layers of the retina [Xi et al., 2003]. The functional roles of crystallins as chaperones, anti-apoptotic proteins, or signal transducers in the retina have also been described [Xi et al., 2003; Sakaguchi et al., 2003; Kapphahn et al., 2003; Kim et al., 2007]. Phosphorylated αB-crystallin directly interacts with Bax and caspase-3 to suppress their pro-apoptotic action, and thus exerts a cytoprotective effect in the retina [Kim YH et al., 2007]. Light-induced up-regulation of αA-crystallin and increased phosphorylation of αA-crystallin in the aged retina have been reported [Kapphahn et al., 2003]. The specific function of each crystallin, particularly α/β-crystallin in the RPE, is still largely unknown, although levels of αB-crystallin are increased after heat shock and oxidative stress, and αB-crystallin immunoreactivity has been found in both rod outer segments and the RPE after light exposure [Sakaguchi et al., 2003].

3. Early proteome changes under oxidative stress

Two-dimensional differential gel electrophoresis (2-D DIGE) is an advanced proteomic technique that labels minor protein samples with fluorescent dyes before 2-D electrophoresis. It enables accurate analysis of differences in protein concentrations between samples. DIGE method reduces experimental variations and technical errors. It is possible to separate up to three different samples within the same 2-D gel using three different fluorescent molecules. However, there are limitations of DIGE methods also, including covalent modifications on cysteine or lysine.

We used two different biological models that include primary bovine RPE cells and human RPE cell line D407, to uncover differential biosignatures under oxidative stress [Davis et al., 1995]. We employed a combination of proteomic technologies, including sensitive fluorescent labeling and TOF-TOF mass spectrometry analysis with high mass accuracy and low tolerance in the range of 50 ppm (0.05 Dalton). Identified proteins were confirmed by quantitative Western blotting. We observed expression changes of cellular signaling related molecules, including intermediate filament, retinoid metabolism, energy metabolism, and antioxidant proteins in bovine RPE cells. Several intermediate filament components, including neurofilament H, M, L proteins and glial fibrillary acidic protein, were up-regulated in bovine RPE cells. Intermediate filament proteins are cytoskeletal components that form fibrils with an average diameter of 10 nm. Neurofilament H, M, and L proteins are specifically expressed in neurons. Glial fibrillary acidic protein is a biomarker in glial cells. Previous studies showed that environmental changes, such as culture conditions, could induce dedifferentiation of RPE cells and give rise to mesenchymal-like cells.

Proteome changes related to energy metabolism were also observed under oxidative stress in bovine RPE cells. Pyruvate dehydrogenase E1 transforms pyruvate into acetyl-CoA that is used in the citric acid cycle to generate ATP. Pyruvate kinase M1 transfers a phosphate group from phosphoenolpyruvate (PEP) to adenosine diphosphate (ADP), to synthesize ATP and pyruvate. Up-regulation of both enzymes may indicate higher energy consumption to compensate oxidative stress-induced faster turnover of proteins in the RPE.

In RPE D407 cells, several molecular chaperones were altered as a result of H_2O_2 treatment. Hsp 90α and Hsp β1 exhibit general protective chaperone properties such as preventing unspecific aggregation of non-native proteins. Calreticulin, up-regulated in bovine RPE cells, is a multifunctional protein that binds to Ca^{2+} and misfolded proteins to export them from the endoplasmic reticulum (ER) to the Golgi apparatus. Elimination of misfolded proteins in the ER affects cellular homeostasis and survival, so chaperone function of heat shock proteins is indispensible under stress conditions.

Retinoid metabolism in primary bovine RPE cells is altered under oxidative stress conditions. Photosensitivity and the steady state of retinoid concentrations are controlled by regeneration of 11-*cis*-retinoid, which is called the visual cycle. RPE65, a peripheral membrane protein of RPE cells, is an all-*trans*-retinyl ester isomerohydrolase. Indeed, we showed that RPE65 in bovine RPE is up-regulated under oxidative stress. Our data demonstrated that RPE65 is cleaved into a 45 kDa and 20 kDa truncation forms under oxidative stress. This data indicates that oxidative stress can influence the visual cycle by up-regulation of RPE65 and cleavage of this protein. Further studies of whether this truncated form might be a biomarker of oxidative stress are currently under investigation. It seems that immortalized human RPE cells suppress RPE65 expressions as a basic regulatory mechanism for the visual cycle that is not essential for survival. Prohibitin, a mitochondrial chaperone involved in oxidative stress and aging, was found to be downregulated under oxidative stress in primary bovine RPE cells.

Antioxidant proteins were upregulated under oxidative stress. Peroxiredoxin is a ubiquitous family of antioxidant enzymes that can be regulated by changes of redox potential in the cell. Thioredoxin-dependent peroxide reductase is an antioxidant enzyme that provides protection mechanism against oxidative stress. It reduces H_2O_2 by hydride provided by thioredoxin, thioredoxin reductase, and NADPH. Upregulation of antioxidants can regulate redox homeostasis in RPE cells and thus protect cells from oxidative stress-induced damage.

Both biological models using primary bovine RPE cells and immortalized D407 cells have advantages and limitations. We observed differences in protein expressions correlated with oxidative stress in two biological models used in our study, which can be attributed, at least partially, to the inherent differences in two different RPE cell types. It has been reported that cytoskeletal remodeling and cell survival factors are differentially expressed in primary culture and immortalized human RPE cells. Dedifferentiated, immortalized human RPE cells results in down-regulation of specific proteins associated with retinoid metabolism. At the same time, they induce the differential expressions related with cytoskeletal organization, cell shape, migration, and proliferation. Thus, we speculate that two different proteome list in two different systems such as primary bovine vs. immortalized human RPE cells is due to different cell type and not due to species difference or detection system.

Oxidative stress alone is the major risk factor of retinal degeneration compared to genetic risk factors. Furthermore, oxidative stress may influence the expression of genetic risk factor, such as complement factor H (CFH). Cellular processes induced by oxidative stress in RPE cells and the molecular mechanisms under the oxidative stress that contribute to retinal degeneration are not clear at this point. We revealed several expression changes in the RPE proteome that is induced by H_2O_2 treatment. Targeting early signaling proteins is a useful therapeutic strategy for the treatment of degenerative diseases of the retina and the RPE.

4. Prohibitin as a new oxidative stress biomarker

It is estimated that every ten minutes in the USA someone becomes blind. More than 4 million Americans have age-related macular degeneration (AMD), the most common cause of legal blindness in those older than fifty five. Even though the role of abnormal angiogenesis in the pathogenesis of AMD has been recently established, we still do not know why the macular deteriorates and why AMD progresses. Our proteomic experiments demonstrate that prohibitin is a shuttling protein primarily expressed in mitochondria, however, it translocalizes to the nucleus under oxidative stress. The extent of prohibitin localization in mitochondria inversely correlates with levels of oxidative stress. Our knockdown approach suggests that prohibitin may have the anti-apoptotic function through Bcl-xL and mitochondrial DNA binding mechanisms. Our data further suggests that specific lipid-binding mechanisms involving altered cardiolipin interactions might be the key element to determine prohibitin shuttling between mitochondria and the nucleus. Mitochondrial dysfunction is associated with AMD and our preliminary studies also suggest specific pathophysiological mechanisms involving altered mitochondrial disruption.

Prohibitin is involved in the alternative pathway of complement C activation. However, the regulatory mechanisms are elusive. Prohibitin is subjected to various post-translational modifications under growth factor stimulation and oxidative stress. Prohibitin induces a conformational change that enhances activation of C3.

Prohibitin is originally known as an anti-proliferative protein [McClung et al., 1989]. It is highly conserved from bacteria to human [Asamoto and Cohen SM, 1994], but its function is not clearly understood. Prohibitin was proposed to have a role as a cell cycle inhibitor [Nuell et al, 1991; McClung et al, 1995], a transcriptional regulator [Wang et al, 1999a; Wang et al, 1999b], an inflammatory modulator [Sharma and Qadri, 2004], a plasma membrane receptor [Kolonin et al, 2004], and a mitochondrial chaperone [Nijtmans et al, 2000; Artal-Sanz et al, 2003; Steglich et al, 1999]. Its chaperone function in mitochondria has recently received more attention as a modulator that responds to oxidative stress [Coates et al., 2001]. Prohibitin is involved in apoptosis and aging by stabilizing newly synthesized respiratory enzymes [Bourges et al, 2004; Nijtmans et al, 2002], however, its presence and function in the eye has never been studied. Our studies demonstrate that prohibitin is a novel protein that shuttles between mitochondria and the nucleus as an anti-apoptotic chaperone as well as a transcriptional regulator under oxidative stress [Arnouk, et al., 2011; Lee et al., 2010; Srinivas et al., 2011].

Prohibitin undergoes phosphorylation at multiple residues under various cellular condition or in response to various stimuli. Phosphorylation of prohibitin facilitate its interaction with SH2 domain containing phospho tyrosine phosphatases Shp1 and Shp2. In a separate study, prohibitin was identified as a substrate for Akt and it has been shown that Akt induced prohibitin phosphorylation at threonine258. While these studies have clearly shown that prohibitin is phosphorylated at multiple residues, however, conditions under which these residues are phosphorylated and functional consequences are not clear. Prohibitin binding proteins were apoptosis related (Bcl-2 like protein), cholesterol homeostasis (PI4K5, diacylglycerol kinase, apolipoprotein B48 receptor, VLDLR), nucleotide binding proteins (guanine exchange factor, endonuclease, cell cycle regulator) and a complement component (Table 2).

5. Anti-apoptotic prohibitin function in mitochondria

We performed loss of function studies using prohibitin-specific small interfering RNA (siRNA) to demonstrate an increase of apoptotic signaling when prohibitin was knockdown. We tested two siRNA constructs that inhibit prohibitin expression compared to a control siRNA that has a random sequence. A solvent vehicle was used as the second negative control also. We chose conditions when prohibitin expressions were reduced by 80-90% compared to random sequence control. We examined whether prohibitin knockdown activates pro-apoptotic AIF, BAK, and caspases. Prohibitin knockdown may control other anti-apoptotic molecules also. Indeed, pro-apoptotic AIF, caspase-9, and BAK increased under prohibitin knockdown condition whereas anti-apoptotic Bcl-xL decreased. Also we examined decreased prohibitin condition cleaves poly (ADP ribose) polymerase (PARP) as a

Prohibitin binding proteins	MW/pI	Function
Vav-1 guanine exchange factor	98 kDa/6.2	proto-oncogene
ATP binding cassette 4	66 kDa/6.9	regulator of cAMP level
DEAD box 32	84 kDa/5.0	RNA helicase
epithelial cell transforming 2	104 kDa/7.5	oncogene
guanine exchange factor	119 kDa/5.9	activation of GTPases
Transglutaminase	93 kDa/6.5	protein aggregation
phosphoinositol-4-phosphate 5 kinase	45 kDa/9.6	epithelial cell morphology actin polymerization
Nei Endonuclease VIII like protein 1	37 kDa/9.2	DNA excision repair
Bcl-2 like protein 14	37 kDa/7.7	apoptosis facilitator
calpastatin	76 kDa/4.9	calpain inhibitor
complement component C6	105 kDa/6.7	membrane complex
cell cycle regulator Mat89Bb homolog	80 kDa/6.2	nucleus-centrosome coupling
diacylglycerol kinase zeta	103 kDa/9.8	phosphatidic acid synthesis
Apolipoportein B48 receptor-like	109 kDa/4.4	carrying cholesterol to tissues
very low density lipoprotein receptor	93 kDa/4.7	regulator of cholesterol levels

Table 2. Prohibitin binding proteins determined by immunoprecipitation.

pro-apoptotic marker because PARP cleavage is an early marker of caspase activation. Transfection of siRNA of prohibitin into ARPE-19 cells resulted in increased cleavage of PARP which represents that an apoptotic signal is induced when prohibitin is down-regulated.

Next we examined whether caspases are also activated as essential markers in apoptosis. The activation of caspase-9, one of the upstream regulators in apoptosis, showed early apoptotic signaling under prohibitin knockdown condition. Our results suggest that knockdown of prohibitin increases caspase-dependent apoptotic signaling. This data implies that prohibitin may act as an anti-apoptotic protein in mitochondria by forming a functional complex with other apoptotic proteins. Prohibitin concentration is inversely correlated with the initiation of apoptosis. Then we asked whether decreased prohibitin disrupts the filamentous reticular network of mitochondria resulting in fragmented mitochondria. Immunocytochemical analysis showed that prohibitin knockdown led to accumulation of fragmented mitochondria. Then we asked whether expression and localization of prohibitin is altered under stress condition.

Emerging evidence suggest that oxidative stress and associated local upregulation of alternative pathway of complement may play a critical role in the progression of AMD. However, the link between oxidative stress. Altered prohibitin function may be a connecting link between oxidative stress and complement activation in AMD. Our studies demonstrate that prohibitin expression in the RPE is altered under oxidative stress *in vitro* and *in vivo*. We tested an advanced proteomic approach using a 2D differential gel electrophoresis (DIGE) technique to label RPE proteome by fluorescent molecules to uncover new biomarkers under stress conditions. We found that prohibitin is a chaperone molecule maintaining mitochondrial structure and function shown by immunoprecipitation and knockdown method.

We have been actively seeking early molecular signaling events under oxidative stress in the retina and RPE using a proteomics and metabolomics approach to identify new biomarkers. This approach demonstrated that prohibitin is involved in oxidative stress signaling *in vitro* and *in vivo* [Lee et al., 2010b; Arnouk et al., 2011; Srinivas et al., 2011]. Prohibitin was proposed as an anti-proliferative protein or a tumor suppressor forming a high molecular complex with prohibitin2 in mitochondria [Steglich et al., 1999]. Localization of prohibitin has been controversial, possibly being mitochondrial, nuclear, or cell surface [Wang et al., 2002; Rivera-Milla et al., 2006].

We examined the cellular localization of prohibitin which is a controversial question. Confluent ARPE19 cells were treated with 200 μM H_2O_2 for 24 hrs and prohibitin localization in response to oxidative stress was investigated using immunocytochemistry. Subcellular organelles and prohibitin were visualized by DAPI (nuclear DNA, blue, 369/460 nm absorbance/emission), MitoTracker (mitochondria, red, 578/599 nm absorbance/emission), and Alexa-488 (prohibitin, green, 495/519 nm absorbance/emission), by taking three color fluorescent images every hour. This kinetic assay confirmed that the signaling pathway was involved in prohibitin transit to the nucleus from mitochondria. H_2O_2 treated cells showed nuclear translocalization of prohibitin, whereas untreated cells showed localization in mitochondria. After 8 hrs, prohibitin showed an accumulation in the nucleus as compared to the control group. After 24 hrs, more nuclear prohibitin was observed and prohibitin didn't show as much colocalization with mitochondria.

To answer whether prohibitin is modified under stress condition, we tested the correlation between oxidative stress and the ratio of soluble vs. membrane-binding prohibitin. Because prohibitin may exist in both detergent-resistant and soluble fractions, we tried to separate prohibitins by longer running time SDS-PAGE. Soluble prohibitin in the cytosolic fraction moved faster when compared to membrane-bound mitochondrial and microsomal prohibitin. Detergent-resistant, membrane-binding prohibitin showed slightly higher molecular weight when compared to soluble prohibitin. We found that the ratio of soluble prohibitin to membrane binding prohibitin decreased under oxidative stress. Under stress condition, soluble prohibitin decreased and membrane-binding prohibitin increased. To answer how long this trend would last under oxidative stress, we performed a kinetic assay under oxidative stress. After 6 hrs, the soluble prohibitin level returned to its control level. It is possible that the membrane-binding and soluble form exists in different subcellular organelles, so we next examined the subcellular localization of prohibitin by fractionation.

Membrane-binding prohibitin showed slightly higher molecular weight when compared to soluble prohibitin. We examined the correlation between oxidative stress and soluble vs. membrane-binding prohibitin and found that the ratio of soluble prohibitin to membrane binding prohibitin decreased under oxidative stress. Soluble prohibitin decreased and membrane-binding prohibitin increased under stress condition. Then we tested how long this trend would last under oxidative stress. After 6 hrs, the soluble prohibitin level returned to its control level. It is possible that the membrane-binding and soluble form exists in different subcellular organelles, so we examined whether prohibitin binds a mitochondrial specific phospholipid, cardiolipin.

6. Prohibitin binds cardiolipin under oxidative stress

We asked whether prohibitin localization could be controlled by membrane lipid binding. We speculated that the localization and trafficking of prohibitin might be determined by mitochondrial-specific lipid such as cardiolipin. Lipid interaction assay demonstrated that mitochondrial prohibitin has a strong affinity at low cardiolipin concentration whereas nuclear prohibitin showed a much weaker affinity to cardiolipin, interacting at higher concentrations. Lipid analysis in ARPE-19 cells by mass spectrometry demonstrated that cardiolipin concentration decreased 20-70% under 200 μM H_2O_2.

This result suggests that membrane lipid and modification may determine prohibitin localization under oxidative stress. When cardiolipin concentration is low under oxidative stress, prohibitin moves to the nucleus. Then we tested whether prohibitin may have preference toward specific lipids when prohibitin is a limiting factor. Under normal condition, prohibitin from ARPE-19 cells demonstrated a strong interaction with phosphatidylinositol 3,4,5 triphosphate (PIP3), PIP2, PIP, and 3-sulfogalactosylceramide, but not with cardiolipin. Lipid binding affinity changed dramatically under oxidative stress. Prohibitin under stress showed a strong affinity toward cardiolipin, phosphatidylserine, and phosphatidic acid. This observation led us to conclude that prohibitin has an affinity towards negatively charged phospholipids, especially cardiolipin under oxidative stress.

To examine prohibitin response under oxidative stress in detail, we then examined protein expression level changes *in vitro* using ARPE-19 cells. We examined whether prohibitin level changes under H_2O_2 in time and dose dependent manner. Protein analysis by SDS-PAGE and Western blot demonstrated that prohibitin is down-regulated under oxidative stress (50-200 μM H_2O_2, 1-24 hrs). Cells treated with 200 μM H_2O_2 showed a 40% decrease of prohibitin, but the levels between treated groups in 24 hrs revealed no significant difference by t-test, indicating that decreased levels of prohibitin under oxidative stress is an acute process that occurs within 2 hrs. This result suggests that the nuclear prohibitin may not be a newly synthesized protein as there was no prohibitin increase for 24 hrs; instead the nuclear prohibitin might be derived from mitochondria since prohibitin was not colocalized with mitochondria after extended H_2O_2 treatment.

Our previous *in vivo* experiments suggest that prohibitin may respond differently in the retina and RPE under oxidative stress conditions, including diabetes and aging. To specify the location of prohibitin in cells, we separated subcellular fractions using serial centrifugations, specific detergents, and polyamines. Subcellular proteins were separated into soluble and insoluble nuclear and mitochondrial proteins as well as cytosolic and microsomal fractions. Denatured and native gel electrophoresis, followed by Western blot of subcellular organelle showed that prohibitin is widely distributed in cells but is centralized in mitochondria.

In mitochondrial fraction, prohibitin showed 32 kDa molecular weight and pI=5.6 as expected. Prohibitin was more acidic in the nucleus showing pI=5.3, possibly due to post-translational modifications such as phosphorylation. Mass spectrometry analysis revealed that S101 and S151 sites are phosphorylated. Cytosolic prohibitin showed very basic spots of pI=6-7 and higher molecular weight as shown in the box.

As each subcellular prohibitin showed different pI values in 2D electrophoresis, we examined potential post-translational modifications, including phosphorylation. Each fraction was separated by electrophoresis and prohibitin was visualized by Western blot using prohibitin and phospho-serine (pSer) antibodies. Only the nuclear fraction showed phosphorylated prohibitin shown by pSer Western blot. Mitochondrial, cytosolic, and microsomal prohibitin did not show phosphorylation. To confirm this data, we performed native gel electrophoresis and received the same result.

7. Neuroprotective erythropoietin (EPO)

Apoptosis is the primary mechanism that results in the abnormal death of photoreceptors, retinal ganglion cells (RGC), or retinal pigment epithelial cells (RPE) in degenerative retinal diseases, including age-related macular degeneration (AMD), retinitis pigmentosa (RP), and glaucoma. Light insults result in increased production of reactive oxygen and nitrogen species that include hydrogen peroxide and nitric oxide, which are involved in an early event of retinal degeneration. In response to intense or constant light triggers, neuroprotective proteins provide an antiapoptotic effect to protect retinal and retinal pigment epithelial (RPE) cells, however, the mechanisms remain elusive. Thus there is a critical need for understanding the intrinsic neuroprotective mechanisms that prevents apoptotic cell death. Our studies suggest that potential degeneration signaling may result from expression changes and phosphorylations of key proteins of EPO downstream. EPO down-regulates caspases and intense light up-regulates caspases, which imply that depleting EPO is one of the major light effects that can cause changes in protein expression through anti-apoptotic mechanisms.

We demonstrated that the retinal expression of EPO and subsequent phosphorylation of Jak2 and Stat3 are tightly linked to the circadian clock after oxidative stress and in anticipation of daily light onset. Our data suggest that the neuroprotective effects of EPO might be involved the regulation of apoptotic signaling molecules, including Bcl-xL, and caspase-3. In the RPE, NO was proposed as a secondary messenger in phagocytosis. Interdependent regulation of NO and EPO has not been examined, even though recent studies imply potential interactions of NO-EPO through the Hif1a pathway.

Retinal injury due to light occurs through oxidative mechanisms. Recently we demonstrated that the recycling reactions of 11-*cis*-retinal, called the visual cycle, is circadian coordinated to effectively protect the retina from the detrimental effects of light-induced and oxygen-dependent damage [Chung et al., 2009, Lee et al., 2010a]. Our data suggested that the retinal expression of EPO and its receptor (EPOR), as well as subsequent Janus kinase 2 (Jak2) phosphorylations, are tightly linked to a time window after oxidative stress and in anticipation of daily light onset. This is consistent with physiological protection against daily light-induced, oxidative mediated apoptosis [Hardeland et al., 2003; Hrushesky 1985; Scheving et al., 1988; Smaaland et al., 1991; Smaaland et al., 1992].

We found that nitric oxide (NO) was generated in RPE cells under light exposure. NO is related to the inhibition of ischemic injury and plays a key role in the delayed cell death following transient retinal ischemia. Thus, NO is proposed as a neuroprotective molecule or neurotoxic reagent based on its local concentration. In the RPE, NO was proposed as a second messenger in phagocytosis. Interdependent regulation of nitric oxide and EPO has not been examined, even though recent studies imply potential interactions of NO-EPO through either HIF1a or arginine metabolism. Appropriate levels of nitric oxide (NO) may cause up-regulation of EPO/EPOR in RPE and thereby assist in limiting retinal degeneration.

EPO has been extensively studied for its neuroprotective role for the past 10 years, but the regulation mechanisms have not been understood at the molecular level [Brines and Cerami, 2005; Calapai et al., 2000; Jelkmann 2007; Kanaan et al., 2006; Kawakami et al., 2001; Li et al., 2007; Mauer 1965; Miyake et al., 1977; Yamaji et al., 1996; Zhong et al., 2007]. Previous approaches using the *in vivo* mice model was not satisfactory, because the EPO knockout mice model is lethal. No approach to date has been effective in moving beyond the addition of EPO *in vitro* and *in vivo*.

The *in vivo* erythropoietic effects of administered EPO are known to depend upon the time of administration [Wood et al, 1998; Bellamy et al., 1988]. Moreover, elevated EPO levels during the proliferative stage may contribute to neovascularization and accelerate pathological angiogenesis, in which EPO showed little therapeutic effect at later stages of retinopathy [Chen et al., 2008]. Light kills retinal cells. In response to light, neuroprotective proteins trigger an anti-apoptotic pathway in the retina to protect cells from light-induced oxidative stress. However, the mechanism that regulates expression of these retinal proteins remains elusive.

Erythropoietin (EPO) is an oxygen-dependent hematopoietic cytokine that stimulates the proliferation, differentiation, and survival of erythroid progenitor cells. EPO protects cells from neuronal damage, including experimental central nervous system models of hypoxic and ischemic insults [Jelkmann and Metzen, 1996; Jelkmann, 2005]. Oxygen dependent mechanisms are derived from models such as traumatic brain injury [Brines et al., 2000], spinal cord injury [Celik et al., 2002], Parkinson's disease [Kanaan et al., 2006], excitotoxicity [Kawakami et al., 2001; Morishita et al., 1997], oxidative stress [Calapai et al., 2000] and chemical neurotoxicity [Genc et al., 2001]. EPO can protect retinal ganglion cells (RGCs) from degeneration induced by acute ischemia reperfusion injury [Liu XT et al., 2006] and axotomy injury [Weishaupt et al., 2004].

EPO promotes survival of RGCs in a glaucoma mouse model [Zhong et al., 2007], and stimulates neurogenesis and post-stroke recovery [Tsai et al., 2006]. *In vitro* models reveal that EPO stimulates neuritic outgrowth by postnatal [Böcker-Meffert et al., 2002] and adult RGCs [Kretz et al., 2005]. EPO is produced in the retina in response to acute hypoxia via Hif-1α stabilization, which confers protection from light-induced retinal degeneration [Grimm et al., 2002]. The specific role of EPO was emphasized in that only EPO gene expression was significantly affected among various angiogenic factors in Hif-1a-Like Factor (HLF) knockdown model [Morita et al., 2003].

However, controversial discussions of EPO in retinal neuroprotection exist. Understanding EPO function in pathological angiogenesis is critical to timing for intervention [Chen et al., 2008]. Our studies demonstrated that EPO and EPOR interactions represent an important retinal shield from physiologic and pathologic light-induced oxidative injury.

To test the hypothesis that EPO is regulated by light *in vivo*, retinas from mice subjected to normal 12 h light/dark cycle were accessed for EPO and EPOR protein content. Retinal EPO increased for 2 h after the light turned on and gradually declined in the late light phase. However, 2 h before the light returned, EPO increased. The 24 h pattern of EPOR followed a similar pattern to EPO. This result suggests that the endogenous circadian clock may regulate EPO and EPOR levels such that they increase just before light onset in anticipation of the daily light period (L/D 22 h). However, under constant dark condition (D/D 22 h), EPO/EPOR were not upregulated.

Our data demonstrated that the circadian organization of retinal EPO and EPOR elaboration is a potentially effective endogenous physiologic strategy for retinal protection from light-induced, oxygen-mediated damage. These findings are consistent with documented circadian regulation of the full range of oxidative damage protecting enzymes or antioxidants, including glutathione (GSH/GSSG).

Then, we tested the hypothesis that oxidative stress, including intense light, hypoxia, and hyperoxia, may induce EPO response in the retina *in vitro*. As early as 15 min after light exposure in retinal cells, EPO expression increased. Immunoblots showed that expressions of EPO increased 1 h after exposure to hypoxia and hyperoxia. In retinal and RPE cells, cells appeared morphologically viable, and no cell death was noticed for 6 hrs under hypoxic and hyperoxic conditions. Under oxidative stress, upregulation of EPO confers a neuroprotective function against retinal degeneration. Our aim was to explicate the role of the light and oxidative stress in the control of neuroprotective EPO expression in the retina and RPE.

We treated EPO (50-200 U) on rat retinal cells and human RPE cells *in vitro* under oxidative stress to examine its protective effect. EPO inhibited caspase-3 activation in retinal cells under stress, indicating that EPO is anti-apoptotic.

As an endpoint analysis, we performed a cell viability assay using a rat retina and human primary RPE cell culture treated with H_2O_2 as an oxidative stress model for a control experiment. At a concentration of 20 μM or higher for 3 hrs, H_2O_2 exerted significant toxicity to retinal cell cultures. H_2O_2-induced retinal cell death was reduced to 40, 46, or 43 %, respectively, by 30 min pretreatment of 50 units of EPO with 40 μM H_2O_2 for 6, 12, and 24 hrs. In contrast, only a mild protective effect (15%) was observed in the RPE exposed to H_2O_2 by EPO treatment in 24 hrs.

To see the protective effect in the RPE, a high dose of EPO (up to 200 U) was required, and was found mildly toxic to the RPE cells. Phase-contrast photomicrographs showed that no significant cell death occurred in sham-washed control or treated human RPE cells with 400 μM H_2O_2 for 12 h. Cell viability was assessed by the amount of lactate dehydrogenase (LDH) release measured from the medium of RPE cultures exposed to H_2O_2 for 3, 6, 12, and 24 hrs.

EPO is a powerful cytoprotective protein against apoptosis. However, elevated levels of EPO are found in the vitreous due to proliferative diabetic retinopathy [Katsura et al., 2005; Watanabe et al., 2005]. In addition, high dose of EPO increased the risk of cardiovascular disease and tumor growth [Singh et al., 2006; Bohlius et al., 2006].

These studies suggest a role of EPO in pathological retinal angiogenesis. The effects of EPO on angiogenesis are not well understood and the role of EPO in vascular stability is not clear. Understanding the functional role of EPO on angiogenesis is beneficial to patients with diabetic retinopathy (DR) and retinopathy of prematurity (ROP). EPO has been known to promote endothelial cell proliferation and vessel growth, however, the influence of EPO on apoptotic signaling and retinopathy is beginning to be understood. To determine the effects of EPO on vessel growth, we explored downstream regulators of EPO under normal physiological condition. VEGFR1 and angiotensin I/II as two major angiogenic factors were examined. VEGFR1 in the retina and angiotensin I/II in RPE increased after EPO treatment (100 U) in 6-12 h, respectively.

Our study suggests that the role of EPO in the development of initial vessel loss via VEGF/VEGFR/angiotensin signaling. This signaling is important in understanding retinal vessel loss that is initiated prior to neovascularization. The initial vessel loss determines the severity of neovascularization. VEGF was downregulated upon EPO knockdown in RPE cells, which may suggest that EPO and VEGF expression is regulated in parallel, and they may interact directly or indirectly.

EPO induces the proangiogenic phenotype in rat retina and human RPE cells. Addition of EPO correlates with the progression of VEGFR and AngiotensinI/II, which suggests that EPO might be an endogenous stimulant of vessel growth during retinal angiogenesis and in the development of neovascularization. Possibly, EPO mediates the renin-angiotensin system (RAS) which may promote neovascularization through local changes in blood flow and production of VEGF. EPO is considered as a proinflammatory agent since it triggers the expression of angiotensin I/II, which may act as an inflammatory agent by enhancing vascular permeability through VEGF. We examined whether the EPO-dependent pathway is up-regulated or down-regulated in various oxygen-imbalance conditions. Along with increased levels of EPO after light exposure, levels of rhodopsin in retinal cells increased as early as 15 min after 5000 lux light exposure in a time-dependent manner. RPE65 cleavage increased after 15 min exposure to 5000 lux light in the RPE. Immunoblots for Bcl-xL and c-Fos showed that the neuroprotective effects of EPO may involve upregulation of these early markers in stress-induced condition. Anti-apoptotic Bcl-xL and c-Fos were also up-regulated in the light. EPO-mediated neuroprotective effects attribute to interaction with Jak2, Bcl-xL, and c-Fos. Other downstream regulators such as Stat3 might be required for anti-apoptotic Bcl-xL induction as shown in the motor neuron [Schweizer et al, 2002]. Jak2 and Stat3 phosphorylations in retinal and RPE cells increased under hypoxia, hyperoxia, and light exposure.

Proangiogenic protein VEGF is up-regulated under hypoxic conditions in the retina and the RPE. Our data demonstrated that EPO and VEGF expressions are regulated in parallel, and they may interact directly or indirectly. We will test our hypothesis that pro-angiogenic signaling of VEGF regulated by EPO.

EPO and EPOR had a similar pattern of distribution in both neurons and astrocytes. Within 3 hrs after exposure to hypoxia, expression of EPO and EPOR in various retinal cells increased. The number of co-localized cells with EPO/EPOR with retinal cell markers also increased in 1% O_2 hypoxic condition. Relative levels of EPO mRNA were determined by real time-PCR in hypoxia. An elevated EPO level was detected after exposure of primary retinal cells to hypoxia (1% O_2) with 6-fold up-regulation after 12 h. We observed intense light induced up-regulation of c-Fos, Bcl-xL, thioredoxin pJak2, pSTAT3 in early passage of human RPE cells. Rat retina cells under bright light up-regulated pJak2, EPO, and EPOR in an hour. pJak2 and pStat3 in the RPE increased in hypoxic condition (1% O_2). Phosphorylation of Jak2 and Stat3 was confirmed as shown by phospho-Western blot. As an upstream regulator of EPO, HIF-1a was examined. HIF-1a increased in light, hyperoxic, and hypoxic conditions.

8. Cytoskeletal reorganization under oxidative stress

Not only intense light but also constant moderate light may trigger induction of anti-apoptotic Bcl-xL, EPO, and pro-apoptotic caspases. We postulate that light may induce post-translational modifications of target proteins. Previously, we identified that serine/threonine protein phosphatase 2A (PP2A) is induced and modified under constant light *in vivo*.

To our knowledge, protein nitration mechanism under various oxidative environmental conditions, including intense light and continuous light, has never been studied in retinal cell cultures, RPE cells, or mouse model system. Our contribution here is expected to be a detailed understanding of how PP2A modification of a subunit is regulated by endogenous signaling molecule, nitric oxide (NO). PP2A and vimentin might be critically involved in the process of light-induced retinal and RPE cell damage. It is expected that what is learned will be equally applicable to anti-apoptotic mechanism. In addition, the research will be of significance because what is learned will contribute to broader understanding of how other phosphatase activity can be modulated as an approach to therapy.

Although the potential importance of protein dephosphorylation as a therapeutic target has been appreciated, no detailed approach has been made targeting PP2A. Abnormalities in PP2A activity and concentrations have been linked to neurodegenerative diseases, including Alzheimer's and Parkinson's. The mechanism by which PP2A activity is regulated under oxidative stress remains largely elusive. Despite recent advances on structural investigation of PP2A, comprehensive understanding of dephosphorylation mechanism is far from complete.

Our data suggests that PP2A and vimentin are critically involved in the process of light-induced damage in the retina and RPE. By modulation of light-induced post-translational modifications of PP2A, vimentin may assist in maintaining the proper filament network in Müller cells, which subsequently supports neuronal survival and architecture in the retina. Dephosphorylation switch by tyrosine nitration will provide new targets for therapeutic interactions in apoptosis-mediated disorders.

Light-induced photoreceptor damage depends on the functional visual cycle, a biochemical regeneration of 11-*cis*-retinal chromophore. The induction of light damage depends on the light condition; acute damage by intense light requires rhodopsin bleaching, whereas constant moderate light involves phototransduction. Recently we showed that the visual cycle is coordinated in a circadian manner as a means of effectively protecting the retina from the detrimental effects of light-induced, oxygen-dependent, free-radical-mediated damage, especially at the times of day when light is more intense [Chung et al, 2009]. RPE65 defects are known to trigger a remodeling of the retina that disrupt photoreceptor homeostasis and induce an apoptotic cascade causing retinal degeneration [Grimm et al., 2000; Wenzel et al., 2005]. As a downstream signal of light-induced signaling, anti-apoptotic proteins, including erythropoietin (EPO) and subsequent Janus kinase 2 (Jak2) phosphorylations, are tightly linked to a specific temporal period after oxidative stress and in anticipation of daily light onset. This is consistent with physiological protection against daily light-induced, oxidative mediated retinal apoptosis [Noell et al., 1966; Chung et al, 2009]. Continuous exposure to bright light (5000 lux) within 60 minutes induced apoptosis in retinal cells by activating caspase-3 signals. This suggests that endogenous neuroprotective proteins may not be sufficient in such intense oxidative stress conditions. Thus, we are seeking to define effective endogenous physiological neuroprotective strategies for anti-apoptosis from light-induced, oxygen-mediated damages that have clinical relevance.

The expression levels of a scaffold subunit of PP2Aa and vimentin are significantly increased when mice are exposed under continuous light for 7 days compared to control in rd 1 degeneration model [Zhang et al., 2010]. When melatonin is administered to animals while they are exposed to continuous light, the levels of vimentin and PP2A return to a normal level. Vimentin is a PP2A target of direct dephosphorylation. Vimentin is present in all mesenchymal cells and often used as a differentiation marker. Like other intermediate filaments, vimentin acts to maintain cellular integrity; further, vimentin may play a role in adhesion, migration, and cellular survival in the RPE. We demonstrated that bright light up-regulates pro-apoptotic signaling by cleavage of caspase-3 and Bcl-xL [Chung et al., 2009].

Exposure to continuous light at intensities ordinarily encountered during daytime causes retinal degeneration. How constant light induces retinal degeneration remains unknown, although potential mechanisms have been proposed, including defects in rhodopsin regeneration, accumulation of free radicals, and a continuous low level of Ca^{2+} resulting from an excessively active phototransduction cascade.

We examined the impact of constant light-exposed proteome changes *in vivo*. We exposed mice to either light (250-300 lux) for 12 hours followed by 12 hours of darkness or the same intensity of continuous light for seven days. Two proteins up-regulated by continuous light were identified as PP2A and vimentin by mass spectrometry. We examined cytoskeletal proteins as potential substrates of PP2A. Cytoskeletal filament proteins were upregulated under constant light condition *in vivo*. Neurofilament, intermediate filament vimentin, tubulin, and actin increased in different levels under constant light exposure. The cytoskeletal target proteins were further analyzed by mass spectrometry to determine their modifications. Site-specific nitration and phosphorylations were found in PP2A and filament proteins.

Protein	Site	Modification
PP2Aa	Y169	nitration
Actin b cytoplasmic 1	T186	phosphorylation
Tubulin b 2B	Y50, Y51, T55	phosphorylation
Tubulin b 5	Y159	nitration
Tubulin b 5	S168, S172	phosphorylation
Vimentin	Y38, S325 ,S412, S420	phosphorylation

Table 3. Modifications of PP2A and filament proteins under constant light *in vivo*

Vimentin is a major component of intermediate filament that spread throughout the cell and serve as signal transducer conveying mechanical and molecular information from cell surface to nucleus and intracellular compartments. Neuronal cytoskeleton is a potential therapeutic target in neurodegenerative diseases. Vimentin phosphorylations were further analyzed by 2D electrophoresis with narrow range of pI for higher resolution. Vimentin phosphorylation decreased under constant light *in vivo*. Modifications of vimentin are essential reactions of filament dynamics. Changes of vimentin phosphorylation are directed to reorganization of the intermediate filament network and altered function of Müller cells.

Hyperphosphorylation of vimentin can disassemble intermediate filament into soluble monomeric form. Müller cells are the major glial cells in the retina and play crucial roles in maintaining neuroretinal architecture and support neuronal survival. Our results suggest that vimentin and Müller cells might be critically involved in the process of light-induced damage in the retina. By reducing the light-induced post-translational modification of vimentin, PP2A may assist to maintain the proper filament network in Müller cells, which subsequently supports neuronal survival and architecture in the retina. To test changes of PP2A and cytoskeletal proteins in RPE *in vitro*, we examined ARPE-19 cells under stress condition. When RPE cells were under oxidative stress (100-250 μM H_2O_2), a catalytic subunit PP2Ac was initially upregulated, then decreased in time and dose dependent manner.

A decrease in cytoskeletal protein turnover leads to the accumulation of large aggregates of actin and tubulin, which triggers an increase in the levels of reactive oxygen species (ROS). Dynamic and differential changes in the cytoskeleton occur in apoptotic cellular processes. Thus, we ask how phosphorylation of vimentin regulates cytoskeletal dynamics and cell survival under stress conditions in RPE. We hypothesize that the modifications of PP2A and vimentin influence the cytoskeletal network through interplay with other cytoskeletal proteins. A stabilized vimentin may act as an antiapoptotic agent when cells are under stress.

Methylation and phosphorylation of PP2A catalytic c subunit are evolutionary conserved mechanisms that critically control the PP2A holoenzyme assembly and substrate specificity. However, interplay of PP2A nitration and phosphorylation that may control subunit binding has never been studied.

Regulation of tyrosine nitration could be a potential intervention of early stage light-induced ocular diseases. We postulate, on the basis of our data, that modifications of PP2A and vimentin influence the cytoskeletal network through interplay with other cytoskeletal proteins, including tubulin and actin. A positive correlation between the levels of PP2A and vimentin under light-induced stress suggests that cytoskeletal dynamics is regulated by dephosphorylation of vimentin as a PP2A substrate.

To examine PP2A and cytoskeletal proteins under oxidative stress, we examined light-induced cytoskeletal changes using ARPE-19 cells. ARPE-19 contains retinal G-protein receptors (RGR) and peropsin as light detecting chromophores. The assembly of the major cytoskeleton proteins, including vimentin, tubulin and actin, are highly interdependent. Thus, we investigated β-tubulin and the interplay of vimentin dynamics with microtubules under light. Tubulin is a highly concentrated building block (10–20 μM) of microtubules. β-tubulin is aggregated as shown by particles (white arrow) under intense light (Figure 5). b-tubulin is colocalized with mitochondria in dark, but changed localization under light condition. Confluent ARPE-19 cells were treated with either dark or 7000 lux white light for 2 hr. Mitochondria was stained by 100 nM MitoTracker Orange. β-tubulin was visualized by Alexa 488 secondary antibody and the nucleus was stained by DAPI. To follow vimentin-tubulin interaction changes in light, we analyzed tubulin polymerization rates and vimentin-tubulin colocalization. β-tubulin is a major component of the microtubule and also an essential component of the cytoskeleton. They play a critical role in cell division and cell motility. Our results demonstrated that actin filament also aggregated in cytosol under intense light condition in RPE. In the dark, β-actin is localized in cytosol, but in light β-actin is aggregated outside of mitochondria. Light-induced modification of cytoskeletal proteins may imply a potential regulatory mechanism in apoptosis. Direct interaction between vimentin and actin has been observed [Esue et al., 2006]. The tail domain of vimentin intermediate filaments interacts directly with actin, which may regulate cytoskeletal crosstalk. Morphologic change and cytoskeletal reorganization of RPE cells were observed under oxidative stress *in vitro*.

9. The visual cycle

The steady-state of retinoid concentration and photosensitivity are controlled by the biosynthetic pathway leading to 11-*cis*-retinal regeneration, which is called the visual cycle. For continued vision, 11-*cis*-retinoid must be regenerated by a series of enzymes, including retinol dehydrogenases (RDHs), lecithin retinol acyltransferase (LRAT), and RPE65 [Saari 2000; Rando 2001; Jahng et al 2002; Jahng et al., 2003a; Jahng 2003b; Bok et al., 2003; Xue et al., 2004; Xue et al., 2006] (Figure 1).

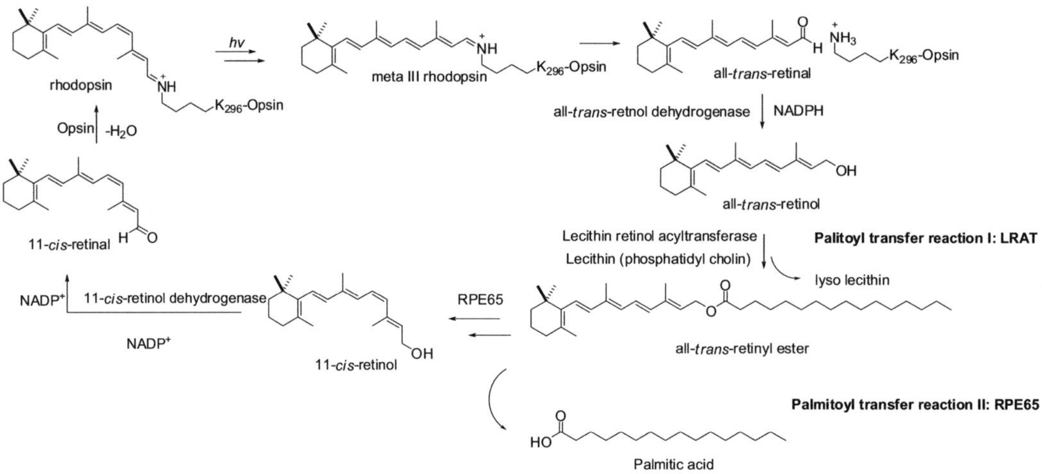

Figure 1. Biochemical reactions in the visual cycle and two palmitoylation transfer steps.

RPE is susceptible to oxidative stress due to its high oxygen consumption, the generation of reactive oxygen species (ROS), the presence of a high percentage of unsaturated fatty acids, and exposure to light [Bok, 1993; Strauss, 2005]. RPE65, a peripheral membrane protein of RPE cells, is thought to be an all-*trans*-retinyl ester isomerohydrolase [Moiseyev et al, 2005; Jin et al, 2005; Redmond et al, 2005]. In conjunction with other proteins, it isomerizes all-*trans*-retinyl ester and hydrolyzes it into 11-*cis*-retinol, the immediate precursor to 11-*cis*-retinal Schiff base chromophore which is enzymatically regenerated in the RPE. RPE65 was originally identified as the putative RPE membrane receptor for the plasma retinol-binding protein, and later shown to be a retinoid binding protein with high affinity toward all-*trans*-retinyl palmitate [Hooks et al, 1989; Bavik et al, 1991; Bavik et al, 1992; Bavik et al, 1993; Hamel et al, 1993a; Hamel et al, 1993b; Tsilou et al, 1997; Ma et al., 2001; Jahng et al., 2003a; Gollapalli et al, 2003; Mata et al, 2004; Xue et al, 2004]. It is homologous to beta-carotene monooxygenase [Kloer et al., 2005].

RPE contains anti-apoptotic and neuroprotective factors to support retina survival and maintenance. With aging, an imbalance occurs between ROS production and the capacity for detoxification resulting in the accumulation of ROS and the diminution of mitochondrial respiratory function. These ROS may contribute to the development of eye diseases such as cataract [Spector, 1995], uveitis [Satici et al, 2003; Bosch-Morell et al, 2002], glaucoma [Osborne et al, 1999; Babizhayev et al, 1989], retinopathy of prematurity [Dani et al, 2004; Head 1999], AMD [Beatty et al, 2000; Spraul 1996], and diabetic retinopathy [Kowluru et al, 1994]. Thus, understanding the mechanism of elevated ROS during aerobic metabolism and the resulting oxidative stress is important to the treatment of eye diseases. Under sub-lethal conditions of oxidative stress, mitochondrial respiratory function is impaired by electron leakage [Yakes and Van Houten, 1997; Melov et al, 1999] leading to decreased ATP production. Moreover, elevated ROS induce mutations in mitochondrial DNA, oxidative damage to cellular macromolecules forming cross-linked aggregates, and accumulation of damaged proteins [Grune et al, 1997].

Several mutations in the *RPE65* gene have been shown to be associated with retinal degenerations, including autosomal recessive childhood-onset severe retinal dystrophy, Leber's congenital amaurosis (LCA), and retinitis pigmentosa [Gu et al., 1997; Chen et al., 2006; Cottet et al., 2006; Hamel et al., 2001; Travis et al., 2007; Felius et al., 2002]. The RPE65 L450M mutant is associated with the reduced concentration of A2E lipofuscin [Kim et al., 2004]. RPE65 is essential for 11-*cis*-retinol biosynthesis *in vivo* and *in vitro* [Redmond et al., 1998; Nicolaeva et al., 2009]. Studies using RPE65 knockout mice demonstrate the importance of RPE65 in 11-*cis*-retinal biosynthesis *in vivo* [Redmond et al, 1998]. The synthesis of 11-*cis*-retinal is eliminated in these mice, while all-*trans*-retinyl esters accumulate as oil droplets in RPE cells. The control elements that regulate the overall biosynthetic pathway to 11-*cis*-retinal under light and oxidative stress are not known. Furthermore, connection between the visual cycle and resulting redox imbalance is in question.

In 1989, Rando proposed that RPE membranes might be the energy source for isomerization of all-*trans*-retinyl ester to 11-*cis*-retinol [Deigner et al., 1989]. In his hypothesis, the free energy of hydrolysis of the retinyl ester is coupled to the endothermic *trans* to *cis* isomerization. However, there are series of questions inlcuding; 1) C11 position is not nucleophilic and palmitate is not a good leaving group; 2) isomerization of the conjugated double bond of the retinoid cannot be explained in this mechanism. In 1999, Palczewsky proposed a carbocation intermediate mechanism [Stecher et al., 1999]. They suggested that the regeneration of 11-*cis* retinal might occur through a retinyl carbocation based on the observation of inhibition by positively charged retinoid as transition state analog. Both hypotheses do not explain the 11-*cis*-specific isomerization reaction of conjugated double bonds. Rather, singlet oxygen may bind to iron (Fe^{2+}) in the active site of RPE65 and catalyze C11 specific isomerization through oxygen radical-mediated epoxide intermediate as shown in Figure 2.

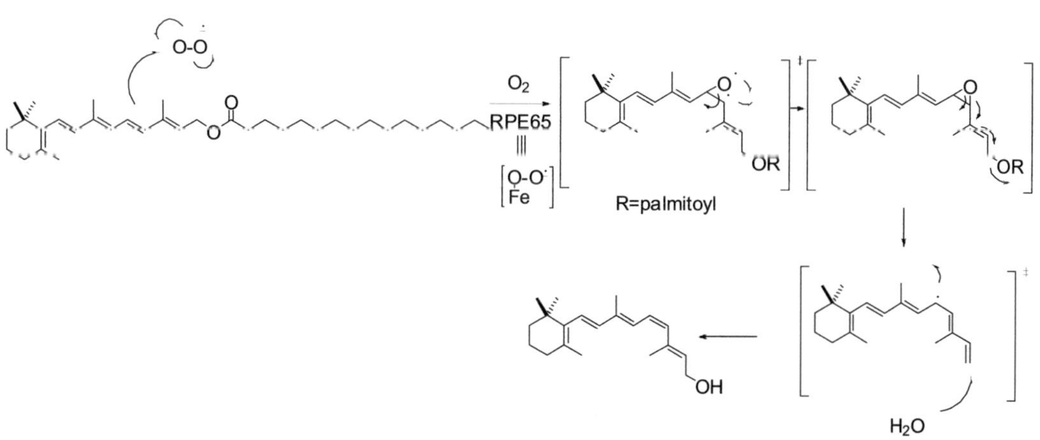

Figure 2. Putative Retinoid Isomerization Mechanism

Recently, we found that levels of RPE65 and RPE45, as a truncated form of RPE65, increased after short-term exposure to intense or constant light in the human RPE cultures [Chung et al., 2009; Lee et al., 2010a]. Also, the level of RPE45 is present in cells exposed to high oxidative stress *in vitro* and *in vivo* [Lee et al., 2010a]. We further suggest that the RPE45 fragment may be generated via ubiquitination involving interaction of specific proteases with RPE65. We also identified that retinaldehyde binding protein (CRALBP1) in the Müller cell showed a reversal of expression under constant light after melatonin treatment compared to constant light only condition (light vs. light+melatonin) [Zhang et al., 2010). Light-induced CRALBP1 may accelerate the retinal damage through higher rate of the visual cycle.

Interestingly, C57BL/6 mice have a gene polymorphism (M450) associated with lower level of RPE65 expression and reduced light-damage sensitivity. We observed a higher threshold for RPE45 appearance when RPE cells were exposed to light and oxidative stress simultaneously compared to cells under oxidative stress alone, suggesting that the protective mechanism may exist to maintain RPE65 concentration under light-induced oxidative stress.

We examined the appearance of RPE45 and RPE20 fragments *in vitro* with different amounts of H_2O_2 (100, 300, 500 and 1000 μM) in order to mimic different levels of oxidative stress on bovine RPE cells. As expected, RPE45 and RPE20 were produced in a dose-dependent manner after H_2O_2 treatment.

To address the functional significance of RPE45, we tested the ability of the RPE45 fragment to bind biotinylated all-*trans*-retinyl chloroacetate (BRCA), an all-*trans* retinyl ester analog used to investigate the retinoid-binding roles of RPE proteins. In this experiment, RPE proteins from bovine RPE cells were incubated with BRCA 50 μM/100 mg RPE proteins and separated by SDS-PAGE. BRCA-labeled proteins were visualized using an avidin-peroxidase antibody and an anti-RPE65 peptide antibody. BRCA-labeled RPE65, RPE45 and LRAT were confirmed by electrospray tandem mass spectrometry and Western-blot analyses, demonstrating that RPE45 binds this all-*trans*-retinyl ester analog.

A defect in RPE65 can trigger a remodeling of the retina that may disrupt photoreceptor homeostasis and induce apoptosis cascades leading to retinal degeneration [Shang and Taylor, 2004]. Light influences the translocation of transducin, arrestin, and recoverin; tyrosinase-mediated light adaptation, and the synthesis of retinoic acid and melatonin. Our studies indicate that oxidative stress and light exposure can influence the visual cycle. The dose-dependent induction of RPE45, a fragment of RPE65 generated in response to H_2O_2 or light exposure by a specific caspase-mediated cleavage suggests that RPE45 is a potential signaling molecule of oxidative stress- and light-induced apoptosis [Chung et al., 2009; Lee et al., 2010a]. Proteolysis after stress is an important signal transduction pathway mediated by caspases, presenilin, and amyloid precursor protein, which can lead to neurodegenerative disorder or inflammation [Martinon and Tschopp 2004; Shi 2004; Haass and Strooper 1999]. We also observed up-regulation of NF-kB and amyloid beta in the RPE under oxidative stress. RPE65 is known as highly uveitogenic and antigenic protein implying involvement in pathogenic autoimmune diseases in the eye [Ham et al, 2002]. Changes in RPE65 expression are also seen *in vivo* during cycles of light and dark and may be mediated by light cues.

In nature, all biochemical reactions are dependent on the coupling of the free energy changes of phosphate- (ATP), thio- (CoA), and oxy- (membrane lipids) esters. For all-*trans*-retinyl ester isomerization/hydrolysis biochemical reactions catalyzed by RPE65, palmitoyl transfer reaction should be coupled with retinyl ester isomerization and retinyl ester hydrolysis energetically and chemically.

We suggest that RPE45 may result from degradation of RPE65 by ROS-induced proteases [Budihardjo et al., 1999; Santoro et al., 1998]. It is likely that RPE cells have a defense mechanism against oxidative stress and we therefore investigated the expression of anti-apoptotic factors in oxidative stress. We found that anti-apoptotic Bcl-xL was increased under intense light [Chung et al., 2009]. The positive correlation between the expression of these anti-apoptotic factors and RPE65 under oxidative stress suggests that RPE65 may have a positive role in apoptotic signaling. Proteolysis after stress is an important signal transduction mediated by caspases, presenilin, and amyloid precursor protein, which can lead to neurological disorder or inflammation in the retina and brain [Martinon and Tschopp 2004, Shi 2004, Haass and Strooper 1999]. RPE65 is known as highly uveitogenic protein implying involvement in pathogenic autoimmune disease in the eye [Ham et al. 2002]. Under oxidative stress, aged cells increase the number of mitochondria and induce anti-oxidant genes [Sitte et al, 2000; Lee et al, 2000]. Retinoid map in the retina and the RPE is shown in Figure 3. Potential target sites to regulate retinoid and A2E are shown in red bars.

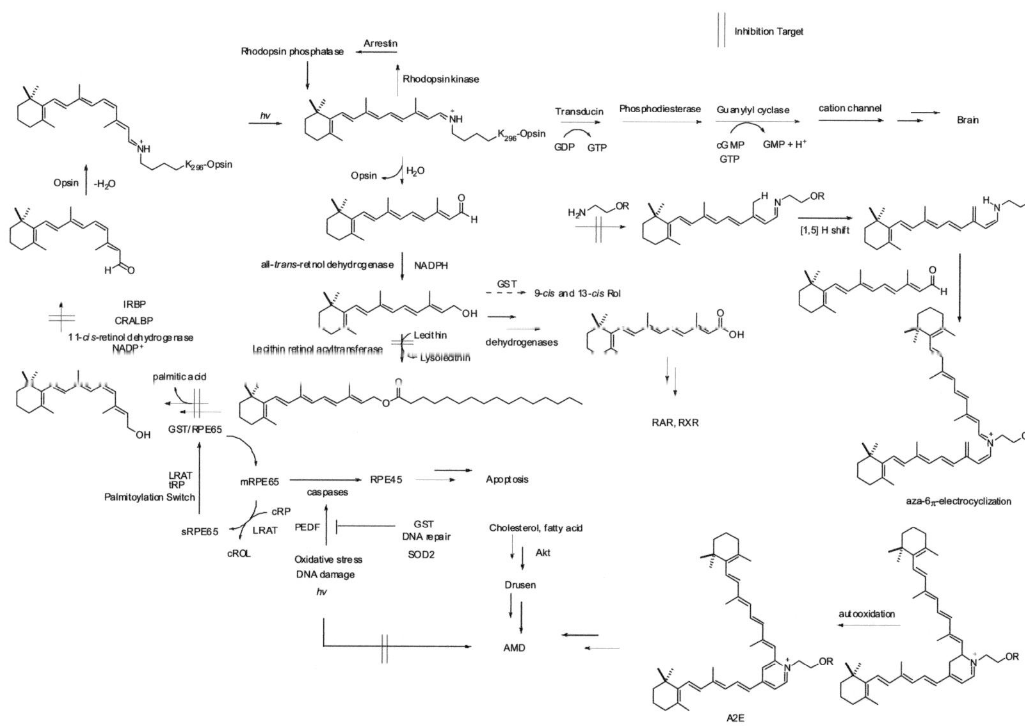

Figure 3. Retinoid Map in the Retina and RPE cells

10. Conclusion

While the end point of apoptosis is well established, there is still a large gap between knowledge of early biochemical events and the end stage of age-related macular degeneration (AMD). Proteome changes under oxidative stress have been studied in regard to the pathogenesis of AMD [Yang et al 2006]. Understanding the molecular mechanism of proteomic signaling will provide a novel insight into apoptotic processes in AMD. It is expected that the knowledge will be equally applicable for understanding the lipid-mediated cell death mechanism.

Light-induced retinal degeneration in animal model occurs only when the visual cycle is functional. Regeneration of 11-*cis*-retinal as a chromophore of rhodopsin is depending on biochemical reactions of retinoid processing enzymes, including lecithin retinol acyltransferase and RPE65 [Xue et al., 2004; Xue et al., 2006; Jahng et al., 2003a; Jahng et al., 2003b; Jahng et al., 2002; Bok et al., 2003]. Activity and expressions of these enzymes might be controlled by circadian regulators or daily light onset [Xue et al., 2004; Chung et al., 2009; Lee et al., 2010a]. A study of RPE65 knockout mice exhibited that light damage only occurs when the retina is supplied with 11-*cis* retinal [Wenzel et al., 2005]. Additional evidence in RPE65 L450M mice showing slow rhodopsin regeneration, halothane anesthesia as inhibition method of 11-*cis*-retinal regeneration, and 13-*cis*-retinoic acid as a putative RPE65 inhibitor imply that continuous regeneration of 11-*cis*-retinal is one of the key steps to induce retina degeneration [Wenzel et al., 2005]. Our goal is to explicate the role of light and time under oxidative stress in the control of neuroprotective protein expressions in the retina and the RPE [Zimmermann et al., 2006]. Our questions include whether antiapoptotic factors, that include prohibitin, nitric oxide, vimentin, PP2A, and erythropoietin can protect retina and RPE cells against oxidative- or light-induced apoptotic neurodegeneration at specific time points.

Our proteomic approaches to understand RPE cell death under stress conditions demonstrate that: 1) crystallins are upregulated and hyperphosphorylated. 2) neuroprotective erythropoietin and subsequent JAK2 phosphorylations are tightly linked to a specific time after oxidative stress and in anticipation of daily light onset. 3) early signaling molecules, including mitochondrial prohibitin, changes their expression, subcellular localization, phosphorylation, and lipid interaction under oxidative stress. 4) relative lipid compositions, including phosphatidylcholine and cholesterol, are altered under oxidative stress. 5) oxidative stress leads to cytoskeletal reorganization through site-specific vimentin phosphorylations that regulate intermediate filaments, resulting in nonfilamentous particles.

AMD is characterized in its early stages by the presence of extracellular deposits, known as drusen, that accumulates between the basal surface of the RPE and Bruch's membrane. During the past decade, compelling evidence has emerged implicating the immune system and the complement system in particular in drusen biogenesis and AMD. A number of the proteins detected in drusen are either complement components or related molecules. Despite these significant advances, the identity of the molecules responsible for triggering activation of the complement cascade, as well as the downstream molecular interactions that promote AMD pathology, remain elusive. Our proteomics studies will provide new insight into the underlying mechanisms involved in the development and progression of AMD and further elucidate the relationship between various risk facotors, including oxidative stress and complemnt activation. Such information are critical for the development of more effective therapeutic strategies for the treatment of retinal degeneration that includes AMD.

Author details

Wan Jin Jahng
Retina Research Laboratory, Department of Petroleum Chemistry, American University of Nigeria, Yola, Nigeria

11. References

Alcazar O, Hawkridge AM, Collier TS, Cousins SW, Bhattacharya SK, Muddiman DC, Marin-Castano ME. Proteomics characterization of cell membrane blebs in human retinal pigment epithelium cells. Mol Cell Proteomics. 2009;8:2201-11

Alge CS, Suppmann S, Priglinger SG, Neubauer AS, May CA, Hauck S, Welge-Lussen U, Ueffing M, Kampik A. Comparative proteome analysis of native differentiated and cultured dedifferentiated human RPE cells. Invest Ophthalmol Vis.Sci. 2003;44: 3629–3641.

Alge CS, Hauck SM, Priglinger SG, Kampik A, Ueffing M. Differential protein profiling of primary versus immortalized human RPE cells identifies expression patterns associated with cytoskeletal remodeling and cell survival. J Proteome Res. 2006;5:862–878.

An E, Lu X, Flippin J, Devaney JM, Halligan B, Hoffman EP, Strunnikova N, Csaky K, Hathout Y. Secreted proteome profiling in human RPE cell cultures derived from donors with age related macular degeneration and age matched healthy donors. J Proteome Res. 2006;5:2599-2610.

Arnouk H, Lee H, Zhang R, Chung H, Hunt RC, Jahng WJ. Early biosignature of oxidative stress in the retinal pigment epithelium. J Proteomics. 2011;74:254-261.

Artal-Sanz M, Tsang WY, Willems EM, Grivell LA, Lemire BD, van der Spek H, Nijtmans LG. The mitochondrial prohibitin complex is essential for embryonic viability and germline function in Caenorhabditis elegans. J Biol Chem. 2003;278:32091-9.

Asamoto M, Cohen SM. Prohibitin gene is overexpressed but not mutated in rat bladder carcinomas and cell lines. Cancer Lett. 1994;83:201-7.

Babizhayev MA, Bunin AYa. Lipid peroxidation in open-angle glaucoma. Acta Ophthalmol (Copenh). 1989;67:371-7.

Bavik CO, Erikson U, Allen RA, and Peterson PA. Identification and partial characterization of a retinal pigment epithelial membrane receptor for plasma retinol-binding protein. J. Biol. Chem. 1991;266:14978-14985.

Bavik CO, Busch C, and Eriksson U. Characterization of a plasma retinol-binding protein membrane receptor expressed in the retinal pigment epithelium. J. Biol. Chem. 1992;267:23035-23042.

Bavik CO, Levy F, Hellman U, Wernstedt C, and Eriksson U. The retinal pigment epithelium membrane receptor for plasma retinol-binding protein. J. Biol. Chem. 1993;268:20540-20546.

Beatty S, Koh H, Phil M, Henson D, Boulton M. The role of oxidative stress in the pathogenesis of age-related macular degeneration. Surv Ophthalmol. 2000;45:115-34.

Bellamy WT, Alberts DS, Dorr RT. 1988. Daily variation in non-protein sulfhydryl levels of human bone marrow. Eur J Cancer Clin Oncol 24: 1759-1762.

Böcker-Meffert S, Rosenstiel P, Röhl C, Warneke N, Held-Feindt J, Sievers J, Lucius R. Erythropoietin and VEGF promote neural outgrowth from retinal explants in postnatal rats. Invest Ophthalmol Vis Sci 2002;43:2021–2026.

Bohlius J, Wilson J, Seidenfeld J, Piper M, Schwarzer G, Sandercock J, Trelle S, Weingart O, Bayliss S, Djulbegovic B, Bennett CL, Langensiepen S, Hyde C, Engert A. Recombinant human erythropoietins and cancer patients: updated meta-analysis of 57 studies including 9353 patients. J Natl Cancer Inst. 2006;98(10):708-14.

Bok D. The retinal pigment epithelium: a versatile partner in vision. J. Cell Sci. 1993;Sup 17:189-195.

Bok D, Ruiz A, Yaron O, Jahng WJ, Ray A, Xue L, Rando RR. Purification and characterization of a transmembrane domain-deleted form of lecithin retinol acyltransferase. Biochemistry. 2003;42(20):6090-8.

Bosch-Morell F, Romá J, Marín N, Romero B, Rodriguez-Galietero A, Johnsen-Soriano S, Díaz-Llopis M, Romero FJ. Role of oxygen and nitrogen species in experimental uveitis: anti-inflammatory activity of the synthetic antioxidant ebselen. Free Radic Biol Med. 2002;33:669-75.

Bourges I, Ramus C, Mousson de Camaret B, Beugnot R, Remacle C, Cardol P, Hofhaus G, Issartel JP. Structural organization of mitochondrial human complex I: role of the ND4 and ND5 mitochondria-encoded subunits and interaction with prohibitin. Biochem J. 2004;383:491-499.

Brines M, Cerami A. Emerging biological roles for erythropoietin in the nervous system. Nat Rev Neurosci 2005;6:484–494.

Brines M L, Ghezzi P, Keenan S, Agnello D, de Lanerolle NC, Cerami C, Itri LM, Cerami A. Erythropoietin crosses the blood-brain barrier to protect against experimental brain injury. Proc Natl Acad Sci USA 2000;97:10526–10531.

Budihardjo, I., Oliver, H., Lutter, M., Luo, X., and Wang, X. Biochemical pathways of caspase activation during apoptosis. Annu. Rev. Cell Dev. Biol. 1999;15:269-290.

Calapai G, Marciano MC, Corica F, Allegra A, Parisi A, Frisina N, Caputi AP, Buemi M. Erythropoietin protects against brain ischemic injury by inhibition of nitric oxide formation. Eur J Pharmacol 2000;401:349–356.

Celik M, Gökmen N, Erbayraktar S, Akhisaroglu M, Konakc S, Ulukus C, Genc S, Genc K, Sagiroglu E, Cerami A, Brines M. Erythropoietin prevents motor neuron apoptosis and neurologic disability in experimental spinal cord ischemic injury. Proc Natl Acad Sci USA 2002;99:2258–2263.

Chen J, Connor KM, Aderman CM, Smith LE. Erythropoietin deficiency decreases vascular stability in mice. J Clin Invest. 2008;118(2):526-33.

Chen, Y., Moiseyev, G., Takahashi, Y., and Ma, J.-x. Impacts of two point mutations of RPE65 from Leber's congenital amaurosis on the stability, subcellular localization and isomerohydrolase activity of RPE65. FEBS Lett. 2006;580:4200-4204.

Chung H, Lee H, Lamoke F, Hrushesky WJ, Wood PA, Jahng WJ. Neuroprotective role of erythropoietin by antiapoptosis in the retina. J Neurosci Res. 2009;87:2365-2374.

Clark JI, Muchowski PJ, Small heat-shock proteins and their potential role in human disease, Curr. Opin. Struct. Biol. 2000;10:52-59.

Coates PJ, Nenutil R, McGregor A, Picksley SM, Crouch DH, Hall PA, Wright EG. Mammalian prohibitin proteins respond to mitochondrial stress and decrease during cellular senescence. Exp Cell Res. 2001;265:262-273.

Cottet, S., Michaut, L., Boisset, G., Schlecht, U., Gehring, W., and Schorderet, D. F. Biological characterization of gene response in RPE65-/- mouse model of Leber's congenital amaurosis during progression of the disease. FASEB J. 2006;20:2036-2049.

Crabb JW, Miyagi M, Gu X, Shadrach K, West KA, Sakaguchi H, Kamei M, Hasan A, Yan L, Rayborn ME, Salomon RG, Hollyfield, JG. Drusen proteome analysis: an approach to the etiology of age-related macular degeneration. Proc Natl Acad Sci U S A. 2002;12:14682-14687.

Dani C, Cecchi A, Bertini G. Role of oxidative stress as physiopathologic factor in the preterm infant. Minerva Pediatr. 2004;56:381-394.

Davis, A.A., Bernstein P.S., Bok, D., Turner, J., Nachtigal, M., and Hunt, R.C. A human retinal pigment epithelial cell line that retains epithelial characteristics after prolonged culture. Invest. Ophthalmol. Vis. Sci. 1995;36:955-964.

Decanini A, Karunadharma PR, Nordgaard CL, Feng X, Olsen TW, Ferrington DA. Human retinal pigment epithelium proteome changes in early diabetes. Diabetologia. 2007;51:1051-1061.

Deigner, P. S., Law, W. C., Canada, F. J., and Rando, R. R. Membranes as the energy source in the endergonic transformation of vitamin A to 11-cis-retinol. Science 1989;244:968-971.

den Engelsman J, Gerrits D, de Jong WW, Robbins J, Kato K, Boelens WC. Nuclear import of {alpha}B-crystallin is phosphorylation-dependent and hampered by hyperphosphorylation of the myopathy-related mutant R120G. J Biol Chem. 2005;280:37139-37148.

Ethen CM, Reilly C, Feng X, Olsen TW, Ferrington DA, The proteome of central and peripheral retina with progression of age-related macular degeneration, Invest. Ophthalmol. Vis. Sci. 2006;47:2280-2290.

Felius J, Thompson DA, Khan NW, Bingham EL, Jamison JA., Kemp JA, and Sieving PA. Clinical course and visual function in a family with mutations in the RPE65 gene. Arch. Ophthalmol. 2002;120:55-61.

Gangalum RK, Atanasov IC, Zhou ZH, Bhat SP. AlphaB-crystallin is found in detergent-resistant membrane microdomains and is secreted via exosomes from human retinal pigment epithelial cells. J Biol Chem. 2011;286:3261-3269.

Genc S, Kuralay F, Genc K, Akhisaroglu M, Fadiloglu S, Yorukoglu K, Fadiloglu M, Gure A. Erythropoietin exerts neuroprotection in 1-methyl-4-phenyl-1,2,3,6-tetrahydropyridinetreated C57/BL mice via increasing nitric oxide production. Neurosci Lett 2001;298:139–141.

Grimm C, Wenzel A, Hafezi F, Yu S, Redmond TM, Reme CE. Protection of Rpe65-deficient mice identifies rhodopsin as a mediator of light-induced retinal degeneration. Nature Genet 2000;25:63–66.

Grimm C, Wenzel A, Groszer M, Mayser H, Seeliger M, Samardzija M, Bauer C, Gassman M, Reme CE. HIF-1 induced erythropoietin in the hypoxic retina protects against light-induced retinal degeneration. Nat Med 2002;8:718–724.

Grune T, Reinheckel T, Davies KJ. Degradation of oxidized proteins in mammalian cells. FASEB J. 1997 ;11:526-34.

Gu, S. M., Thompson, D.A., Srikumari, C.R., Lorenz, B., Finckh, U., Nicoletti, A., Murphy, K.R., Rathmann, M., Kumaramanickavel, G., Denton, M.J., and Gal, A. Mutations in RPE65 cause autosomal recessive childhood-onset severe retinal dystrophy. Nat. Genetics 1997;17:194-197.

Haass, C., and Strooper, B. D. The presenilins in Alzheimer's disease-proteolysis holds the key. Science 1999;286:916-919.

Ham DI, Gentleman S, Chan CC, McDowell JH, Redmond TM, Gery I. RPE65 is highly uveitogenic in rats. Invest Ophthalmol Vis Sci. 2002;43:2258-2263.

Hamel, C. P., Tsilou, E., Harris, E., Pfeffer, B. A., Hooks, J. J., Detrick, B., and Redmond, T. M. A developmentally regulated microsomal protein specific for the pigment epithelium of the vertebrate retina. J. Neuroscience Res. 1993a;34:414-425.

Hamel, C. P., Tsilou, E., Pfeffer, B. A., Detrick, B., and Redmond, T. M. Molecular cloning and expression of RPE65, a novel retinal pigment epithelium-specific microsomal protein that is post-transcriptionally regulated in vitro. J. Biol. Chem. 1993b;268:15751-15757.

Hamel, C. P., Griffoin, J.-M., Lasquellec, L., Bazalgette, C., and Arnaud, B. Reinal dystrophies caused by mutations in RPE65: assessment of visual functions. Br. J. Ophthalmol. 2001;85:424-427.

Hardeland R, Coto-Montes A, Poeggeler B. Circadian rhythms, oxidative stress, and antioxidative defense mechanisms. Chronobiol Int. 2003;20:921-62.

Head KA. Natural therapies for ocular disorders, part one: diseases of the retina. Altern Med Rev. 1999 Oct;4(5):342-59.

Hrushesky WJ. 1985. Circadian timing of cancer chemotherapy. Science 228:73-5.

Hooks, J. J., Detrick, B., Percopo, C., Hamel, C., Siraganian, R. P. Development and characterization of monoclonal antibodies directed against the retinal pigment epithelial cells. Invest. Ophthalmol. Vis. Sci. 1989;30:2106-2113.

Jahng WJ, Cheung E, Rando RR. Lecithin retinol acyltransferase forms functional homodimers. Biochemistry. 2002;41(20):6311-9.

Jahng WJ, David C, Nesnas N, Nakanishi K, Rando RR. A cleavable affinity biotinylating agent reveals a retinoid binding role for RPE65. Biochemistry. 2003a;42(20):6159-68.

Jahng WJ, Xue L, Rando RR. Lecithin retinol acyltransferase is a founder member of a novel family of enzymes. Biochemistry. 2003b;42(44):12805-12.

Jelkmann W, Metzen E. Erythropoietin in the control of red cell production. Ann Anat 1996;178:391–403.

Jelkmann W. Effects of erythropoietin on brain function. Current Pharmaceutical Biotech 2005;6:65–79.

Jelkmann W. Erythropoietin after a century of research: younger than ever. Eur J Haematol 2007;78:183–205.

Jin, M., Li, S., Moghrabi, W.N., Sun, H. and Travis, G.H. Rpe65 is the retinoid isomerase in bovine retinal pigment epithelium. Cell 2005;122:449-459.

Kanaan NM, Collier TJ, Marchionini DM, McGuire SO, Fleming MF, Sortwell CE. Exogenous erythropoietin provides neuroprotection of grafted dopamine neurons in a rodent model of Parkinson's disease. Brain Res 2006;1068:221–229.

Kapphahn RJ, Ethen CM, Peters EA, Higgins L, Ferrington DA, Modified alpha A crystallin in the retina: altered expression and truncation with aging, Biochemistry 2003;42:15310-15325.

Katsura Y, Okano T, Matsuno K, Osako M, Kure M, Watanabe T, Iwaki Y, Noritake M, Kosano H, Nishigori H, Matsuoka T. Erythropoietin is highly elevated in vitreous fluid of patients with proliferative diabetic retinopathy. Diabetes Care. 2005;28(9):2252-4.

Kawakami M, Sekiguchi M, Sato K, Kozaki S, Takahashi M. Erythropoietin receptor-mediate d inhibition of exocytotic glutamate release confers neuroprotection during chemical ischemia. J Biol Chem 2001;276:39469–39475.

Kim, SR., Fishkin, N., Kong, J., Nakanishi, K., Allikmets, R., and Sparrow, J. R. Rpe65 Leu450Met variant is associated with reduced levels of the retinal pigment epithelium lipofuscin fluorophores A2E and iso-A2E. 2004;101:11668-11672.

Kim T, Kim SJ, Kim K, Kang UB, Lee C, Park KS, Yu HG, Kim Y. Profiling of vitreous proteomes from proliferative diabetic retinopathy and nondiabetic patients. Proteomics. 2007;7:4203-4215.

Kim YH, Choi MY, Kim YS, Han JM, Lee JH, Park CH, Kang SS, Choi WS, Cho GJ, Protein kinase C delta regulates anti-apoptotic alphaB-crystallin in the retina of type 2 diabetes, Neurobiol. Dis. 2007;28:293-303.

Kloer, D. P., Ruch, S., Al-Babili, S., Beyer, P., and Schulz, G. E. The structure of a retinal-forming carotenoid oxygenase. Science 2005;308:267-269.

Kolonin MG, Saha PK, Chan L, Pasqualini R, Arap W. Reversal of obesity by targeted ablation of adipose tissue. Nat. Med. 2004;10:625-632.

Kretz A, Happold CJ, Martick, JK, Isenmann S. Erythropoietin promotes regeneration of adult CNS neurons via Jak2/Stat3 and PI3K/AKT pathway activation. Mol Cell Neurosci 2005;29:569–579.

Lee H, Chung H, Arnouk H, Lamoke F, Hunt RC, Hrushesky WJ, Wood PA, Lee SH, Jahng WJ. Cleavage of the retinal pigment epithelium-specific protein RPE65 under oxidative stress. Int J Biol Macromol. 2010a;47:104-108.

Lee H, Arnouk H, Sripathi S, Chen P, Zhang R, Hunt RC, Hrushesky WJ, Chung H, Lee SH, Jahng WJ. Prohibitin as an oxidative stress biomarker in the eye. Int J Biol Macromol. 2010b;47:685-690.

Lee H, Chung H, Lee SH, Jahng WJ. Light-induced phosphorylation of crystallins in the retinal pigment epithelium. Int J Biol Macromol. 2011;48:194-201.

Lee HC, Yin PH, Lu CY, Chi CW, Wei YH. Increase of mitochondria and mitochondrial DNA in response to oxidative stress in human cells. Biochem J. 2000;348:425-32.

Li Y, Lu Z, Keogh CL, Yu SP, Wei L. 2007. Erythropoietin-induced neurovascular protection, angiogenesis, and cerebral blood flow restoration after focal ischemia in mice. J. Cereb. Blood. Flow Metab. 2007;27:1043-1054.

Liu X, Shen J, Jin Y, Duan M, Xu J. 2006. Recombinant human erythropoietin (rhEPO) preconditioning on nuclear factor-kappa B (NF-kB) activation & proinflammatory cytokines induced by myocardial ischaemi a-reperfusion. Indian J Med Res124:343–354.

Ma, J-x., Zhang, J., Othersen, K. L., Moiseyev, G., Ablonczy, Z., Redmond, T. M., Chen, Y., Crouch, R. K. Expression, purification, and MALDI analysis of RPE65. Invest. Ophthalmol. Vis. Sci. 2001;42:1429-1435.

Madigan MC, Penfold PL, Provis JM, Balind TK, Billson FA. Intermediate filament expression in human retinal macroglia. Histopathologic changes associated with age-related macular degeneration. Retina. 1994;14(1):65-74.

Martinon, F., and Tschopp, J. Inflammatory caspases: linking an intracellular innate immune system to autoinflammatory diseases. Cell 2004;117:561-574.

Mata NL, Moghrabi WN, Lee JS, Bui TV, Radu RA, Horwitz J, Travis GH. Rpe65 is a retinyl ester binding protein that presents insoluble substrate to the isomerase in retinal pigment epithelial cells. J. Biol. Chem. 2004;279:635-643.

Mauer AM. Diurnal variation of proliferative activity in the human bone marrow. Blood 1965;26:1-7.

McClung, J. K., Danner, D. B., Stewart, D. A., Smith, J. R., Schneider, E.L., Lumpkin, C. K., Dell'Orco, R. T., Nuell, M. J. Isolation of a cDNA that hybrid selects antiproliferative mRNA from rat liver. Biochem. Biophys. Res. Commun. 1989;164:1316-1322.

McClung JK, Jupe ER, Liu XT, Dell'Orco RT. Prohibitin: potential role in senescence, development, and tumor suppression. Exp Gerontol. 1995;30:99-124.

Melov S, Coskun P, Patel M, Tuinstra R, Cottrell B, Jun AS, Zastawny TH, Dizdaroglu M, Goodman SI, Huang TT, Miziorko H, Epstein CJ, Wallace DC. Mitochondrial disease in superoxide dismutase 2 mutant mice. Proc Natl Acad Sci U S A. 1999;96:846-51.

Miyake T, Kung CKH, Goldwasser E. Purification of human erythropoietin. J Biol Chem1977;252:5558–5564.

Morishita E, Masuda S, Nagao M, Yasuda Y, Sasaki R. Erythropoietin receptor is expressed in rat hippocampal and cerebral cortical neurons, and erythropoietin prevents in vitro glutamate-induced neuronal death. Neuroscience 1997;76:105–116.

Morita M, Ohneda O, Yamashita T, Takahashi S, Suzuki N, Nakajima O, Kawauchi S, Ema M, Shibahara S, Udono T, Tomita K, Tamai M, Sogawa K, Yamamoto, M, Fujii-Kuriyama Y. HLF/HIF-2alpha is a key factor in retinopathy of prematurity in association with erythropoietin. EMBO J 2003;22:1134–1146.

Moiseyev, G., Chen, Y., Takahashi, Y., Wu, B.X. and Ma, J.-x. RPE65 is the isomerohydrolase in the retinoid visual cycle. Proc. Natl. Acad. Sci. USA. 2005;102:12413-12418.

Nikolaeva O, Takahashi Y, Moiseyev G, Ma JX. Purified RPE65 shows isomerohydrolase activity after reassociation with a phospholipid membrane. FEBS J. 2009;276:3020-3030

Nijtmans LG, de Jong L, Artal Sanz M, Coates PJ, Berden JA, Back JW, Muijsers AO, van der Spek H, Grivell LA. Prohibitins act as a membrane-bound chaperone for the stabilization of mitochondrial proteins. EMBO J. 2000;19:2444-2451.

Nijtmans LG, Artal SM, Grivell LA, Coates PJ. The mitochondrial PHB complex: roles in mitochondrial respiratory complex assembly, ageing and degenerative disease. Cell Mol Life Sci. 2002;59:143-55.

Nordgaard CL, Berg KM, Kapphahn RJ, Reilly C, Feng X, Olsen TW, Ferrington DA, Proteomics of the retinal pigment epithelium reveals altered protein expression at progressive stages of age-related macular degeneration, Invest. Ophthalmol. Vis. Sci. 2006;47:815-822.

Nordgaard CL, Karunadharma PP, Feng X, Olsen TW, Ferrington DA. Mitochondrial proteomics of the retinal pigment epithelium at progressive stages of age-related macular degeneration. Invest Ophthalmol Vis Sci. 2008;49:2848-55.

Nuell MJ, Stewart DA, Walker L, Friedman V, Wood CM, Owens GA, Smith JR, Schneider EL, Dell' Orco R, Lumpkin CK, et al. Prohibitin, an evolutionarily conserved intracellular protein that blocks DNA synthesis in normal fibroblasts and HeLa cells. Mol Cell Biol. 1991;11:1372-81.

Organisciak D, Darrow R, Barsalou L, Rapp C, McDonald B, Wong P. Light induced and circadian effects on retinal photoreceptor cell crystallins. Photochem Photobiol. 2011;87:151-159.

Osborne NN, Ugarte M, Chao M, Chidlow G, Bae JH, Wood JP, Nash MS. Neuroprotection in relation to retinal ischemia and relevance to glaucoma. Surv Ophthalmol. 1999;43 Suppl 1:S102-28.

Rando, R. R. The biochemistry of the visual cycle. Chem. Rev. 2001;101:1881-1896.

Redmond, T. M., Yu, S., Lee, E., Bok, D., Hamasaki, D., Chen, N., Goletz, P., Ma, J.-x., Crouch, R. K., Pfeifer, K. Rpe65 is necessary for production of 11-cis-vitamin A in the retinal visual cycle. Nature Genet. 1998;20:344-351.

Redmond, T.M., Poliakov, E., Shirley, Y., Tsai, J.-Y., Lu, Z. and Gentleman, S. Mutation of key residues of RPE65 abolishes its enzymatic role as isomerohydrolase in the visual cycle. Proc. Natl. Acad. Sci. USA. 2005;102:13658-13663.

Rivera-Milla, E., Stuermer, C. A., Málaga-Trillo, E. Ancient origin of reggie (flotillin), reggie-like, and other lipid-raft proteins: convergent evolution of the SPFH domain. Cel.l Mol. Life Sci. 2006;63:343-357.

Saari, JC. Biochemistry of visual pigment regeneration. Invest. Ophthalmol. Vis. Sci. 2000;41:337-348.

Sakaguchi H, Miyagi M, Darrow RM, Crabb JS, Hollyfield JG, Organisciak DT, Crabb JW, Intense light exposure changes the crystallin content in retina, Exp. Eye. Res. 2003;76:131-133.

Santoro MF, Annand RR, Robertson MM, Peng YW, Brady MJ, Mankovich JA, Hackett MC, Ghayur T, Walter G, Wong WW, Giegel DA. Regulation of protein phosphatase 2A activity by caspase-3 during apoptosis. J Biol Chem. 1998; 273:13119-13128.

Satici A, Guzey M, Gurler B, Vural H, Gurkan T. Malondialdehyde and antioxidant enzyme levels in the aqueous humor of rabbits in endotoxin-induced uveitis. Eur J Ophthalmol. 2003 Nov-Dec;13(9-10):779-83.

Scheving L, Tsai T, Sothern R, Hrushesky W. 1988. Circadian susceptibility-resistance cycles to radiation and their manipulability by methylene blue (a non-toxic, in vivo oxidation-reduction complex). Pharmacology and Therapeutics 1988;39:397-402.

Schlunck G, Martin G, Agostini HT, Camatta G, Hansen LL. Cultivation of retinal pigment epithelial cells from human choroidal neovascular membranes in age related macular degeneration. Exp Eye Res. 2002;74:571-6.

Schütt F, Völcker HE, Dithmar S. N-acetylcysteine improves lysosomal function and enhances the degradation of photoreceptor outer segments in cultured RPE cells. Klin Monatsbl Augenheilkd. 2007;224:580-584.

Schweizer U, Gunnersen J, Karch C, Wiese S, Holtmann B, Takeda K, Akira S, Sendtner M. Conditional gene ablation of Stat3 reveals differential signaling requirements for survival of motoneurons during development and after nerve injury in the adult. J Cell Biol 2002;156:287–297.

Shang, F., and Taylor, A. Function of the ubiquitin proteolytic pathway in the eye. Exp. Eye Res. 2004;78:1-14.

Sharma A, Qadri A. Vi polysaccharide of Salmonella typhi targets the prohibitin family of molecules in intestinal epithelial cells and suppresses early inflammatory responses. Proc Natl Acad Sci U S A. 2004;101:17492-17497.

Singh AK, Szczech L, Tang KL, Barnhart H, Sapp S, Wolfson M, Reddan D; CHOIR Investigators. Correction of anemia with epoetin alfa in chronic kidney disease. N Engl J Med. 2006;355(20):2085-98.

Sitte N, Huber M, Grune T, Ladhoff A, Doecke WD, Von Zglinicki T, Davies KJ. Proteasome inhibition by lipofuscin/ceroid during postmitotic aging of fibroblasts. FASEB J. 2000;14:1490-8.

Smaaland R, Laerum OD, Lote K, et al. DNA synthesis in human bone marrow is circadian stage dependent. Blood 1991;77: 2603-2611.

Smaaland R, Abrahamsen JF, Svardal AM, Lote K, Ueland PM. DNA cell cycle distribution and glutathione (GSH) content according to circadian stage in bone marrow of cancer patients. Br J Cancer. 1992 Jul;66(1):39-45.

Spector A. Oxidative stress-induced cataract: mechanism of action. FASEB J. 1995 Sep;9(12):1173-82.

Spraul CW, Lang GE, Grossniklaus HE. Morphometric analysis of the choroid, Bruch's membrane, and retinal pigment epithelium in eyes with age-related macular degeneration. Invest Ophthalmol Vis Sci 1996; 37:2724-35.

Sreekumar PG, Kannan R, Kitamura M, Spee C, Barron E, Ryan SJ, Hinton DR. αB crystallin is apically secreted within exosomes by polarized human retinal pigment epithelium and provides neuroprotection to adjacent cells. PLoS One. 2010;5:e12578.

Sripathi SR, He W, Atkinson CL, Smith JJ, Liu Z, Elledge BM, Jahng WJ. Mitochondrial-Nuclear Communication by Prohibitin Shuttling under Oxidative Stress. Biochemistry. 2011;50:8342-51.

Stecher H, Gelb MH, Saari JC, Palczewski K. Preferential release of 11-cis-retinol from retinal pigment epithelial cells in the presence of cellular retinaldehyde-binding protein. J Biol Chem. 1999;274:8577-85.

Steglich G, Neupert W, Langer T. Prohibitins regulate membrane protein degradation by the m-AAA protease in mitochondria. Mol Cell Biol. 1999;19:3435-3442.

Strauss, O. The retinal pigment epithelium in visual function. Physiol. Rev. 2005;85:845-881.

Taniguchi CM, Emanuelli B, Kahn CR, Critical nodes in signalling pathways: insights into insulin action, Nat. Rev. Mol. Cell. Biol. 2006;7:85-96.

Tao WA, Wollscheid B, O'Brien R, Eng JK, Li XJ, Bodenmiller B, Watts JD, Hood L, Aebersold R, Quantitative phosphoproteome analysis using a dendrimer conjugation chemistry and tandem mass spectrometry, Nat. Methods. 2005;2:591-598.

Tezel G, Yang X, Cai J. Proteomic identification of oxidatively modified retinal proteins in a chronic pressure-induced rat model of glaucoma. Invest Ophthalmol Vis Sci. 2005;46:3177-3187.

Travis, G. H., Golczak, M., Moise, A. R., Palczewski, K. Diseases caused by defects in the visual cycle: retinoids as potential therapeutic agents. Annu. Rev. Pharmocol. Toxicol. 2007;47:8.1-8.44.

Tsai PT, Ohab JJ, Kertesz N, Groszer M, Matter C, Gao J, Liu X, Wu H, Carmichael ST. A critical role of erythropoietin receptor in neurogenesis and post-stroke recovery. J Neurosci 2006;26;1269 –1274.

Tsilou, E., Hamel, C. P., Yu, S., and Redmond, T. M. RPE65, the major retinal pigment epithelium microsomal membrane protein, associates with phospholipids liposomes. Arch. Biochem. Biophys. 1997;346:21-27.

Wang S, Nath N, Fusaro G, Chellappan S. Rb and prohibitin target distinct regions of E2F1 for repression and respond to different upstream signals. Mol Cell Biol. 1999b;19:7447-60.

Wang, S., Fusaro, G., Padmanabhan, J., Chellappan, S. P. Prohibitin co-localizes with Rb in the nucleus and recruits N-CoR and HDAC1 for transcriptional repression. Oncogene 2002;21:8388-8396.

Warburton S, Davis WE, Southwick K, Xin H, Woolley AT, Burton GF, Thulin CD. Proteomic and phototoxic characterization of melanolipofuscin: correlation to disease and model for its origin. Mol Vis. 2007;13:318-329.

Watanabe D, Suzuma K, Matsui S, Kurimoto M, Kiryu J, Kita M, Suzuma I, Ohashi H, Ojima T, Murakami T, Kobayashi T, Masuda S, Nagao M, Yoshimura N, Takagi H. Erythropoietin as a retinal angiogenic factor in proliferative diabetic retinopathy. N Engl J Med. 2005;353(8):782-92.

Weishaupt JH, Rohde G, Pölking E, Siren AL, Ehrenreich H, Bähr M. Effect of erythropoietin axotomy-induced apoptosis in rat retinal ganglion cells. Invest Ophthalmol Vis Sci 2004;45:1514–1522.

Wenzel A, Grimm C, Samardzija M, and Reme CE. Molecular mechanisms of light-induced photoreceptor apoptosis and neuroprotection for retinal degeneration. Prog Retinal Eye Res 2005;24:275–306.

West KA, Yan L, Miyagi M, Crabb JS, Marmorstein AD, Marmorstein L, Crabb JW. Proteome survey of proliferating and differentiating rat RPE-J cells. Exp Eye Res. 2001 Oct;73(4):479-91.

Wood PA, Hrushesky WJM, Klevecz R. 1998. Distinct circadian time structures characterize myeloid and erythroid progenitor and multiprogenitor clonogenicity as well as marrow precursor proliferation dynamics. Exp Hematol 26:523-533.

Xi J, Farjo R, Yoshida S, Kern TS, Swaroop A, Andley UP, A comprehensive analysis of the expression of crystallins in mouse retina, Mol. Vis. 2003;28:410-419.

Xue L, Gollapalli DR, Maiti P, Jahng WJ, Rando RR. A palmitoylation switch mechanism in the regulation of the visual cycle. Cell. 2004;117(6):761-71.

Xue L, Jahng WJ, Gollapalli D, Rando RR. Palmitoyl transferase activity of lecithin retinol acyl transferase. Biochemistry. 2006;45(35):10710-8.

Yakes FM, Van Houten B. Mitochondrial DNA damage is more extensive and persists longer than nuclear DNA damage in human cells following oxidative stress. Proc Natl Acad Sci U S A. 1997;94:514-9.

Yamaji R, Okada T, Moriya M, Naito M, Tsuruo T, Miyatake K, and Nakano Y. Brain capillary endothelial cells express two forms of erythropoietin receptor mRNA. Eur. J. Biochem. 1996;239, 494-500.

Yang P, Peairs JJ, Tano R, Jaffe GJ, Oxidant-mediated Akt activation in human RPE cells, Invest. Ophthalmol. Vis. Sci. 2006;47:4598-4606.

Yen SH, Gaskin F, Fu SM. Neurofibrillary tangles in senile dementia of the Alzheimer type share an antigenic determinant with intermediate filaments of the vimentin class. Am J Pathol. 1983;113:373-381.

Yu KR, Hijikata T, Lin ZX, Sweeney HL, Englander SW, Holtzer H. Truncated desmin in PtK2 cells induces desmin-vimentin-cytokeratin coprecipitation, involution of intermediate filament networks, and nuclear fragmentation: a model for many degenerative diseases. Proc Natl Acad Sci U S A. 1994;91:2497-2501.

Zhang R, Hrushesky WJ, Wood PA, Lee SH, Hunt RC, Jahng WJ. Melatonin reprogrammes proteomic profile in light-exposed retina in vivo. Int J Biol Macromol. 2010;47:255-60.

Zhong L, Bradley J, Schubert W, Ahmed E, Adamis AP, Shima DT, Robinson GS, Ng YS. Erythropoietin promotes survival of retinal ganglion cells in DBA/2J glaucoma mice. Invest Ophthalmol Vis Sci. 2007;48(3):1212-8.

Zhou H, Ye H, Dong J, Han G, Jiang X, Wu R, Zou H, Specific phosphopeptide enrichment with immobilized titanium ion affinity chromatography adsorbent for phosphoproteome analysis, J. Proteome. Res. 2008;7:3957-3967.

Zigler JS Jr, Zhang C, Grebe R, Sehrawat G, Hackler L Jr, Adhya S, Hose S, McLeod DS, Bhutto I, Barbour W, Parthasarathy G, Zack DJ, Sergeev Y, Lutty GA, Handa JT, Sinha D. Mutation in the βA3/A1-crystallin gene impairs phagosome degradation in the retinal pigmented epithelium of the rat. J Cell Sci. 2011;124(Pt 4):523-531.

Zimmermann MB, Biebinger R, Rohner F, Dib A, Zeder C, Hurrell RF, Chaouki N. Vitamin A supplementation in children with poor vitamin A and iron status increases erythropoietin and hemoglobin concentrations without changing total body iron. Am J Clin Nutr 2006;84:80–586.

Chapter 7

Recent Advances in Ocular Nucleic Acid-Based Therapies: The Silent Era

Covadonga Pañeda, Tamara Martínez, Natalia Wright and Ana Isabel Jimenez

Additional information is available at the end of the chapter

http://dx.doi.org/10.5772/48454

1. Introduction

The central dogma of biology describes the transfer of biological information from DNA through to protein (1). In the first phase, known as transcription, DNA is converted into a complementary sequence of messenger RNA (mRNA). This mRNA allows the genetic message to be communicated outside of the cell nucleus, to other areas of the cell, where it is then translated into protein by ribosomes. Post-transcriptional regulatory events take place after an RNA molecule is formed; thereafter the resulting RNA molecule is decoded to produce a specific protein. Protein production depends on the length of survival of RNA in a cell and the efficiency of its utilizations.

Since Paterson et al. first demonstrated the utility of nucleic acids in modulating gene expression over 30 years ago (2), and in 1978 Zamecnik and Stephenson showed the capacity of antisense molecules to inhibit viral replication (3, 4), nucleic acids have emerged as a potent force both as R&D tools and as therapeutic agents.

Indeed, the field of nucleic acid therapeutics has evolved considerably with numerous gene targets and methods having been applied *in vitro* and *in vivo* in a variety of contexts with varying degrees of success. Strategies have included ribozymes, DNA enzymes (DNAzymes), antisense oligonucleotides (ASON), decoys, aptamers and siRNAs, all of which attenuate gene expression by interfering with cytosolic mRNA or translated protein. Currently, a number of these approaches are being evaluated in human and animal trials and are poised to offer considerable inroads and additions to our current therapies.

Ribozymes are catalytically active RNA molecules capable of site-specific cleavage of target mRNA and can occur naturally (5). They must contain antisense sequences that will bind to the target, and also a sequence that will fold into a structure with ribonuclease activity. Such sequences are found in natural hammerhead or hairpin ribozymes. Consequently, ribozymes don't depend on cellular nucleases for activity (6). The possibility of designing ribozymes to cleave any specific target RNA has rendered them valuable tools in both basic research and therapeutic applications.

DNAzymes, like ribozymes, may be perceived as gene-specific molecular scissors. They appeared as a development in the study of ribozymes using analogous deoxyoligonucleotides, given that catalytic DNA has not been observed in nature (7). All existing molecules have been derived by *in vitro* selection processes similar to those used to identify aptamers (see below). The most well-characterized DNAzyme is the "10-23" subtype comprising a cation-dependent catalytic core of 15 desoxyribonucleotides that binds to and cleaves its target RNA. This core is flanked by complementary binding arms of 6 to 12 nucleotides in length that confer target mRNA Specificity (8).

ASONs are single-stranded segments of DNA or RNA generally 15 to 25 nucleotides in length designed to mirror specific mRNA sequences and block protein production. Although their precise mechanism of action is not fully understood, their function is mediated by interaction with target mRNA via hydrogen bonding, blocking translation into protein by steric hindrance of ribosomal movement or by activation of endogenous RNase H for targeted destruction of the DNA/RNA heteroduplex, resulting in mRNA degradation (9). Unmodified ASONs molecules are prone to degradation, and their negative charge makes cellular membrane penetration inefficient. As such, these molecules have evolved with a variety of modifications that enhance stability and efficacy. Around 50 clinical studies have used antisense strategies spanning a variety of disease processes, including cancer, cardiovascular disease, inflammation and infection (10). Fomivirsen or Vitravene®, which targets the immediate-early RNA encoded by human cytomegalovirus (CMV) DNA, has been approved by the FDA for use in humans for treatment of CMV retinitis (11).

In contrast to antisense approaches that target mRNA, oligonucleotide decoys are short, double-stranded DNA molecules that contain binding elements for a variety of protein targets that competitively inhibit promoter binding and gene expression. Although several types of decoys have been developed there are important issues to take into account affecting the potential clinical use of these molecules, including susceptibility to nuclease degradation, propensity to induce a host immunological response, and cell transfection difficulties with higher concentration requirements (12). Currently, decoy oligonucleotides are not pursued as aggressively as other forms of therapeutic oligonucleotides (13).

Aptamers are single-stranded oligonucleotides which may fold into complex secondary and tertiary structures and bind their target protein with high affinity and specificity, inhibiting its function. They are derived by *in vitro* selection from a combinatorial library of nucleic acid sequences (14). Recent developments demonstrate that aptamers are valuable tools for diagnostics, purification processes, target validation, drug discovery and therapeutics. Macugen® is an aptamer approved by the FDA for treatment of wet AMD (15).

RNA interference (RNAi) is one of the gene silencing strategies which has received most attention in recent times. Its initial discovery in 1998 by Nobel laureates Fire and Mello (16) in *Caenorhabditis elegans*, led to the subsequent finding of the mechanism in mammalian cells and the understanding that it was triggered by small double stranded RNA duplexes of 19-23 nucleotides in length (17). In the following decade siRNA (short interfering RNA) have become widely used tools for silencing gene expression, as they make use of a naturally occurring regulatory mechanism that uses these molecules to direct homology-dependent mRNA degradation via a multienzymatic complex termed RISC (RNA-induced silencing complex). Cells use their own small RNA duplexes as a form of gene regulation. These novel molecules have enormous therapeutic potential and at present there are close to 20 compounds which have reached clinical trials (18).

2. Ocular diseases addressable by nucleic acid–based drugs

2.1. Glaucoma

Glaucoma is the second leading cause of blindness globally (19). By year 2020 almost 80 million people are estimated to be affected by primary open-angle glaucoma (POAG), the most common type of glaucoma. Glaucoma is defined as the process of ocular tissue destruction caused by a sustained elevation of intra ocular pressure (IOP) above its normal physiological limits (20). In open angle glaucoma (OAG), elevated IOP causes a progressive optic neuropathy due to loss of retinal ganglion cells that ultimately leads to blindness (21). In angle-closure glaucoma the sudden high rise in IOP often renders the eye blind. Blindness in glaucoma is caused by a degenerative process of the retina and optic nerve, but is functionally associated with impairments in the balance between aqueous humor (AH) secretion and outflow. Mechanistically, the changes observed in the trabecular meshwork include loss of cells as well the deposition and accumulation of extracellular debris including protein plaque-like material (22). The loss of vision is not usually evident until significant nerve damage has occurred. For this reason, up to half of glaucoma sufferers are unaware of their condition. Because of this, early diagnosis and treatment is crucial in halting the progression of this pathological condition (23). Risk factors associated with glaucoma include high intraocular pressure, advanced age, family history of glaucoma, African ancestry myopia, hypertension, morphologic features of the optic disc, thinness of the cornea, eye trauma, concomitant use of drugs, diabetes mellitus, hypothyroidism, cardiovascular and haematological abnormalities (24-28). Treatment of glaucoma is mainly focused on lowering IOP. The first line of treatment is medication, followed by surgical and laser treatment. Pharmacological compounds for treating glaucoma fall into four main classes of drugs: parasympathomimetics, antagonists of α and β-adrenoreceptors, inhibitors of carbonic anhydrases and prostaglandin analogues. Clinicians prescribe medications in a stepwise manner to achieve the target goal of IOP and maintain a balance between medication effectiveness, tolerability and safety. Beta blockers and prostaglandins are the standard first line treatment for POAG (29). Both groups of drugs are very efficient in lowering IOP but beta blockers are not recommended in patients with cardiovascular and respiratory problems and prostaglandin-analogs have local tolerability issues (30, 31). Second-line drugs of choice include alpha-2-adrenergic agonists and carbonic anhydrase inhibitors. When IOP is not adequately regulated with monotherapy it is common to combine different antiglaucoma drugs, these combinations appear to have the advantage of greater efficacy, better cost and safety, but limit the individualization of dosing. The efficacy of current IOP-lowering therapies is relatively short lived, requiring repetitive dosing throughout the day and in some cases the efficacy decreases with time. Such negative effects may lead to decreased patient compliance or to the end of treatment. If no efficacy in reducing IOP is achieved with any of these drugs, laser therapy may be applied to the trabecular meshwork in order to increase AH outflow. The last therapeutic resource is surgical intervention to create a new route for AH outflow (32).

Novel nucleic-based therapies seek improving the limitations of current antiglaucoma treatment. These are the goals pursued by Sylentis' SYL040012, an siRNA-based drug for the treatment of glaucoma, currently in phase II clinical trial. SYL040012 is a chemically synthesized double-stranded oligonucleotide, specifically designed to target and inhibit synthesis of β_2-adrenergic receptors. The compound has proven efficacious in inhibiting the expression of its target in cell cultures and in lowering IOP in normotensive and hypertensive rabbits (Martínez et al, unpublished results). The efficacy of SYL040012 in reducing IOP is similar to that of commercially available drugs (34). On the other hand, when commercial drugs are used, sustained reduction of IOP relies on the continuous application of the drugs. This is not the case with SYL040012, whose effect in animal models not only lasts 15 times longer than the effect of current treatments, but is also able to maintain the reduction in IOP levels even when the compound is not administered for a period of up to 72 hours. This feature is very attractive since it would protect against the eventual optic damage caused by a reboot effect on IOP in case of poor compliance with the treatment. Moreover, SYL040012 is stable up to 24 h in rabbit aqueous humour, but stability rapidly decreases in rabbit serum. The stability properties of SYL040012 support the use of a siRNA-based therapeutic approach for glaucoma since the compound should be stable enough to exert its effect in the eye but should be rapidly degraded when reaching general circulation, hence anticipating low systemic side effects.

Using a completely different approach, Quark pharmaceuticals is developing QPI-1007, a synthetic chemically modified siRNA designed to temporarily inhibit the expression of the pro-apoptotic protein Caspase 2. QPI-1007 is currently undergoing clinical trials for optic nerve atrophy and non-arteritic ischemic optic neuropathy, but the company has expressed interest in developing adequate delivery systems for the potential use of this drug as a neuroprotectant for glaucoma (35).

2.2. Age-Related Macular Degeneration (AMD)

Age-related macular degeneration (AMD) is the leading cause of severe vision loss in the Western world, it occurs primarily among individuals over 50 years of age (36). AMD was a rare disorder in the 19th century but increase in life expectancy together with changes in life-style have enormously affected the prevalence of this disease (37). According to the 2005-2008 National Health and Nutrition Examination Survey 6.5% of the US population over 40 years of age had signs of AMD (38). Extensive epidemiologic and genetic studies indicate that development of AMD is the result of a combination of several aspects such as genetic predisposition and environmental factors. Tobacco smoking seems to be the most consistent and modifiable risk factor (39). Other risk factors include hypertension, cardiovascular disease and high body mass index (40). Among the genetic factors that confer susceptibility to developing AMD are variants in several genes encoding complement pathway proteins (41).

The underlying cause for AMD seems to be accumulation of residual material produced by the renewal process of the external part of the photoreceptors of the retina in the retinal pigment epithelium (RPE). The accumulation of this undegraded material, known as *drusen* in the RPE leads to production of inflammatory mediators that cause photoreceptor degeneration in the central retina, or macula (42). The center of the macula, named fovea, mediates high acuity vision; hence its degeneration causes severe vision loss. In the early stages of the disease the accumulations of *drusen* are small and often observed along with hypo- or hyperpigmentation of the RPE. As the disease progresses both the size and the amount of *drusen* increase. Advanced AMD is characterized by the presence of large or several medium size *drusen* and loss of central vision and can take two forms: dry or wet. The dry form is characterized by a sharply delineated area of RPE atrophy along with loss of photoreceptors and changes in pigmentation of the RPE. In the wet form, or choroidal neovascularisation (CNV), fragile blood vessels of the choriocapillaris grow into the RPE and frequently leak blood and fluid that accumulate between RPE and the choriocapillaris. As a result of these abnormal growths, dense scars are formed in the macula. Detachment of the RPE is also a frequent feature of this form of AMD. The wet form is more severe than the dry form and sometimes dry AMD can develop into wet AMD.

Great advances have been made in recent years in the treatment of wet AMD; on the other hand treatment options for dry AMD are currently limited to dietary supplements and life-style changes. Several pharmaceutical companies are developing compounds for dry AMD by targeting different aspects of the physiopathological progress of the disease. As mentioned above, inflammatory mediators are generated during the process leading to dry AMD, for this reason it has been suggested that antioxidants may play a role in minimizing progression of the disease. The Age-Related Eye Disease Study (AREDS) demonstrated that oral supplementation of antioxidants in patients with unilateral intermediate or advanced AMD reduced vision loss by 19%. In addition these patients showed a decrease of 25% in the chances of developing AMD in the other eye (43, 44).

Other therapeutic approaches for dry AMD currently in clinical development are aimed towards reducing the accumulation of toxic metabolites, diminishing activation of the complement system or avoiding loss of neurons in the retina using neuroprotectants.

As of March 2012 there were approximately 10 clinical studies for pharmaceuticals under development to treat dry AMD registered at www.clinicaltrials.gov with status "recruiting" or "active". Among these clinical trials, only one is using an oligonucleotide based approach to treat dry AMD. ARC1905 is a pegylated aptamer that is currently in phase I study sponsored by Ophtotech Corporation. This compound antagonizes the cleavage of complement component C5 into C5a and C5b, thus inhibiting complement activation.

ARC1905 has shown to be safe when administered by intravitreal injection in combination with ranibizumab for wet AMD (45).

Perhaps one of the facts preventing more oligonucleotide based therapies being developed for dry AMD is that doublestrand RNAs as short as 21 base pair are able to bind and activate Toll Like Receptor 3; and activation of this receptor has been associated with progress of dry AMD (46, 47).

Wet AMD is characterized by the invasion of leaky blood vessels into the RPE. This mechanism is mediated by the action of vascular endothelial growth factor (VEGF). The biological activity of this growth factor has been the target of several therapeutic strategies in the past few years and the pharmaceuticals developed under these programs are the current first line treatment for wet AMD.

Pegaptanib sodium (Macugen®) is a 28-base pegylated aptamer designed to target VEGF (48) by Gilead Pharmaceuticals, licensed to Eyetech Pharmaceuticals/OSI. This drug was approved by the FDA in December 2004 for the treatment of all subtypes of wet AMD by intravitreal injection every six weeks. Pegaptanib specifically binds to $VEGF_{165}$, the most pathogenic of the four isoforms of VEGF that are generated by alternative splicing of a common mRNA. The union of pegaptanib to VEGF prevents activation of either of the two receptors for VEGF (VEGFR-1 and VEGFR-2) present on the surface of epithelial cells; hence inhibiting its biological activity. The VEGF Inhibition Study in Ocular Neovascularizations trial demonstrated that pegaptanib sodium injection reduced the risk of moderate vision loss from 70% to 55% and of severe vision loss from 22% to 10% without serious systemic effects and a low rate of serious ocular adverse events (49).

In July 2006 the second drug based on anti-VEGF therapy was approved by the FDA. Ranibizumab (Lucentis®) is a recombinant, humanised, monoclonal anti-VEGF antibody fragment with high affinity for all isoforms of VEGF developed by Genentech that is administered by intravitreal injection. Two clinical trials (MARINA and ANCHOR) support the safety and efficacy of ranibizumab for wet AMD (50, 51). The results of these trials showed that almost 95% of patients receiving the drug avoided moderate visual loss versus the 62.2% that managed to do so in the control group (receiving veteporfin). In addition, ranibizumab was not only able to stall progression of wet AMD but even to improve visual acuity in 35.7% of the patients treated with the low dose and in 40.3% of the patients treated with the high dose.

The third anti-VEGF compound currently used in the clinic for treatment of wet AMD is bevacizumab (Avastin®). Bevacizumab is a full-length monoclonal antibody that binds to and inhibits all isoforms of VEGF also developed by Genentech. Bevacizumab is in fact the full length antibody that was modified to develop ranibizumab. Ranibizumab was developed because preliminary results indicated that the size of the full length antibody would not allow for appropriate distribution within the retina. Additionally, the longer half life of bevacizumab raised concerns in terms of systemic toxicity. Bevacizumab is currently approved for the treatment of metastatic colorectal cancer and several other malignancies, and it is used off-label for wet AMD (52). The reduced cost of bevacizumab compared to ranibizumab has extended the off-label use of this drug, for this reason several clinical trials have started in the last four years in order to gather evidence on the efficacy of bevacizumab in wet AMD (53, 54).

In addition to pegaptanib, several other attempts have been made to treat wet AMD with oligonucleotides. Bevasiranib was the first small interfering RNA agent developed for this condition. Developed by OPKO Health, this agent is a naked 21-nt siRNA designed to target VEGF administered by intravitreal injection (55). The results of clinical trials conducted for phases I and II were positive and OPKO Health initiated a phase III clinical trial to examine the safety and efficacy of the combination of bevasiranib with ranibizumab. In March 2009 OPKO terminated the phase III trial because the primary endpoint was not likely to be met: improved efficacy over ranibizumab.

Following the same VEGF-inhibition strategy Sirna Therapeutics (now Merck) developed Sirna-027; a modified siRNA that targets one of the receptors for VEGF, VEGFR-1 (56). In vivo studies demonstrated that Sirna-027 was able to reduce the mRNA and protein levels of VEGFR-1 and to reduce the areas of neovascularation in a mouse model of ischemic retinopathy. An inverted sequence with the same chemical modifications as Sirna-027 was used as control and was shown not to have an effect on any of the parameters analysed (56). The control used in this study demonstrated that the effect of Sirna-027 was sequence specific; this was relevant due to the controversy generated by the results of a study published in 2008 that stated that angiogenesis could be suppressed by 21-nt siRNAs in a sequence-independent manner via TLR3 (57). Further clinical development of Sirna-027 was sponsored by Merck in collaboration with Allergan but, again, clinical trials for this compound were halted because the primary endpoint of efficacy trials was not met.

Using a different strategy Quark developed PF-655, now developed in collaboration with Pfizer, a 19-nt 2'O-methyl-stabilized siRNA designed against RTP801, a newly discovered target that is rapidly and sharply upregulated in hypoxia and promotes apoptosis of neural cells (58, 59). In addition to its anti-apoptotic effect, this compound cooperates with VEGF inhibitors to reduce retinal neovascularisation. Although full results of the clinical trial have not yet been made public, in March 2011 Quark announced that their compound was not superior to ranibizumab, thus expectations for the phase IIb initiated by Quark alone are somewhat low.

With two of the candidates already halted and a third most likely to be so, the fate of siRNAs in AMD is at least uncertain. Reports supporting that siRNAs 21 nt or longer activate TLR3 have certainly had a say in the matter. Activation of TLR3 in the RPE seems to induce RPE cell death and contribute to development of dry AMD (47), therefore tackling any form of AMD with double stranded RNA has to be achieved with shorter compounds and target specificity should be thoroughly studied.

2.3. Diabetic retinopathy

Diabetic retinopathy (DR) is a microvascular complication secondary to diabetes mellitus that leads to structural and functional changes in the retina, this complication is the leading cause of visual loss in working-age individuals (60). The overall prevalence of this complication among individuals with diabetes is 34.6% (61) and it accounted for 2.4 million cases of blindness worldwide in 2002 (60). Hyperglycemia is a decisive factor in the development of DR because of its damaging effects *per se;* it also serves as a biomarker for control on the disregulation of metabolism that occurs in diabetes.

In the initial phases of DR the vessels that irrigate the retina show microaneurysms and small leakages, this initial step of the disease is frequently referred to as nonproliferative DR. The changes observed in this phase are result of thickening of the capillary basement membrane as well as apoptosis and migration of pericytes. As the disease progresses the capillaries become permeable due to loss of interaction between endothelial cells and pericytes, and eventually macular edema can develop due to accumulation of fluids in the macula. The progressive occlusion of capillaries in the retina leads to tissue ischemia. As a result of the hypoxia caused by ischemia angiogenic factors such as VEGF are upregulated and capillaries grow into the retina, this stage is also known as proliferative DR (62). The new veins formed in response to the changes seen in the diabetic retina are fragile and permeable and some of them can break through the optic nerve leaking into the vitreous cavity or into the preretinal space. The process of neovascularisation is also associated with accumulation of a fibrous component that when contracted can lead to retinal detachment severely impairing vision (63).

Currently, the gold-standard for treating DR is laser photocoagulation (64); this procedure seeks to mitigate damage but has no effect on the underlying causes of the disease. In addition, steroids can be intravitreally administered into the eye to reduce accumulation of fluids within the retina. Sometimes, the accumulation of blood in the vitreous humour can physically impede laser photocoagulation; in these cases a vitrectomy can be performed in order to remove the blood accumulated in the vitreous prior to laser photocoagulation.

As mentioned previously, the action of angiogenic factors plays an important role in the development of DR. In this sense, several VEGF-inhibitors currently used for the treatment of AMD, are being studied for DR (see section 2.2 for details). Most of them are in late clinical trials and are expected to reach market authorization shortly.

In the oligonucleotide-based field, some of the compounds initially developed for AMD have undergone clinical trials for different forms of diabetic retinopathy as well. Opko Health's bevasiranib is one of these cases. A phase II clinical trial for diabetic macular edema was completed in 2008, and although positive results were reported, further development has not been announced. iCo Therapeutics is using a different approach with their lead compound iCo-007. iCo-007 is a chemically modified ASON inhibiting c-raf; a downstream mediator of several growth factors, including VEGF. In 2011 a phase II clinical trial was started for diabetic retinopathy in which two different doses of iCo-007 are to be assayed, either as a monotherapy or in combination with ranibizumab or laser photocoagulation. Preliminary results of this trial are expected in the second half of 2012. Another antisense alternative is being developed by Antisense Therapeutics, in this case a novel antisense compound ATL1103 which targets growth hormone receptor and has successfully completed a phase I clinical trial. This compound is being developed for treatment of acromegaly and also diabetic retinopathy (65).

2.4. Dry eye pain

Dry eye disease (DED) or keratoconjunctivitis sicca (KCS) is a multifactorial ocular condition resulting from tear film instability that can eventually lead to ocular surface damage. Typical symptoms of DED include ocular discomfort, visual disturbance, itching, burning, sensation of foreign body, light sensitivity; inflammation and pain. Factors contributing to DED are insufficient tear secretion; excessive evaporation and alteration in the composition of the tear film. The tear film has three essential components: aqueous layer, secreted by the lachrymal glands; mucus layer, produced by the globet cells of the conjunctiva and by epithelial cells of the cornea and conjunctiva and finally a lipid layer, secreted by the meibomian glands. Changes in the tear film can be temporary causing an acute form of DED or long-lasting leading to chronic DED; damage to the ocular surface is usually more severe in the chronic forms than in the acute ones. DED is frequent in some conditions such as Sjögren's disease, or lachrymal gland dysfunction, but it can also be caused by vitamin deficiency, contact lens wear and use of several prescription drugs. As such, it is not surprising that DED is a very frequent condition; the prevalence varies tremendously depending on the study, and the condition is more frequent in patients with autoimmune diseases, postmenopausal women and elderly population (66).

Treatment of DED depends on the etiology of the condition. The first line treatment is usually use of lubricants such as artificial tears and avoidance of preservatives such as BAK if other eye treatments are required. Other treatment options include procedures that favour tear retention: punctal occlusion, moisture chamber spectacles and contact lenses; pharmacologic agents that stimulate tear secretion or anti-inflammatory therapy.

Although some advances have been made towards alleviating some of the symptoms of DED, pain associated to this condition is not usually addressed. Sylentis is currently developing an siRNA, SYL1001, for the treatment of pain associated to DED. The compound targets TRPV1, a very well known target for pain, which is highly expressed in the cornea and trigeminal ganglion. SYL1001 is applied in eye drops, contains no preservatives and has recently shown favourable local and systemic tolerance results in a phase IA study.

2.5. Corneal neovascularitation associated with corneal graft rejection

Optimal vision is contingent upon transparency of the cornea. Corneal neovascularization, trauma and surgical procedures such as photorefractive keratectomy and graft rejection after penetrating keratoplasty (PKP) can lead to corneal opacification (67). Corneal neovascularization, regardless of the underlying cause, leads to decreased vision, recurrent corneal erosion, and incompetent barrier function thus presenting a serious clinical problem for which treatment is poor (68). When transparency of the native cornea cannot be maintained at a functional level corneal transplantation is often the next intervention. Once transplanted, the major cause of corneal graft failure is allograft rejection. Despite this fact, corneal transplantation has a very high success rate. Over 90% of low-risk corneal transplants retain clarity years after transplantation using only local immunosuppression. Blocking access of the host immune system to the donor cornea is the first line of defense against corneal allograft rejection, of which corneal avascularity is an essential component. Corneal graft rejection is primarily a cell-mediated immune response controlled by T cells (69). Normal corneal immune privilege can be eroded by neovascularisation, especially if it is accompanied by ocular inflammation and increased intraocular pressure. New vessels generated by neovascularisation provide a route of entry for immune-mediating cells to the graft, while the growth of new lymphatic vessels enables the exit of APCs and antigenic material from the graft to regional lymph nodes. The cornea consequently becomes infiltrated with and sensitized to immune reaction mediators. Therefore, neovascularisation may induce an immune response that can lead to immunological corneal graft rejection (70, 71). In normal low risk grafts it is a general practice to avoid exposing suture knots and ends which may stimulate neovascularization, and to treat neovascularization aggressively using topical steroids (67).

Due to the crucial role of VEGF in neovascularisation (see section 2.2), many have suggested that VEGF inhibition may prevent corneal transplant rejection. Despite the efforts made in recent years on the use of anti-VEGF compounds for corneal rejection it is still not clear whether the treatment is adequate (72, 73).

Several nucleic-based therapies are currently being developed with the hope of filling this uncovered therapeutic gap. Although the molecular mechanisms that control neovascularization are not well understood, inflammation has been found to frequently precede corneal neovascularisation. For this reason, many studies have concentrated their efforts on targeting humoral and corneal-derived inflammatory mediators. Among these mediators are arachidonic-acid derived eicosanoids of the cytochrome P450 monooxygenase (CYP) pathways. Seta and collaborators designed specific siRNAs targeting CYP4B1a, CYP4B1b and CYP4B1c and demonstrated that silencing the expression of CYP4B1 diminished corneal vascular response and greatly attenuated VEGF mRNA levels in an animal model of inflammatory neovascularization (68). One of the most advanced nucleic-based therapies is GS-101 (Aganirsen). GS-101, developed by the Swiss company GeneSignal, is a 25-mer phosphorothioate ASON that inhibits the expression of Insulin Receptor Substrate-1 (IRS-1). IRS-1 is a cytoplasmic adapter protein without intrinsic kinase activity. The main function of this protein is to recruit other proteins to their receptors and induce the organization of intracellular signalling cascades (74). IRS-1 interacts with the VEGF-receptor complex in angiogenesis (75) and it promotes lymphangiogenesis by interacting with integrins (76, 77). Downregulation of IRS-1 results in prevention of neovascular growth and has been reported to prevent the angiogenic process in preclinical *in vivo* and *in vitro* experiments (78, 79). Phase I clinical studies demonstrated excellent safety and tolerability of GS-101 when applied as eyedrops three times a day. In April 2007 the EMA granted orphan drug designation for GS-101 for the treatment of corneal graft rejection associated to corneal neovascularisation. After successfully completing a phase II trial GS-101 is about to enter phase III clinical trials (80).

2.6. Ophthalmic infections

There are several sight-threatening diseases caused by viral infections. Infections caused by virus imply the use of the cellular machinery by the virus to replicate. Hence, all infected cells will have foreign nucleic acids encoding viral specific proteins inside them. Given that oligonucleotide based therapies pursue downregulating expression of genes it seems obvious to target viral specific genes. In the following section several approaches using this rationale will be explained focusing on antivirals developed for treating viral infections in the eye. The first success case of oligonucleotide-based therapies came precisely in this field, fomivirsen was the first compound based on oligonucleotides to be approved by the FDA.

Citomegalovirus-induced retinitis is among the most common opportunistic infections in severely immunocompromised patients (81). In AIDS patients, CMV infection is associated with gastrointestinal disorders and retinitis. An estimated 15 to 40% of AIDS patients will suffer CMV-induced retinitis. This condition if left untreated leads to blindness within six months (82). Three systemic compounds are available for the treatment of this disease: ganciclovir, foscarnet, and cidofovir. The mechanism of action of these three compounds is inhibition of the CMV DNA polymerase. However, these treatments have some drawbacks such as limited efficacy, poor oral bioavailability, toxicity and emergence of multidrug resistant strains due to mutations in the target gene (83). Because of this, effective therapy usually implies alternation between the three available antivirals or different combinations of them, along with intraocular drug injections. This approach, known as highly active antiretroviral therapy (HAART), reduces 55%-95% the number of new cases of CMV (81). Without acute therapy, retinitis spreads throughout the entire retina causing total retinal destruction and blindness; without chronic suppressive maintenance therapy relapse of the retinitis occurs promptly (84). Looking for an alternative approach Isis Pharmaceuticals Inc. developed an ASON that targets the *immediate-early* (*IE*) gene of human CMV. Fomivirsen, (Vitravene®) is a phosphorothioate oligonucleotide (ISIS-2922) developed by Isis in partnership with CIBA vision, for the treatment of newly diagnosed and advanced CMV retinitis in AIDS patients and was the first oligonucleotide based drug approved by the FDA in 1998. Administered by intravitreal injection it has shown good clinical activity against this disease (85).

Acute Retinal Necrosis (ARN) is a type of retinitis that affects both healthy and immuno-compromised patients (86). This inflammatory disease is caused by several members of the herpesvirus family including herpes simplex virus (HSV-1), varicela zoster virus (VZV) and citomegalovirus (CMV) (87, 88). The disease usually starts with signs of uveitis: red eyes, light sensitivity, eye pain and blurred vision. Detailed examination of the eyes of these patients show infiltration of inflammatory cells in the anterior and posterior segments in all retinal layers (89). As the disease progresses retinal necrosis and occlusive arteriolar retinopathy are found. Current treatment for this condition includes antiviral therapy and topical cortosteroids (89). There is no treatment that can prevent the establishment or persistence of latent infection. Reactivation of HSV-1 infections, are currently controlled clinically with long term administration of acyclovir or its derivatives.

Antiviral drugs can quell symptoms resulting from reactivation outbreaks but cannot eliminate latent virus. Furthermore, long-term usage of antiviral drugs can lead to development of drug-resistant viruses (90). Several authors have designed specific ASON targeting the proinflammatory cytokine tumor necrosis factor alpha (TNFα) (91, 92). TNFα is known to possess many cell-activating and proinflammatory activities. TNFα mRNA and protein are up-regulated in eyes infected with HSV-1 (93). Moreover, experiments using DNA microarrays have shown that TNFα and its receptors are upregulated in eyes of mice with HSV-1 retinitis (94). The results of these experiments show that either intravitreal or subconjunctival injections of TNFα-ASON provide local therapeutic effects without systemic adverse effects. Another strategy uses morpholino oligomers specifically designed to reduce viral mRNA trough steric blocking. Moerdyk-Schauwecker and collaborators have developed five phosphoro- diamidate morpholino oligomers (PMO) that target three HSV-1 genes: *ICP0*, *ICP4* and *ICP27*. Their experimental results demonstrated that PMO targeting HSV-1 mRNAs not only inhibited viral replication in cell cultures but also in mouse models of the disease (90).

HSV-1 not only causes ARN it is also responsible for Herpetic Stromal keratitis (HSK) a well- defined immune mediated blinding corneal disease (95). There is profound evidence that the corneal inflammation in HSK is orchestrated by CD4+ T cells and is accompanied by uncontrolled development of blood vessels within the eye (96). The corneal infiltration contains abundant polymorphonuclear cells. These cells, although important for controlling virus replication, are also responsible for damage to the cornea (97, 98). Due to the relevant role of TNF-α and IFNγ in the progress of HSK, targeting TNF-α and IFNγ has been proposed as a therapeutic approach (99). Wasmuth and collaborators demonstrated that topical administration of ASONs targeting either TNF-α or IFNγ were capable of reducing their target in mice infected by HSV-1 without altering antiviral immune response (100, 101). In addition to the production of proinflammatory cytokines, neovascularization of the cornea is observed in this pathogenesis. As in other diseases in which neovascularisation plays a role, VEGF seems to be at least in part, responsible for the process. Validation of this theory has been performed by inhibiting HSV induced angiogenesis in mice with either a VEGF neutralizing antibody or an siRNA designed against this target (102).

Acute Hemorrhagic Conjuntivitis (AHC) is a highly contagious eye disease caused primarily by enterovirus 70 (EV70) or coxackievirus A24 (CVA24) infection. Thus, several authors attempted to develop novel siRNA-based anti-AHC agent effective against both EV70 and CVA24. Resulting siRNAs showed excellent cytoprotective effects and dramatic decreases in viral replication and protein synthesis in primary human conjunctival cells, MRC5 and HeLa cells (103) or in Rabdomyosarcoma cells (104).

2.7. Chronic optic nerve atrophy and ischemic optic neuropathy

Ischemic optic neuropathy is defined as vision loss due to lack of blood supply to the optic disc (infarction). Decreased visual acuity and visual field are usually the only symptoms of ischemic optic neuropathy regardless of the underlying cause. Ischemic optic neuropathy is primarily of two types: Anterior (AION) and posterior (PION) involving the optic nerve head (ONH) and the rest of the optic nerve, respectively (105). AION can be arteritic (A-AION) and non-arteritic (NA-AION). In the management of AION, it is crucial to identify the form of AION. A-AION is an ophthalmic emergency and requires urgent treatment with high-dose steroid therapy to prevent further visual loss to both the affected eye and the sometimes asymptomatic Contralateral eye. NA-AION is the most common form of the disease and it is usually detected due to unilateral painless visual loss along with edema to the optic nerve. It is more frequent in patients between 40 and 70 years of age and vision loss is usually less severe than in the A-AION. Systemic risk factors particularly nocturnal arterial hypotension, play major roles in the development of NA-AION. NA-AION patients treated with high doses of systemic steroid therapy showed significant improvement in visual acuity and visual field. (106).

Given that the loss of vision in these conditions is due to loss of retinal ganglion cells (RGC) neuroprotection seems a rational approach. Focusing on this line of thought, Quark Pharmaceuticals is currently developing a nucleic-acid based therapy, specifically a siRNA-based therapy: QPI-1007. QPI-1007 is a synthetic siRNA designed to temporarily inhibit expression of the pro-apoptotic protein caspase 2 that is currently in clinical trials for the treatment of NA-AION. Ahmed and colleagues in collaboration with Quark pharmaceuticals have shown that caspase-2 contributes loss of RGC in rat models of the condition and have demonstrated that intravitreal injections of QPI-1007 are effective in protecting against the death of RGC (35). Quark Pharmaceuticals is conducting a Phase I-dose escalation safety study using QPI-1007 in patients suffering from Optic Nerve Atrophy and NA-AION. Caspase 2 isn't the only interesting target that offers a potential avenue for treatment in optic neurophaty. Helen and collaborators have focused on the action of another protein: connexin 43 (Cx43). Preclinical results show that an ASONs designed to specifically reduce upregulated levels of Cx43 in a model of optic ischemia has therapeutic potential (107)

2.8. Inherited ocular diseases: Retinitis Pigmentosa (RP) and Ocular Albinism (OA)

Retinitis pigmentosa (RP) is a class of diseases involving progressive degeneration of the retina and a leading cause of inherited blindness. RP is a heterogeneous disorder that starts in mid-periphery and advances towards the macula and fovea. Typical symptoms include night blindness followed by decreasing visual field, leading to tunnel vision and eventually legal blindness or in many cases complete blindness (108). This disorder involves photoreceptor-cell degeneration and affects ~ 1 in 3000 people (109). On the cellular level the rod photoreceptor system is predominantly affected but in later stages of the disease cone photoreceptors can also be affected (108). More than 40 causative genes have been implicated in RP, although mutations in rhodopsin gene (RHO) account for 15% of all types of RP. Great efforts have been made to explore new gene therapies for RP, but inter and intragenic heterogeneity represent significant barriers to therapeutic development. For example more than 100 mutations in the human RHO gene, which encodes the photosensitive pigment in rod photoreceptors, have been identified in autosomal dominantly inherited RP (110). Development of therapies for each individual mutation would be technically difficult to achieve and not economically viable; thus a therapeutic approach that circumvents mutational diversity would be of great value. At present, there is one treatment which has reached the clinic for the treatment of Leber's congenital amaurosis form 2 (LCA2), a type of RP, based on adenoviral (AAV) delivered gene therapy. Three years ago, Maguire and colleagues reported results in 12 patients who were treated with gene-replacement therapy. LCA2 is associated with mutations in *RPE65*, which encodes a protein requisite for the isomerohydrolase activity of the retinal pigment epithelium. This activity produces 11-*cis*-retinal, the natural ligand and chromophore of the opsins of rod and cone photoreceptors, the opsins cannot capture light and transduce it into electrical responses to initiate vision. In this study patients received one subretinal injection of AAV2-hRPE65v2 (a viral vector encoding RPE65 protein). Visual improvement was observed in all 12 patients with the greatest gains among younger patients (111).

Still in early research stages are different approaches to the treatment of RP based on the administration of AAV-delivered RNA interfering compounds. Amongst these, both the University of Florida and Smurfit Institute of Genetics have achieved interesting results *in vivo* by silencing the expression of RHO in mouse models (112). More recent studies by Jiang and collaborators show how using an AVV2/8 vector to develop an RNAi-based therapy in a dominant retinal degeneration mouse model expressing bovine GCAP1 (Y99C), significantly improved photoreceptor survival, delaying disease onset and increasing visual function (113). There are also several studies that target inosine 5'-monophosphate dehydrogenase 1 (IMPDH1) with viral delivered siRNA for the treatment of RP10 form of autosomal dominant RP(114). Another interesting approach based on RNAi therapy uses siRNAs to facilitate transplantation of rod photoreceptors, by disrupting junctional proteins and enhance donor cell integration in the retina (115).

Ocular albinism type 1 is a group of X-linked or autosomal genetic disorders characterized by partial or total lack of melanin pigmentation in the eyes due to mutations in genes encoding proteins involved in melanogenesis. Eyes may be severely affected with photophobia and reduced visual acuity. Nystagmus or strabismus, are often associated and the irides and fundus are depigmented. Many forms of albinism, more or less severe, have been described. Some forms also affect skin and hair. As in other forms of albinism, these patients suffer loss of stereoscopic vision due to reduction of the ipsilateral component of the optic tract (116). General prevalence of albinism is 1/15,000 inhabitants. Treatment is exclusively symptomatic. Vetrini and collaborators have described an intronic point mutation in ocular albinism type 1 (OA1) gene in a family with the X-linked form of ocular albinism. Interestingly the mutation creates a new acceptor splice in intron 7 of the OA1 gene leading to aberrant protein expression. In addition to low levels of normally spliced mRNA product of the OA1 gene, patient samples contained aberrant spliced mRNA. OA1 expression was rescued in the patient's melanocytes with an antisense morpholino modified oligonucleotide (MO) complementary to the mutant sequence. The MO was able to rescue OA1 expression and restore the protein level in the patient's melanocyte by skipping the aberrant inclusion (116).

Compound	Indication	Company	Type of compound	Target	Stage
SYL040012	Glaucoma	Sylentis	Naked siRNA	ADRB2	Ph II
QPI-1007	Glaucoma	Quark Pharmaceuticals	Modified siRNA	Caspase 2	R&D
	NA-ION				Ph I
ARC1905	Dry AMD	Ophthotech Corporation	Pegylated aptamer	Complement component C5	Ph I
	Wet AMD (in combination with ranibizumab)				Ph I
E10030	Wet AMD (in combination with ranibizumab)	Ophthotech Corporation	Aptamer	PDGF	Ph II
Pegaptanib	Wet AMD	Eyetech/OSI Eyetech/Pfizer	Pegylated aptamer	VEGF	Approved
	Diabetic Macular Edema				Ph III
Bevasiranib	Wet AMD	OPKO Health	Naked siRNA	VEGF	Ph III (Term.)
	Diabetic Macular Edema				Ph II
Sirna-027	Wet AMD	Merck/Allergan	Modified siRNA	VEGF	Ph II (Term.)
PF-655	Wet AMD	Quark/Pfizer	Modified siRNA	RTP801	Ph IIb
iCO-007	Diabetic Macular Edema	iCO Therapeutics	Modified antisense	c-raf	Ph II
ALT1103	Diabetic retinopathy	Antisense Therapeutics	Antisense	GHR	R&D
SYL1001	Dry eye pain	Sylentis	Naked siRNA	TRPV1	Ph I
GS-101	Corneal graft rejection associated to corneal neovascularization	GeneSignal	Phosphorothioate antisense	IRS-1	Ph III
Fomivirsen	Advanced CMV infection in AIDS patients	Isis/CIBA	Phosphorothioate antisense	IE gene CMV	Approved

Table 1. Compounds based on oligonucleotides under development for the treatment of ocular diseases.

3. Safety issues

3.1. Immunotoxicity

As part of the defensive duties of the innate immune system it needs to discriminate between foreign and endogenous genetic material. Destruction of exogenous genetic material is an essential part of protection against microorganisms, but can be a hurdle when trying to introduce synthetic genetic material for therapeutic purposes. The immune system responds to microbial RNA and DNA by producing type I interferon and proinflammatory cytokines. The chain reaction leading to production of these immune mediators is initiated by detecting conserved motifs of pathogens; this job is performed by several cell membrane and cytoplasmic receptors present at low levels in most cells. Toll-like receptors (TLR) are present in either the cell surface or in intracellular endocytic organelles and activation of these receptors leads to increase in the presenting capacity of dendritic cells and production of type I interferon. The TLRs responsible for detecting oligonucleotides are present exclusively in endosomes and are TLR3 that senses dsRNA (117), TLR7/8 that sense ssRNA (118) and TLR9 that senses ssDNA (119). TLRs are mainly expressed in immune cells; but foreign material has to be detected in non-immune cells as well; this task is performed by cytosolic sensor proteins. The dsRNA-dependent protein kinase (PKR) is a cytoplasmic sensor of RNA. Upon activation by binding to dsRNA, PKR forms a homodimer that acquires phosphorilation activity. Among the phosphorilation targets of PKR is eIF-2α; phosphorilation of this transcription factor leads translation inhibition and apoptosis (120). A second cytosolic sensor of dsRNAs is 2′-5′ oligoadenylate synthetase (OAS). Activation of this protein promotes the activation of ribonucleases that degrade endogenous and exogenous RNA, again leading the cell to apoptosis (121). Other cytosolic sensors of dsRNA are the retinoic acid-inducible gene-I (RIG-I)-like receptors (RLRs) (122). RLRs are DExD/H RNA helicases. Two members of this family, RIG-I and MDA-5, have in addition to the helicase domain, two caspase activation and recruiting domains. Binding of dsRNA to RIG-I or MDA-5 activates a complex signalling cascade that ultimately leads to interferon-β production and apoptosis (123). As reviewed above, the immune system is prepared to react when foreign biological material is detected inside the body; several strategies can be used to bypass or modulate the response of the immune system:

- Avoidance of sequence motifs or structures that are specifically recognized by the oligonucleotide sensors of the innate immunity. Lowering the number of uridines in a given RNA seems to lower the likelihood of an immune response; completely replacing the uridines by adenosines completely abrogates immune activation (124). Also, avoiding blunt ends on siRNAs could help reducing the immune response. RIG-I recognizes siRNAs with or without 2-base 3′ overhangs, but only those with blunt ends are able to trigger its ATPase activity and subsequent downstream signalling (125).
- Introducing chemical modifications in nucleotides and/or their backbones to avoid activation of the immune response. 2′OMe and pseudouridine are modifications frequently present in mammalian RNAs; these modifications help avoiding triggering the immune response. Other modifications such as 2′F and LNA can also help evade immune detection (124). Whenever modifications are introduced into an oligonucleotide the modified molecule should be tested in order to make sure that the silencing activity has not been abolished.
- Use targeted delivery of oligonucleotides (126) or delivery techniques that avoid the endosome routes for sequences that could activate TLRs. Use of inhibitors of

endosomal maturation such as chloroquine and bafilomycin A1 can also abrogate the immune response (125).

- Use of immunomodulators to impair or abolish the immune response.

Some of the first therapeutic approaches using oligonucleotides were made in the field of ophthalmology. The eye is an immune privileged site, and this fact is one of the rationales behind the election of this site for the first trials. Several overlapping mechanisms contribute to establishing and maintaining immune privilege: the eye has a high content of immunosuppressive factors; it has a low expression of MHCII, hence limiting antigen presentation; stromal cells of the iris, ciliary body and retina are able to convert immune T cells to regulatory (Treg) cells, and retinal epithelial pigment cells are able to inhibit primed T cells; and finally death receptors such as FasL and PDL-1 are expressed by stromal cells that are able to induce apoptosis in immune cells that enter the eye (127). These advantages should not be interpreted as a free pass in terms of immunity for oligonucleotide therapies in the eye. In this regard, it has been shown that some siRNAs are able to activate TLR3 in a sequence-independent manner. Activation of this receptor by dsRNA has been found to suppress angiogenesis (57) and to induce retinal cell death; thus promoting atrophic AMD (46).

3.2. Non immune off target effects

The interaction of therapeutic oligonucleotides with their intended target RNAs is, with the exception of aptamers, highly sequence-specific. However, binding of one of these molecules to a non-target sequence requires only homology with a few base pairs. The result of this undesired interaction could be the inhibition of an unintended gene or an *off target effect* (OTE). Off-targeting is mostly mediated by the interaction between certain regions of the therapeutic molecule and complementary sites in the unintended target rather than overall homology between the two molecules (128). Careful comparison of candidate sequences with the entire transcriptome, attempting to avoid long stretches of homology, still remain necessary but are inadequate on their own to predict the actual risk of OTEs. Use of chemical modifications and improvement in oligonucleotide design has been successfully employed to reduce the likelihood of OTEs.

The specificity of a sequence can be improved taking into account some important designing parameters such as thermodynamic stability of the duplex and 5′ and 3′-ends, the Tm value of the interaction region between the therapeutic oligonucleotide and possible off-targets (129) When dealing with knock down of mRNAs using siRNAs or antisense oligonucleotides the target position should be selected choosing regions that are as far away as possible from the initiation codon (130). The silencing effect of oligonucleotides is in general concentration-dependent, considerable success in reducing siRNA/antisense off-targeting has been achieved optimizing doses of the therapeutic oligonucleotide (131). Improvements in specificity achieved by altering sequences and/or introducing chemical modifications as well as in delivery of the molecule have also shown to have an impact on reducing potential off-target effects. Placing a 2′OMe at position 2 of the guide strand of a siRNA (132), or incorporating a destabilizing UNA at position 7 are examples of modifications that reduce OTEs (131).

3.3. Oversaturation of endogenous RNAi-silencing complex (RISC)

Bioactive drugs that rely on cellular processes to exert their functions face the risk of saturating endogenous pathways. This may be the case with RNAi-based drugs. Naturally occurring, small RNAs have undergone the process of evolution because of selection pressure and they exist in a perfect balance with their precursors and targets, as well as with the associated machinery involved in this process. Gene Silencing is performed by introducing artificially synthesized small RNAs into the cell or by expressing siRNAs/shRNAs within the cell, which enter the endogenous RNAi pathway at different levels. shRNAs and siRNAs are very similar to miRNA precursors before and after Dicer processing, respectively, relying on endogenous miRNA machinery to achieve target silencing. If the siRNA design parameters are not optimal they might cause an imbalance of the endogenous small RNA mediated pathways resulting in various and deleterious unwanted effects in the cells. It becomes therefore crucial to optimize the siRNA/shRNA design parameters and work at the lowest possible concentrations to mitigate the potential of side effects.

4. Advantages of RNAi-based therapeutics and challenges ahead

This new revolutionary technology presents many advantages for therapeutic development with respect to classical compounds, mainly:

- They are based on an endogenous mechanism, thus involving the administration of a type of molecule already present in the cells, and hence, in principle, less hazardous: cells should have the capacity to handle resulting breakdown products.
- As with antisense molecules before them, RNAi molecules can potentially address any pathological target, this means that even diverse intracellular molecules can be the object of these therapies. However, one must bear in mind that in practice, some genes are harder to target than others, and further more sophisticated algorithms must be developed to address this issue.
- Also in comparison to antisense, RNAi is considerably more potent (133) and consequently may be used at lower concentrations. It is believed also to have a more persistent pharmacological action than traditional drugs because it blocks protein synthesis and hence, the cell will have to re-synthesise the protein from scratch to return to its previous state. Thus allowing the use of lower or less frequent doses.
- Given the selectivity and specificity of these compounds, coupled with the fact of their *in silico* design and analysis they will have potentially less harmful side effects.
- Another main advantage from an industry perspective is their much shorter pharmacological development, the estimate being 2-3 years vs 4-6 years from proof of concept. This can be attributed among other things, to the fact that the compound can be designed against homologous regions of the human gene sequence between the

different animal models used for preclinical studies, thus simplifying toxicology studies.

- Finally, despite being novel entities they are easy to manufacture using a nucleotide synthesiser which simplifies large scale production. Additionally, this means the compounds are chemical entities rather than biological products, greatly helping the regulatory process for approval of these medicaments.

Nevertheless, RNAi still has certain hurdles to overcome before its full potential can be exploited. The main obstacle is delivery of siRNAs to the desired tissue, and although many advances have been made in this area, much work still remains for therapeutic possibilities to be fully exploited. On the other hand, in a clinical setting, RNAi can only be used to treat pathologies caused by expression or overexpression of a given protein or by the presence of exogenous organisms, as its mechanism works through suppression of protein expression; i.e. it is only of use when the therapeutic option requires a loss of function. Furthermore, although any gene is a potential target for RNAi, in practice not all mRNAs are as easily silenced and new more sophisticated algorithms will need to be developed to overcome this issue. And last but not least, as discussed in the previous section the issue of off-target effects resulting from siRNAs silencing unwanted genes can lead to important safety considerations when developing new medicaments.

From the perspective of ocular disorders, the eye is a relatively isolated compartment which makes it an ideal target organ for gene silencing. Local delivery of the compound to the eye limits exposure to the rest of the body and reduces the amount that is needed. siRNA injected into the vitreous cavity readily diffuses throughout the eye and is detectable for at least five days (56), the amounts used for intraocular injections are small compared to those used for systemic application and so as siRNA gets out of the eye it is diluted and is difficult to detect. This allows local silencing of a gene with little chance for an effect on the same gene outside the eye, reducing concern of remote effects in other tissues complicating observations in the eye. The sequence specificity of siRNA resulting in targeting of a single gene combined with local administration in the relatively isolated confines of the eye provides an ideal way to study eye-specific effects of gene disruption (34). While the development of siRNA-based therapies has promise for all tissues, the unique characteristics of the eye provide advantages which explain why the first siRNA compounds to advance through clinical trials were for the treatment of wet AMD, a disease affecting the back of the eye.

5. Prospects for current therapies based on nucleic-based strategies

The clinical progress of oligonucleotide drugs has been slow because realizing them requires inventing a new model for pharmaceutical development that allows large, highly charged molecules to be synthesized economically, distribute to target tissues, enter cells, and function within acceptable limits for toxicity. Oligonucleotides are large, unlike traditional small molecule drugs (<500-700 molecular weight), and much effort has been required to understand their properties and optimize them. However, considering RNAi was discovered just over a decade ago, this technology has advanced towards clinical trials with amazing speed. Both for antisense molecules and RNAi compounds initial most advanced therapies were developed taking advantage of the environment within the interior of the eye. One antisense oligonucleotide has been approved by the FDA in 1998: Vitravene® or fomivirsen developed by Isis Pharmaceuticals for the treatment of cytomegalovirus retinitis in immunocompromised patients. Initial most advanced siRNAs were designed to treat wet age-related macular degeneration (AMD) taking advantage of the relatively RNAse free environment of the interior of the eye. These therapies were based on intravitreal injection, a form of administration which allows bypassing on of the main rate-limiting issues for therapeutic oligonucleotides, that of delivery to the required target tissue.

Delivering oligonucleotides in whole organisms requires crossing many barriers. Degradation by serum nucleases, clearance by the kidney, or inappropriate biodistribution can prevent the oligonucleotide from ever reaching its target organ. Generally, the oligonucleotide must pass through the blood vessel wall and navigate the interstitial space and extracellular matrix. Finally, if the oligonucleotide succeeds in reaching the appropriate cell membrane, it will usually be taken up into an endosome, from which it must escape to be active. Antisense oligonucleotides are usually delivered in saline and rely on chemical modifications to enable uptake. Their phosphorothioate backbone binds to serum proteins, slowing excretion by the kidney (134). The aromatic nucleobases also interact with other hydrophobic molecules in serum and on cell surfaces; many types of cells in vivo express surface receptors that actively take up oligonucleotides.

Delivery is even more challenging for siRNAs, where all the aromatic nucleobases are on the inside, leaving heavily hydrated phosphates on the outside of the duplex. This hydrated surface interacts poorly with cell surfaces and is rapidly excreted in the urine. Hence, except for direct injection in targets such as the eye where they are also delivered in saline, researchers have invested heavily in the development of delivery vehicles for siRNA. Various delivery strategies include nanoparticles, cationic lipids, antibodies, cholesterol, aptamers and viral vectors for short hairpin RNAs. In this case, the delivery system most clinically validated is that based on SNALP (stable nucleic acid lipid particle) technology developed by Tekmira for systemic administration of siRNAs. However, although it is being used to formulate at least 4 different siRNAs currently undergoing clinical trials, it has yet to be used more extensively before victory can be claimed on the battle of delivery.

The field of oligonucleotide therapeutics has often swung from irrational optimism to irrational despair. This is true for industry, but in the laboratory as well, gene knockdown experiments have fallen in and out of favour with researchers. In reality, oligonucleotides are useful tools with strengths and weaknesses (135). The promise of RNAi as a powerful new approach for therapeutic treatment of diseases has propelled early stage clinical testing of siRNAs for a variety of diseases. However, it is still too soon to evaluate whether or not RNAi based therapeutics will live up to their expectations. Given the mood swings in this area, with big pharma investing large sums in the technology at one point and then backing out only two or three years later, the industry has been in a turmoil which is now beginning to even out. This relative calm should bring about maturity in the field with the science becoming more solid as we gain more knowledge of the biology of these compounds. From an industry perspective, it is foreseeable that Big Pharma's involvement will continue the later trend of product-specific licensing and co-development rather than the purchase of platform technologies from smaller biotech experts performed in the early days of the technology. This is also in line with structural changes in the industry towards the outsourcing of research (136).

Author details

Covadonga Pañeda*, Tamara Martínez, Natalia Wright and Ana Isabel Jimenez
Sylentis SAU, R&D department, PCM c/Santiago Grisolía, Madrid, Spain

6. References

[1] Crick F. Central dogma of molecular biology. Nature. 1970 Aug 8;227(5258):561-3.

[2] Paterson BM, Roberts BE, Kuff EL. Structural gene identification and mapping by DNA-mRNA hybrid-arrested cell-free translation. Proc Natl Acad Sci U S A. 1977 Oct;74(10):4370-4.

[3] Stephenson ML, Zamecnik PC. Inhibition of Rous sarcoma viral RNA translation by a specific oligodeoxyribonucleotide. Proc Natl Acad Sci U S A. 1978 Jan;75(1):285-8.

[4] Zamecnik PC, Stephenson ML. Inhibition of Rous sarcoma virus replication and cell transformation by a specific oligodeoxynucleotide. Proc Natl Acad Sci U S A. 1978 Jan;75(1):280-4.

[5] Bhindi R, Fahmy RG, Lowe HC, Chesterman CN, Dass CR, Cairns MJ, et al. Brothers in arms: DNA enzymes, short interfering RNA, and the emerging wave of small-molecule nucleic acid-based gene-silencing strategies. Am J Pathol. 2007 Oct;171(4):1079-88.

[6] Goodchild J. Therapeutic oligonucleotides. Methods Mol Biol.764:1-15.

[7] Schlosser K, Li Y. Biologically inspired synthetic enzymes made from DNA. Chem Biol. 2009 Mar 27;16(3):311-22.

[8] Santoro SW, Joyce GF. A general purpose RNA-cleaving DNA enzyme. Proc Natl Acad Sci U S A. 1997 Apr 29;94(9):4262-6.

[9] Bennett MR, Schwartz SM. Antisense therapy for angioplasty restenosis. Some critical considerations. Circulation. 1995 Oct 1;92(7):1981-93.

[10] Crooke ST. Progress in antisense technology. Annu Rev Med. 2004;55:61-95.

[11] Persidis A. Antisense therapeutics. Nat Biotechnol. 1999 Apr;17(4):403-4.

[12] Lee IK, Ahn JD, Kim HS, Park JY, Lee KU. Advantages of the circular dumbbell decoy in gene therapy and studies of gene regulation. Curr Drug Targets. 2003 Nov;4(8):619-23.

[13] Tomita N, Morishita R, Tomita T, Ogihara T. Potential therapeutic applications of decoy oligonucleotides. Curr Opin Mol Ther. 2002 Apr;4(2):166-70.

* Corresponding Author

[14] Thiel KW, Giangrande PH. Therapeutic applications of DNA and RNA aptamers. Oligonucleotides. 2009 Sep;19(3):209-22.

[15] Fraunfelder FW. Pegaptanib for wet macular degeneration. Drugs Today (Barc). 2005 Nov;41(11):703-9.

[16] Fire A, Xu S, Montgomery MK, Kostas SA, Driver SE, Mello CC. Potent and specific genetic interference by double-stranded RNA in Caenorhabditis elegans. Nature. 1998 Feb 19;391(6669):806-11.

[17] Elbashir SM, Harborth J, Lendeckel W, Yalcin A, Weber K, Tuschl T. Duplexes of 21-nucleotide RNAs mediate RNA interference in cultured mammalian cells. Nature. 2001 May 24;411(6836):494-8.

[18] Martinez T, Wright N, Pañeda C, Jimenez A, Lopez-Fraga M. RNA Interference-Based Therapeutics: Harnessing the Powers of Nature In: Rundfeldt C, editor. Drug Development - A Case Study Based Insight into Modern Strategies: InTech; 2011. p. 265-312.

[19] Varma R, Lee PP, Goldberg I, Kotak S. An assessment of the health and economic burdens of glaucoma. Am J Ophthalmol. 2011 Oct;152(4):515-22.

[20] Quigley H. Glaucoma. Lancet. 2011;377((9774)):1367-77.

[21] Weinreb RN, Khaw PT. Primary open-angle glaucoma. Lancet. 2004 May 22;363(9422):1711-20.

[22] Marquis RE, Whitson JT. Management of glaucoma: focus on pharmacological therapy. Drugs Aging. 2005;22(1):1-21.

[23] Kaur IP, Kakkar S. Newer therapeutic vistas for antiglaucoma medicines. Crit Rev Ther Drug Carrier Syst. 2011;28(2):165-202.

[24] Gordon MO, Beiser JA, Brandt JD, Heuer DK, Higginbotham EJ, Johnson CA, et al. The Ocular Hypertension Treatment Study: baseline factors that predict the onset of primary open-angle glaucoma. Arch Ophthalmol. 2002 Jun;120(6):714-20; discussion 829-30.

[25] Kass MA, Heuer DK, Higginbotham EJ, Johnson CA, Keltner JL, Miller JP, et al. The Ocular Hypertension Treatment Study: a randomized trial determines that topical ocular hypotensive medication delays or prevents the onset of primary open-angle glaucoma. Arch Ophthalmol. 2002 Jun;120(6):701-13; discussion 829-30.

[26] Jonas JB, Martus P, Horn FK, Junemann A, Korth M, Budde WM. Predictive factors of the optic nerve head for development or progression of glaucomatous visual field loss. Invest Ophthalmol Vis Sci. 2004 Aug;45(8):2613-8.

[27] Kroese M, Burton H. Primary open angle glaucoma. The need for a consensus case definition. J Epidemiol Community Health. 2003 Sep;57(9):752-4.

[28] Martus P, Stroux A, Budde WM, Mardin CY, Korth M, Jonas JB. Predictive factors for progressive optic nerve damage in various types of chronic open-angle glaucoma. Am J Ophthalmol. 2005 Jun;139(6):999-1009.

[29] De Natale R, Le Pen C, Berdeaux G. Efficiency of glaucoma drug regulation in 5 European countries: a 1995-2006 longitudinal prescription analysis. J Glaucoma. Apr-May;20(4):234-9.

[30] Servat JJ, Bernardino CR. Effects of common topical antiglaucoma medications on the ocular surface, eyelids and periorbital tissue. Drugs Aging. Apr 1;28(4):267-82.

[31] Han JA, Frishman WH, Wu Sun S, Palmiero PM, Petrillo R. Cardiovascular and respiratory considerations with pharmacotherapy of glaucoma and ocular hypertension. Cardiol Rev. 2008 Mar-Apr;16(2):95-108.

[32] Francis BA, Singh K, Lin SC, Hodapp E, Jampel HD, Samples JR, et al. Novel glaucoma procedures: a report by the American Academy of Ophthalmology. Ophthalmology. 2011 Jul;118(7):1466-80.

[33] Martinez T, Gonzalez V, Panizo G, Wright N, Pañeda C, Jimenez A. In vitro and in vivo efficacy of SYL040012, a novel siRNA compound for treatment of glaucoma. Submitted. 2012.

[34] Campochiaro PA. Potential applications for RNAi to probe pathogenesis and develop new treatments for ocular disorders. Gene Ther. 2006 Mar;13(6):559-62.

[35] Ahmed Z, Kalinski H, Berry M, Almasieh M, Ashush H, Slager N, et al. Ocular neuroprotection by siRNA targeting caspase-2. Cell Death Dis. 2011;2:e173.

[36] Smith W, Assink J, Klein R, Mitchell P, Klaver CC, Klein BE, et al. Risk factors for age-related macular degeneration: Pooled findings from three continents. Ophthalmology. 2001 Apr;108(4):697-704.

[37] Rattner A, Nathans J. Macular degeneration: recent advances and therapeutic opportunities. Nat Rev Neurosci. 2006 Nov;7(11):860-72.

[38] Klein R, Chou CF, Klein BE, Zhang X, Meuer SM, Saaddine JB. Prevalence of age-related macular degeneration in the US population. Arch Ophthalmol. Jan;129(1):75-80.

[39] Thornton J, Edwards R, Mitchell P, Harrison RA, Buchan I, Kelly SP. Smoking and age-related macular degeneration: a review of association. Eye (Lond). 2005 Sep;19(9):935-44.

[40] Clemons TE, Milton RC, Klein R, Seddon JM, Ferris FL, 3rd. Risk factors for the incidence of Advanced Age-Related Macular Degeneration in the Age-Related Eye Disease Study (AREDS) AREDS report no. 19. Ophthalmology. 2005 Apr;112(4):533-9.

[41] Khandhadia S, Cipriani V, Yates JR, Lotery AJ. Age-related macular degeneration and the complement system. Immunobiology. Feb;217(2):127-46.

[42] Bird AC. Therapeutic targets in age-related macular disease. J Clin Invest. 2010 Sep;120(9):3033-41.

[43] A randomized, placebo-controlled, clinical trial of high-dose supplementation with vitamins C and E, beta carotene, and zinc for age-related macular degeneration and vision loss: AREDS report no. 8. Arch Ophthalmol. 2001 Oct;119(10):1417-36.

[44] SanGiovanni JP, Chew EY, Clemons TE, Ferris FL, 3rd, Gensler G, Lindblad AS, et al. The relationship of dietary carotenoid and vitamin A, E, and C intake with age-related macular degeneration in a case-control study: AREDS Report No. 22. Arch Ophthalmol. 2007 Sep;125(9):1225-32.

[45] Cousins SW, Group OS. Targeting Complement Factor 5 in combination with Vascular Endothelial Growth Factor (VEGF) Inhibition for Neovascular Age Related Macular

Degeneration (AMD): Results of a Phase 1 Study ARVO Meeting abstracts. 2010;51:1251.

[46] Yang Z, Stratton C, Francis PJ, Kleinman ME, Tan PL, Gibbs D, et al. Toll-like Receptor 3 and Geographic Atrophy in Age-Related Macular Degeneration. N Engl J Med. 2008 Aug 27.

[47] Zhou P, Fan L, Yu KD, Zhao MW, Li XX. Toll-like receptor 3 C1234T may protect against geographic atrophy through decreased dsRNA binding capacity. FASEB J. Oct;25(10):3489-95.

[48] Ruckman J, Green LS, Beeson J, Waugh S, Gillette WL, Henninger DD, et al. 2'-Fluoropyrimidine RNA-based aptamers to the 165-amino acid form of vascular endothelial growth factor (VEGF165). Inhibition of receptor binding and VEGF-induced vascular permeability through interactions requiring the exon 7-encoded domain. J Biol Chem. 1998 Aug 7;273(32):20556-67.

[49] Gragoudas ES, Adamis AP, Cunningham ET, Jr., Feinsod M, Guyer DR. Pegaptanib for neovascular age-related macular degeneration. N Engl J Med. 2004 Dec 30;351(27):2805-16.

[50] Brown DM, Kaiser PK, Michels M, Soubrane G, Heier JS, Kim RY, et al. Ranibizumab versus verteporfin for neovascular age-related macular degeneration. N Engl J Med. 2006 Oct 5;355(14):1432-44.

[51] Rosenfeld PJ, Brown DM, Heier JS, Boyer DS, Kaiser PK, Chung CY, et al. Ranibizumab for neovascular age-related macular degeneration. N Engl J Med. 2006 Oct 5;355(14):1419-31.

[52] Avery RL, Pieramici DJ, Rabena MD, Castellarin AA, Nasir MA, Giust MJ. Intravitreal bevacizumab (Avastin) for neovascular age-related macular degeneration. Ophthalmology. 2006 Mar;113(3):363-72 e5.

[53] Patel PJ, Bunce C, Tufail A. A randomised, double-masked phase III/IV study of the efficacy and safety of Avastin(R) (Bevacizumab) intravitreal injections compared to standard therapy in subjects with choroidal neovascularisation secondary to age-related macular degeneration: clinical trial design. Trials. 2008;9:56.

[54] Tufail A, Patel PJ, Egan C, Hykin P, da Cruz L, Gregor Z, et al. Bevacizumab for neovascular age related macular degeneration (ABC Trial): multicentre randomised double masked study. BMJ. 2010;340:c2459.

[55] Dejneka NS, Wan S, Bond OS, Kornbrust DJ, Reich SJ. Ocular biodistribution of bevasiranib following a single intravitreal injection to rabbit eyes. Mol Vis. 2008;14:997-1005.

[56] Shen J, Samul R, Silva RL, Akiyama H, Liu H, Saishin Y, et al. Suppression of ocular neovascularization with siRNA targeting VEGF receptor 1. Gene Ther. 2006 Feb;13(3):225-34.

[57] Kleinman ME, Yamada K, Takeda A, Chandrasekaran V, Nozaki M, Baffi JZ, et al. Sequence- and target-independent angiogenesis suppression by siRNA via TLR3. Nature. 2008 Apr 3;452(7187):591-7.

[58] Shoshani T, Faerman A, Mett I, Zelin E, Tenne T, Gorodin S, et al. Identification of a novel hypoxia-inducible factor 1-responsive gene, RTP801, involved in apoptosis. Mol Cell Biol. 2002 Apr;22(7):2283-93.
[59] Lee DU, Huang W, Rittenhouse KD, Jessen B. Retina Expression and Cross-Species Validation of Gene Silencing by PF-655, a Small Interfering RNA Against RTP801 for the Treatment of Ocular Disease. J Ocul Pharmacol Ther. 2012 Feb 3.
[60] Resnikoff S, Pascolini D, Etya'ale D, Kocur I, Pararajasegaram R, Pokharel GP, et al. Global data on visual impairment in the year 2002. Bull World Health Organ. 2004 Nov;82(11):844-51.
[61] Yau JW, Rogers SL, Kawasaki R, Lamoureux EL, Kowalski JW, Bek T, et al. Global prevalence and major risk factors of diabetic retinopathy. Diabetes Care. 2012 Mar;35(3):556-64.
[62] Qian H, Ripps H. Neurovascular interaction and the pathophysiology of diabetic retinopathy. Exp Diabetes Res. 2012;2011:693426.
[63] Willard AL, Herman IM. Vascular complications and diabetes: current therapies and future challenges. J Ophthalmol. 2012;2012:209538.
[64] Photocoagulation treatment of proliferative diabetic retinopathy. Clinical application of Diabetic Retinopathy Study (DRS) findings, DRS Report Number 8. The Diabetic Retinopathy Study Research Group. Ophthalmology. 1981 Jul;88(7):583-600.
[65] http://www.antisense.com.au/product-pipeline/atl1103-for-growth-sight-disorders/. [cited]; Available from.
[66] Gayton JL. Etiology, prevalence, and treatment of dry eye disease. Clin Ophthalmol. 2009;3:405-12.
[67] Qazi Y, Wong G, Monson B, Stringham J, Ambati BK. Corneal transparency: genesis, maintenance and dysfunction. Brain Res Bull. 2010 Feb 15;81(2-3):198-210.
[68] Seta F, Patil K, Bellner L, Mezentsev A, Kemp R, Dunn MW, et al. Inhibition of VEGF expression and corneal neovascularization by siRNA targeting cytochrome P450 4B1. Prostaglandins Other Lipid Mediat. 2007 Nov;84(3-4):116-27.
[69] Panda A, Vanathi M, Kumar A, Dash Y, Priya S. Corneal graft rejection. Surv Ophthalmol. 2007 Jul-Aug;52(4):375-96.
[70] Murthy RC, McFarland TJ, Yoken J, Chen S, Barone C, Burke D, et al. Corneal transduction to inhibit angiogenesis and graft failure. Invest Ophthalmol Vis Sci. 2003 May;44(5):1837-42.
[71] Cursiefen C, Chen L, Dana MR, Streilein JW. Corneal lymphangiogenesis: evidence, mechanisms, and implications for corneal transplant immunology. Cornea. 2003 Apr;22(3):273-81.
[72] Bachmann BO, Bock F, Wiegand SJ, Maruyama K, Dana MR, Kruse FE, et al. Promotion of graft survival by vascular endothelial growth factor a neutralization after high-risk corneal transplantation. Arch Ophthalmol. 2008 Jan;126(1):71-7.
[73] Gerten G. Bevacizumab (avastin) and argon laser to treat neovascularization in corneal transplant surgery. Cornea. 2008 Dec;27(10):1195-9.

[74] Hos D, Saban DR, Bock F, Regenfuss B, Onderka J, Masli S, et al. Suppression of inflammatory corneal lymphangiogenesis by application of topical corticosteroids. Arch Ophthalmol. 2011 Apr;129(4):445-52.

[75] Miele C, Rochford JJ, Filippa N, Giorgetti-Peraldi S, Van Obberghen E. Insulin and insulin-like growth factor-I induce vascular endothelial growth factor mRNA expression via different signaling pathways. J Biol Chem. 2000 Jul 14;275(28):21695-702.

[76] Vuori K, Ruoslahti E. Association of insulin receptor substrate-1 with integrins. Science. 1994 Dec 2;266(5190):1576-8.

[77] Dietrich T, Onderka J, Bock F, Kruse FE, Vossmeyer D, Stragies R, et al. Inhibition of inflammatory lymphangiogenesis by integrin alpha5 blockade. Am J Pathol. 2007 Jul;171(1):361-72.

[78] Al-Mahmood S, Colin S, Farhat N, Thorin E, Steverlynck C, Chemtob S. Potent in vivo antiangiogenic effects of GS-101 (5'-TATCCGGAGGGCTCGCCATGCTGCT-3'), an antisense oligonucleotide preventing the expression of insulin receptor substrate-1. J Pharmacol Exp Ther. 2009 May;329(2):496-504.

[79] Andrieu-Soler C, Berdugo M, Doat M, Courtois Y, BenEzra D, Behar-Cohen F. Downregulation of IRS-1 expression causes inhibition of corneal angiogenesis. Invest Ophthalmol Vis Sci. 2005 Nov;46(11):4072-8.

[80] http://www.genesignal.com/index.php?id=23.

[81] Jabs DA, Griffiths PD. Fomivirsen for the treatment of cytomegalovirus retinitis. Am J Ophthalmol. 2002 Apr;133(4):552-6.

[82] Kuppermann BD. Therapeutic options for resistant cytomegalovirus retinitis. J Acquir Immune Defic Syndr Hum Retrovirol. 1997;14 Suppl 1:S13-21.

[83] Chou S, Miner RC, Drew WL. A deletion mutation in region V of the cytomegalovirus DNA polymerase sequence confers multidrug resistance. J Infect Dis. 2000 Dec;182(6):1765-8.

[84] Jabs DA. Ocular manifestations of HIV infection. Trans Am Ophthalmol Soc. 1995;93:623-83.

[85] Orr RM. Technology evaluation: fomivirsen, Isis Pharmaceuticals Inc/CIBA vision. Curr Opin Mol Ther. 2001 Jun;3(3):288-94.

[86] Silverstein BE, Conrad D, Margolis TP, Wong IG. Cytomegalovirus-associated acute retinal necrosis syndrome. Am J Ophthalmol. 1997 Feb;123(2):257-8.

[87] Atherton SS. Acute retinal necrosis: insights into pathogenesis from the mouse model. Herpes. 2001 Nov;8(3):69-73.

[88] Ganatra JB, Chandler D, Santos C, Kuppermann B, Margolis TP. Viral causes of the acute retinal necrosis syndrome. Am J Ophthalmol. 2000 Feb;129(2):166-72.

[89] Mei H, Xing Y, Yang J, Wang A, Xu Y, Heiligenhaus A. Influence of antisense oligonucleotides targeting tumor necrosis factor-alpha on experimental herpetic-induced chorioretinitis of mouse eye. Pathobiology. 2009;76(1):45-50.

[90] Moerdyk-Schauwecker M, Stein DA, Eide K, Blouch RE, Bildfell R, Iversen P, et al. Inhibition of HSV-1 ocular infection with morpholino oligomers targeting ICP0 and ICP27. Antiviral Res. 2009 Nov;84(2):131-41.

[91] Grajewski RS, Li J, Wasmuth S, Hennig M, Bauer D, Heiligenhaus A. Intravitreal treatment with antisense oligonucleotides targeting tumor necrosis factor-alpha in murine herpes simplex virus type 1 retinitis. Graefes Arch Clin Exp Ophthalmol. 2011 Feb;250(2):231-8.
[92] Li J, Wasmuth S, Bauer D, Baehler H, Hennig M, Heiligenhaus A. Subconjunctival antisense oligonucleotides targeting TNF-alpha influence immunopathology and viral replication in murine HSV-1 retinitis. Graefes Arch Clin Exp Ophthalmol. 2008 Sep;246(9):1265-73.
[93] Zheng M, Atherton SS. Cytokine profiles and inflammatory cells during HSV-1-induced acute retinal necrosis. Invest Ophthalmol Vis Sci. 2005 Apr;46(4):1356-63.
[94] Zheng M, Qian H, Joshi RM, Nechtman J, Atherton SS. DNA microarray analysis of the uninoculated eye following anterior chamber inoculation of HSV-1. Ocul Immunol Inflamm. 2003 Sep;11(3):187-95.
[95] Streilein JW, Ksander BR, Taylor AW. Immune deviation in relation to ocular immune privilege. J Immunol. 1997 Apr 15;158(8):3557-60.
[96] Kim B, Tang Q, Biswas PS, Xu J, Schiffelers RM, Xie FY, et al. Inhibition of ocular angiogenesis by siRNA targeting vascular endothelial growth factor pathway genes: therapeutic strategy for herpetic stromal keratitis. Am J Pathol. 2004 Dec;165(6):2177-85.
[97] Tang Q, Chen W, Hendricks RL. Proinflammatory functions of IL-2 in herpes simplex virus corneal infection. J Immunol. 1997 Feb 1;158(3):1275-83.
[98] Thomas J, Gangappa S, Kanangat S, Rouse BT. On the essential involvement of neutrophils in the immunopathologic disease: herpetic stromal keratitis. J Immunol. 1997 Feb 1;158(3):1383-91.
[99] Inoue T, Inoue Y, Kosaki R, Nishida K, Shimomura Y, Tano Y, et al. Immunohistological study of infiltrated cells and cytokines in murine herpetic keratitis. Acta Ophthalmol Scand. 2001 Oct;79(5):484-7.
[100] Wasmuth S, Bauer D, Yang Y, Steuhl KP, Heiligenhaus A. Topical treatment with antisense oligonucleotides targeting tumor necrosis factor-alpha in herpetic stromal keratitis. Invest Ophthalmol Vis Sci. 2003 Dec;44(12):5228-34.
[101] Wasmuth S, Bauer D, Steuhl KP, Heiligenhaus A. Topical antisense-oligonucleotides targeting IFN-gamma mRNA improve incidence and severity of herpetic stromal keratitis by cytokine specific and sequence unspecific effects. Graefes Arch Clin Exp Ophthalmol. 2008 Mar;246(3):443-51.
[102] Zheng M, Deshpande S, Lee S, Ferrara N, Rouse BT. Contribution of vascular endothelial growth factor in the neovascularization process during the pathogenesis of herpetic stromal keratitis. J Virol. 2001 Oct;75(20):9828-35.
[103] Jun EJ, Won MA, Ahn J, Ko A, Moon H, Tchah H, et al. An antiviral small-interfering RNA simultaneously effective against the most prevalent enteroviruses causing acute hemorrhagic conjunctivitis. Invest Ophthalmol Vis Sci. 2011 Jan;52(1):58-63.
[104] Tan EL, Marcus KF, Poh CL. Development of RNA interference (RNAi) as potential antiviral strategy against enterovirus 70. J Med Virol. 2008 Jun;80(6):1025-32.
[105] Hayreh SS. Ischemic optic neuropathy. Prog Retin Eye Res. 2009 Jan;28(1):34-62.

[106] Hayreh SS. Management of ischemic optic neuropathies. Indian J Ophthalmol. 2011 Mar-Apr;59(2):123-36.
[107] Danesh-Meyer HV, Huang R, Nicholson LF, Green CR. Connexin43 antisense oligodeoxynucleotide treatment down-regulates the inflammatory response in an in vitro interphase organotypic culture model of optic nerve ischaemia. J Clin Neurosci. 2008 Nov;15(11):1253-63.
[108] Ferrari S, Di Iorio E, Barbaro V, Ponzin D, Sorrentino FS, Parmeggiani F. Retinitis pigmentosa: genes and disease mechanisms. Curr Genomics. 2011 Jun;12(4):238-49.
[109] Farrar GJ, Kenna PF, Humphries P. On the genetics of retinitis pigmentosa and on mutation-independent approaches to therapeutic intervention. EMBO J. 2002 Mar 1;21(5):857-64.
[110] O'Reilly M, Palfi A, Chadderton N, Millington-Ward S, Ader M, Cronin T, et al. RNA interference-mediated suppression and replacement of human rhodopsin in vivo. Am J Hum Genet. 2007 Jul;81(1):127-35.
[111] Maguire AM, Simonelli F, Pierce EA, Pugh EN, Jr., Mingozzi F, Bennicelli J, et al. Safety and efficacy of gene transfer for Leber's congenital amaurosis. N Engl J Med. 2008 May 22;358(21):2240-8.
[112] Gorbatyuk M, Justilien V, Liu J, Hauswirth WW, Lewin AS. Suppression of mouse rhodopsin expression in vivo by AAV mediated siRNA delivery. Vision Res. 2007 Apr;47(9):1202-8.
[113] Wang JJ, Zeng ZW, Xiao RZ, Xie T, Zhou GL, Zhan XR, et al. Recent advances of chitosan nanoparticles as drug carriers. Int J Nanomedicine. 2011;6:765-74.
[114] Tam LC, Kiang AS, Kennan A, Kenna PF, Chadderton N, Ader M, et al. Therapeutic benefit derived from RNAi-mediated ablation of IMPDH1 transcripts in a murine model of autosomal dominant retinitis pigmentosa (RP10). Hum Mol Genet. 2008 Jul 15;17(14):2084-100.
[115] Pearson RA, Barber AC, West EL, MacLaren RE, Duran Y, Bainbridge JW, et al. Targeted disruption of outer limiting membrane junctional proteins (Crb1 and ZO-1) increases integration of transplanted photoreceptor precursors into the adult wild-type and degenerating retina. Cell Transplant. 2010;19(4):487-503.
[116] Vetrini F, Tammaro R, Bondanza S, Surace EM, Auricchio A, De Luca M, et al. Aberrant splicing in the ocular albinism type 1 gene (OA1/GPR143) is corrected in vitro by morpholino antisense oligonucleotides. Hum Mutat. 2006 May;27(5):420-6.
[117] Alexopoulou L, Holt AC, Medzhitov R, Flavell RA. Recognition of double-stranded RNA and activation of NF-kappaB by Toll-like receptor 3. Nature. 2001 Oct 18;413(6857):732-8.
[118] Heil F, Hemmi H, Hochrein H, Ampenberger F, Kirschning C, Akira S, et al. Species-specific recognition of single-stranded RNA via toll-like receptor 7 and 8. Science. 2004 Mar 5;303(5663):1526-9.
[119] Krug A, Towarowski A, Britsch S, Rothenfusser S, Hornung V, Bals R, et al. Toll-like receptor expression reveals CpG DNA as a unique microbial stimulus for plasmacytoid

dendritic cells which synergizes with CD40 ligand to induce high amounts of IL-12. Eur J Immunol. 2001 Oct;31(10):3026-37.

[120] Gil J, Esteban M. Induction of apoptosis by the dsRNA-dependent protein kinase (PKR): mechanism of action. Apoptosis. 2000 Apr;5(2):107-14.

[121] Samuel CE. Antiviral actions of interferons. Clin Microbiol Rev. 2001 Oct;14(4):778-809, table of contents.

[122] Yoneyama M, Fujita T. RNA recognition and signal transduction by RIG-I-like receptors. Immunol Rev. 2009 Jan;227(1):54-65.

[123] Kato H, Takeuchi O, Sato S, Yoneyama M, Yamamoto M, Matsui K, et al. Differential roles of MDA5 and RIG-I helicases in the recognition of RNA viruses. Nature. 2006 May 4;441(7089):101-5.

[124] Sioud M. Single-stranded small interfering RNA are more immunostimulatory than their double-stranded counterparts: a central role for 2'-hydroxyl uridines in immune responses. Eur J Immunol. 2006 May;36(5):1222-30.

[125] Sioud M. RNA interference and innate immunity. Adv Drug Deliv Rev. 2007 Mar 30;59(2-3):153-63.

[126] Song E, Zhu P, Lee SK, Chowdhury D, Kussman S, Dykxhoorn DM, et al. Antibody mediated in vivo delivery of small interfering RNAs via cell-surface receptors. Nat Biotechnol. 2005 Jun;23(6):709-17.

[127] Stein-Streilein J. Immune regulation and the eye. Trends Immunol. 2008 Nov;29(11):548-54.

[128] Jackson AL, Linsley PS. Recognizing and avoiding siRNA off-target effects for target identification and therapeutic application. Nat Rev Drug Discov. 2009 Jan;9(1):57-67.

[129] Ui-Tei K, Naito Y, Takahashi F, Haraguchi T, Ohki-Hamazaki H, Juni A, et al. Guidelines for the selection of highly effective siRNA sequences for mammalian and chick RNA interference. Nucleic Acids Res. 2004;32(3):936-48.

[130] Yuan B, Latek R, Hossbach M, Tuschl T, Lewitter F. siRNA Selection Server: an automated siRNA oligonucleotide prediction server. Nucleic Acids Res. 2004 Jul 1;32(Web Server issue):W130-4.

[131] Bramsen JB, Kjems J. Chemical modification of small interfering RNA. Methods Mol Biol. 2011;721:77-103.

[132] Jackson AL, Burchard J, Leake D, Reynolds A, Schelter J, Guo J, et al. Position-specific chemical modification of siRNAs reduces "off-target" transcript silencing. Rna. 2006 Jul;12(7):1197-205.

[133] Bertrand JR, Pottier M, Vekris A, Opolon P, Maksimenko A, Malvy C. Comparison of antisense oligonucleotides and siRNAs in cell culture and in vivo. Biochem Biophys Res Commun. 2002 Aug 30;296(4):1000-4.

[134] Levin AA. A review of the issues in the pharmacokinetics and toxicology of phosphorothioate antisense oligonucleotides. Biochim Biophys Acta. 1999 Dec 10;1489(1):69-84.

[135] Watts JK, Corey DR. Silencing disease genes in the laboratory and the clinic. J Pathol. 2012 Jan;226(2):365-79.

[136] Haussecker D. The business of RNAi therapeutics. Hum Gene Ther. 2008 May;19(5):451-62.